"In an era where Social Work is increasingly governed by standardised protocols, the academic study of ethics and philosophy may seem both daunting and an unnecessary luxury. However, few tasks are more complex than promoting the well-being, dignity and autonomy of vulnerable and increasingly diverse service users. One of the greatest strengths of *The Ethical Foundations of Social Work* (Revised Edition) is its ability to challenge the myth that care, protection and promoting autonomy and dignity are simply 'common sense' tasks and that Social Work is purely a practical profession.

This book not only provides a clear introduction to ethical principles and reasoning but also encourages readers to engage with the real-world ethical dilemmas that Social Workers face in ever-changing social and cultural contexts. By situating Social Work within broader historical and geopolitical landscapes, Pullen Sansfaçon and Cowden offer a vital resource that fosters critical thinking, ethical reflexivity and political awareness – an essential resource for both students and practitioners."

Dr Gurnam Singh, *Associate Professor of Sociology, University of Warwick and Visiting Professor of Social Work, Liverpool Hope University, UK*

"*The Ethical Foundations of Social Work* is an essential text, inviting reflexivity and reflection on one's own positionality. This book is a must for Social Work students, professors, and practitioners, as its pedagogically approached theoretical content invites critical reflection on contemporary socio-political issues. The chapters on epistemic injustice, radicalisation, decolonial ethics and the ethics of recognition are valuable additions to this edition because of their topicality and relevance."

Hélène Albert, *Professor of Social Work, The Université de Moncton, Canada*

"Since the first edition of this text the world has radically changed, this updated edition is vitally needed spotlighting ethical thinking and challenges faced globally including social injustice, oppression, conflict, climate change and far right radicalisation. This accessible book, based on the authors' own research and teaching expertise, advances insight into ethical perspectives and social theories. It is essential reading for students and practitioners, with opportunities to apply learning from the book to complex case studies aiding a depth of learning which will aid Social Work practice. The text will support students and Social Workers from across the world to intervene in complex situations developing and actively utilising ethical and critical thinking skills. It is a crucial time for Social Work to continue to ask the question 'is this ethical' promoting social justice, ethical practice and criticality in complex situations, this text is a must read."

Davy Hambling, *Senior Lecturer in Social Work, University of Gloucestershire, UK*

"The new edition of Pullen Sansfaçon and Cowden is a must for teaching ethics in every Social Work programme. The authors have successfully renewed and significantly enhanced their work, by integrating contemporary critical ethical theories, particularly the notions of epistemic justice, radicalisation, and decolonial ethics. The manuscript provides concrete interpretive lenses for Social Work students and echoes the fact that in a world undergoing upheavals, the ethical practice of Social Work enables resistance and change."

Marie-Joëlle Robichaud, *Professor at the Department of Psychoeducation and Social Work, and Head of Social Work Programs, Université du Québec à Trois-Rivières, Canada*

The Ethical Foundations of Social Work

The Ethical Foundations of Social Work offers an engaging, theoretically rigorous and practice-orientated grounding in Social Work ethics.

Fully revised and expanded, with the addition of four new chapters on Decolonial Ethics, Social Work and Radicalisation, the Ethics of Recognition and Epistemic Injustice, this book examines when, how and why principles and debates have historically emerged, and explicitly maps them onto everyday ethical challenges and situations in Social Work practice. By presenting and explaining key theories and applying them to real-world practice examples from different regions, *The Ethical Foundations of Social Work* guides Social Work students and practitioners in developing ethical reasoning to support ethical decision-making in diverse contexts.

Promoting an ethically 'conscious' approach in which principles are integrated flexibly and confidently as tools for critical problem solving, this book serves as a core or supplemental textbook for Social Work Ethics courses at undergraduate or postgraduate levels.

Annie Pullen Sansfaçon is Full Professor of Social Work at the University of Montreal in Canada, and holds the Canada Research Chair RePar E on Partnership Research and the Empowerment of Vulnerable Young People.

Stephen Cowden, PhD, is a senior lecturer in Social Work at the University of Gloucestershire. His research interests are diverse but include Social Work Ethics, Critical Pedagogy, and Radicalisation and Safeguarding.

The Ethical Foundations of Social Work

Second Edition

Annie Pullen Sansfaçon and Stephen Cowden

Routledge
Taylor & Francis Group
LONDON AND NEW YORK

Designed cover image: Getty image number 1185856904

Second edition published 2025
by Routledge
4 Park Square, Milton Park, Abingdon, Oxon, OX14 4RN

and by Routledge
605 Third Avenue, New York, NY 10158

Routledge is an imprint of the Taylor & Francis Group, an informa business

First edition published by Routledge 2012

British Library Cataloguing-in-Publication Data
A catalogue record for this book is available from the British Library

Library of Congress Cataloging-in-Publication Data
Names: Pullen-Sansfaçon, Annie author | Cowden, Stephen author
Title: The ethical foundations of social work / Annie Pullen Sansfaçon and Stephen Cowden.
Description: Second edition. | Abingdon, Oxon ; New York, NY : Routledge, 2025. | First edition published by Routledge 2012. | Includes bibliographical references and index. |
Identifiers: LCCN 2025009095 (print) | LCCN 2025009096 (ebook) | ISBN 9781032603551 hardback | ISBN 9781032603544 paperback | ISBN 9781003458715 ebook
Subjects: LCSH: Social service—Moral and ethical aspects
Classification: LCC HV10.5 .P85 2025 (print) | LCC HV10.5 (ebook) | DDC 174/.93613—dc23/eng/20250522
LC record available at https://lccn.loc.gov/2025009095
LC ebook record available at https://lccn.loc.gov/2025009096

ISBN: 978-1-032-60355-1 (hbk)
ISBN: 978-1-032-60354-4 (pbk)
ISBN: 978-1-003-45871-5 (ebk)

DOI: 10.4324/9781003458715

Typeset in Sabon LT Pro
by codeMantra

Stephen dedicates this book to his partner Jacqui, who is the person who makes his writing possible in so many ways.

Annie dedicates this book to her partner, her family and her close friends. Thank you for being there and for continuing to encourage me to stay true to my Social Work values, even when it gets challenging.

Together, we dedicate this book to all Social Workers who continue to keep alive the project of practical humanitarian social change.

Contents

Figures

Tables

About the Authors

Annie Pullen Sansfaçon is Full Professor of Social Work at the University of Montreal in Canada, and holds the Canada Research Chair ReParE on Partnership Research and the Empowerment of Vulnerablized Youth. She is the Co-founder and Co-director of CRI-JaDE, the Interdisciplinary Research Center on Intersectional Justice, Decolonization and Equity. Her research programme aims at understanding how different structures and contexts affect the wellbeing of gender and sexually diverse youth. Rooted in anti-oppressive and trans affirmative perspectives, she proposes interventions and methodologies that support their empowerment.

Stephen Cowden, PhD, is a senior lecturer in Social Work at the University of Gloucestershire. His research interests are diverse but include Social Work Ethics, Critical Pedagogy, and Radicalisation and Safeguarding. He is a member of the 'Feminist Dissent' collective. His most recent publications are 'Reconciling a Broken Heritage: Developing Mental Health Social Work in Guyana' *International Journal of Environmental Research and Public Health*, 2023, 20, 6931. https://doi.org/10.3390/ijerph20206931, with Coya Halley, and 'Contested Narratives of the Pandemic Crisis: the Far Right, Anti-Vaxxers and Freedom of Speech' *Feminist Dissent Issue* 6. https://doi.org/10.31273/fd.n6.2022.1264, with Nira Yuval-Davis.

Barbara Neale is a registered Social Worker who has worked in adult safeguarding in the UK for several decades, in both hospital and community settings. She has also taught and researched Social Work for a number of UK universities, the most recent being the University of Gloucestershire where she was MA Social Work Programme Director and subsequently Academic Programme Lead for Social Work. Her research interests are focused on forms of education that enhance the understanding of power and injustice so as to develop the knowledge, values and skills of the Social Work profession.

Acknowledgements

We extend our gratitude to Charlotte St-Pierre, who assisted us in updating some of the sources for this revised edition. During the manuscript revision process, Charlotte was completing her master's degree in Social Work at the University of Montreal.

We also wish to thank Barbara Neale who co-authored the chapter on Epistemic Injustice with us.

Preface to the Second Edition

We are excited to present this completely revised and extended edition of *The Ethical Foundations of Social Work*, first published in 2012. When we began the first edition of this book, we were both working as senior lecturers at Coventry University in the United Kingdom. We jointly developed a module to teach Social Work ethics to undergraduate Social Work students. At the centre of our pedagogical approach in the module was the desire to make complex theoretical material on ethics accessible and relevant to students. This was a very successful teaching experience, and the book grew out of that.

We decided to publish a revised edition because the book continues to be something that Social Work students have told us that they find accessible and relevant in thinking about ethical issues in Social Work.

Our situation has also changed. Annie returned to her home country of Canada and is now working at the University of Montreal, and Stephen has been at the University of Gloucestershire since 2021. In this sense, we wanted a book that didn't reflect such a strong United Kingdom focus as in the first edition. But even more importantly, since the publication of the first edition, the world we live in has radically changed. We wrote the first edition during what we would be called the 'New Labour' years in the UK: the years following the removal of Margaret Thatcher's Conservative Party from office and the election of Tony Blair as British prime minister. While the neoliberal economics that developed during the Thatcher years was largely retained by 'New Labour', there were big increases in spending on health and education, and many initiatives developed in the universities around teaching. Our work was situated in what now seems to be a relatively hopeful period. However, all of this optimism came crashing down with the global banking crisis of 2007–2008. This began on Wall Street but, given the global interconnectedness of the banking system and its centrality to the neoliberal economic model, these problems spread across the world. Severe financial depression followed shortly after, but waves of austerity policies were also imposed globally. Many countries in the Global South had borrowed money to fund growth and investment during the late 1990s and early 2000s. They now found themselves unable to pay their debts and turned to international bodies like the International Monetary Fund (IMF), which provided money for loans and unpaid debts. However, in return, the IMF required these countries to introduce reforms that favoured the further development of neoliberal free-market capitalism, which further aggravated social inequalities, poverty and reductions in social spending. Across the world, these reforms therefore had profound effects on vulnerable communities as well as on the Social Work role and social welfare more generally. At the same time, we saw an attempt at the marketisation of public services, including universities, with the aim to remake them into the image of private businesses.

But all of this was met with resistance in many places in the world. For example, in Canada in March 2012, the Quebec provincial government tabled a bill that promised to increase University tuition fees by 75%. The announcement of this bill attracted strong protests by major student associations. This incident was referred to as the 'Maple Spring', and up to 240,000 students engaged in a movement that lasted six months, and which ended when the government announced that tuition fees would finally be frozen. A general election was called shortly thereafter (Pullen Sansfaçon, 2013). Similar protests associated with anti-austerity movements emerged in Greece and in Spain. At this time, some governments were also elected on the basis of their anti-austerity platform, like the Labour party of Jeremy Corbyn in the United Kingdom. However, this wave of opposition to austerity was unable to build momentum. Extreme-right parties began to emerge, exploiting the growing sense of insecurity and social precariousness that arose during the austerity period.

Another key development that followed in the early 2020 was the COVID-19 pandemic, which exposed both the weaknesses and the necessity of global public health systems. Conspiracy theories opposing COVID-19 vaccines were effectively spread by right-wing political groups and leaders, including President Jair Bolsonaro in Brazil and President Donald Trump in the United States, undermining efforts to control the spread of the virus (Cowden and Yuval-Davis, 2022). The pandemic, in addition to affecting the economy, causing increased financial burden for many, also brought dramatic changes to how we communicate, including within Social Work, with significant increases in the use of online platforms and systems.

Over the past decade, we have also witnessed attacks on basic human rights that were, until those recent social changes, guaranteed by judgements from the highest levels of the legal system. For example, in the United States, the right to abortion is no longer guaranteed at the federal level following the overturning of the *Roe v. Wade* Supreme Court judgement. This resulted in many states forbidding medical and social care professionals from providing medical services, advice and support, which had a highly detrimental impact on many vulnerable women, who were no longer able to access these services. Europe and, to a lesser extent, North America have also witnessed attempts by the extreme right to turn international migration into a major political crisis, which have had a major impact on political agendas on every continent.

Another development of massive significance is the increasing global climate change and the impact it has on communities by causing significant hardship and suffering. Global climate change has required Social Workers to adapt and respond to disasters, such as catastrophic floods and other forms of human displacement caused by climate change. The secretary-general of the International Federation of Social Work (IFSW), Rory Truell, recently noted,

> Nature is telling us that we have to do things differently... Social work has started a paradigm shift based on a vision co-evolved with communities... for a new balanced and harmonised eco-social world. Within this new paradigm, social workers are deepening their partnerships with others beyond the traditional role prescribed by governments. We are all moving from reactive models responding to individual need, to sustainable co-existence between peoples and nature. As social workers experienced in transformation, we know this can be done.
>
> (BASW, 2024, pp. 3–6)

In writing this revised edition, we have sought to respond to some of the changes that happened since the publication of the first edition. The revisited edition includes four new chapters. In addition to having undertaken a thorough revision of the chapters from the first edition, we included a new chapter on epistemic injustice, which appears to us as a particularly important concept for understanding how some people experience injustice in a global world, and where the voices of some groups are understood and considered more or less important than others. We also included a new chapter on the role that Social Worker can play in understanding and counteracting radicalisation. In this chapter, we also discuss the rise of the extreme right and its implications for Social Work practice.

Despite intense pressures on Social Work in the developed capitalist world, it is now a global profession which is developing rather than diminishing across the world. To respond to the fact that many Social Work values remain anchored in a Eurocentric view of the profession, we have added a new chapter on decolonial ethics as a framework for working with Indigenous populations. We have also developed a chapter on the ethics of recognition, which allows us to analyse and understand not only how social injustice can be felt at personal, social and political levels but also how Social Work can facilitate the development of a more just society that fosters recognition for everyone.

As in the first edition, this revised edition continues to adopt a different approach to ethics, one that examines ethical theories in their original form and applies them to real contemporary social issues. We felt that, by explaining how these theories historically emerged, what they were trying to address at the time that they were originally articulated, and how they continue to relate to current debates can help students and practitioners to become better-equipped to deal with practical complex situations in Social Work. We also felt that this would allow students and practitioners to better situate some of the foundations of contemporary Codes of Practice and Codes of Ethics that we often draw upon. As academics who still engage in teaching and research, we continue to think it is helpful for Social Workers to draw on ethical theories to think through and around a problem. We also incorporated insights from sociology and social theory into our approach – again, not to see these as a source of technical expertise but as tools which aim to provide students with a better grasp of the complexities of ethical concepts and situations. The revised edition of this book continues to focus on the importance of the relationship between theory and practice, particularly the capacity to understand how situations in Social Work practice, as well as in life in general, practically embody the concerns addressed by ethical theories.

Finally, as the first edition of *The Ethical Foundations of Social Work* was written with United Kingdom Social Work students in mind and we became aware that many people found the book to be useful in other contexts, we have reviewed it in a way that it can also appeal to a global audience. Therefore, for the second edition, we decided to expand the scope of the book and show the relevance of understanding ethical and social theory beyond the United Kingdom. As a result, we also drew from case studies and policies from India, Canada, Australia, the United States and other European countries to illustrate how critically understanding the ethical foundations of Social Work equips Social Workers to intervene in complex situations wherever we are located.

We are grateful to the Social Work students and practitioners who have been using this book over the past decade, and we hope that this new edition will continue to support the development of ethical, practical and critical thinking while sparking new insights into how Social Work can contribute to building a more socially just society.

Annie Pullen Sansfaçon and Stephen Cowden

Introduction

The Importance of Situating the Ethical Social Work Project in a Global, Changing World

For thousands of years, philosophers have proposed ethical theories to guide people on how to identify good actions from bad actions and on how they should live the 'good' life. According to Aristotle, as well as other philosophers who came after him. This concerned the question of how we should think and act in a rational manner.

But what is 'ethics' in the context of Social Work? While ethics is generally understood as the study of what is good or bad or right or wrong (Banks, 2020), it can be articulated in two different ways in a professional context (Clark, 2000). This gives us the conception of ethics as a prescription, which is concerned with what is allowed and not allowed in the context of professional behaviour. People often think of this type of ethics when they refer to their Code of Ethics or Code of Conduct. This way of engaging with ethics is very important in professional practice because it provides people with principles, orientations and even legal guidelines on how to behave in complex practice situations.

Ethics, on the other hand, can also be understood as *discipline*, that is, a process which can be used to examine the foundations, principles and arguments that underpin what we find in Codes of Ethics and Codes of Conduct or to question the assumptions underlying a given decision. *The Ethical Foundations of Social Work* is based on this second way of understanding ethics, as it sheds light on principles and assumptions at the core of Social Work, such as social justice, power, self-determination and empowerment. The aim is to help students develop a greater awareness of the various aspects that shape interventions and decision making in Social Work practice. Throughout this book, we seek to examine different concepts and theories of ethics in order to facilitate a process in which students and readers can critically engage with the complexity of practice situations and the underlying assumptions which we make in assessing and evaluating what is happening in them.

In the Global North, Social Work is a largely regulated profession, while in the Global South, there is still an important process taking place in which Social Workers are seeking professional recognition. Because the demand to be seen as a profession is significant in both of these contexts, we included various standards and norms that are relevant to the profession in the discussions presented in this book while remaining critical about these, even if they are legitimised through a political or bureaucratic process (Clifford and Burke, 2009). Indeed, the fact that an 'authority' establishes norms, principles and concepts does not mean that these must be accepted as ethical (Pullen Sansfaçon, 2013; Clifford and Burke, 2009). As we previously argued, rather than unconditionally following Codes of Conduct, ethical practice should encourage Social Workers to engage in a constant process of self-reflexivity and critical reflection to the point where these values

DOI: 10.4324/9781003458715-1

become part of the professional identity expressed throughout a person's life (Pullen Sansfaçon, 2011).

Self-Reflexivity: The Importance of Critically Reflecting on the 'Self' in the Ethical Social Work Project

Social Work is a relational profession. That is, Social Workers have to foster the development of professional relationships with service users, groups and communities in order to successfully advance their work. At the core of this endeavour is the understanding that it requires Social Workers to critically reflect on how they, as professionals, will shape this relationship and, ultimately, the resulting intervention. 'Use of Self', as some label it, is the process of developing self-knowledge, with the aim of drawing on these personal characteristics – the positionalities and values for Social Workers to professionally intervene (Walsh, 2021). The Manitoba College of Social Workers expressed this aspiration as follows:

> Self-reflecting practice is a guiding principle in social work practice. It entails familiarity with one's social location and privilege afforded to them. It is an ongoing process requiring social workers to identify their own values, culture, attitudes, beliefs, motivations, roles, emotions, and capacities as they relate to others in the social work relationship. Self-reflective practice includes social workers as part of the problem-solving process rather than separated from it.
>
> (Manitoba College of Social Workers, 2021, p. 7)

This definition indicates that Social Workers' values and beliefs, as well as those of wider society, are intrinsically linked to their interventions. In other words, although there are many theories, approaches and techniques in Social Work, no two Social Workers will use these in exactly the same way and with the same results. Indeed, an implicit element of this relational dimension between the professional and the service user is the impact that it can have – positively or negatively – on the success of the intervention. Therefore, as a start to ethical reflection, it is crucial for Social Workers to be able to examine their particular social location and values and reflect on their potential impact on the intervention.

The Importance of Situating Ourselves and to Reflect on our Social Location

Social location refers to a Social Worker's personal characteristics, such as age, race, sexual orientation, immigrant status and gender identity, and their motivation or intention to engage in a specific subject or work with various populations (Holmes, 2020; Hurley and Jackson, 2020). Reflecting on social location may help Social Workers gain a better understanding of the complex relationships between institutions and the people whom they work with or between themselves and service users, groups and/or communities (Bilge, 2009). For example, a white Social Worker of European descent may engage differently with Indigenous or black service users, compared to a Social Worker who shares some of this positionality. This issue of positionality is itself complex; we may share some positionalities (e.g. race) but not others (e.g. age or social class), with all of the impact which this has on our professional practice.

To engage in a more meaningful reflection on positionalities, an intersectional analysis may be helpful, as it allows us to examine and situate social categories within a broader scheme of power and hierarchies (Anthias, 2013). Thus, it helps us to consider how our social location can be multifaceted and influence our practice experience, particularly in the context of power relationships which are inherent to the Social Work profession. Emerging from Black feminist movements and their reflections on the intersection of race and gender, intersectionality as a concept provides one way of understanding the complexity and multiplicity of identities and social inequalities (Bilge, 2009). It offers a way of deconstructing forms of social division such as sex, gender, belonging, class, disability and sexual orientation in a way that recognises the imbrication and interaction of sources of oppression in people's lives at both the micro- and macrosocial levels (Crenshaw, 1991; hooks, 1989). Intersectionality also points to various forms of oppression that service users experience, as well as how we, as professionals, may also be part of these systems of oppression. At the same time, there have been significant critiques of the concept of intersectionality. For instance, the Canadian black feminist writer Humani Bannerji noted,

> This combination of 'race', gender and class is often expressed through the concept of 'intersectionality' in which three particular strands of social relations and ideological practices of difference and power are seen as arising in their own specific social terrain, and then criss-crossing each other 'inter-sectionally' or aggregatively. It is a coming together of social issues to create a moment of social experience. Yet, speaking of experience, both non-white and white people living in Canada/the West know that this social experience is not, as lived, a matter of intersectionality. Their sense of being in the world, textured through myriad social relations and cultural forms, is lived or felt or perceived as being all together and all at once. A working class non-white woman's (Black, South Asian, Chinese, etc.) presence in the usual racialized environment is not divisible separately and serially. The fact of her blackness, her sex and gender neutral personhood of being working class blend into something of an identity simultaneously and instantaneously. This identification is both in the eye of the beholder and her own sense of social presence captured by this gaze. The same goes for a white woman, yet when confronted with this question of "being" and experience we are hard put to theorize them in terms of a social ontology.
>
> (2011, pp. 41–42)

Bannerji indicates that our social being or 'ontology' is a complex thing, and it is because of this that the process of developing the capacity for critical reflection needs to be at the heart of anti-oppressive Social Work. Whether a Social Worker shares their positionality or not with service users, groups or communities does not guarantee any positive or negative outcomes, but it may have an impact on how they see the world and service users and how service users see them.

Values

Values are strong beliefs that people adhere to. These values can be personal, professional, social or even philosophical and are influenced by a multitude of factors, such as social location, political awareness or affiliation and experience (Moss, 2007). Thus, different people may carry different values that have been forged through their life experiences.

When thinking about Social Work ethics, it is important to not only reflect on one's social location, because it has an impact on the relationships that one develops with service users, but also one's values, as they form the basis of what motivates and even transcend one's actions since they serve as standards (Schwartz, 1992). While people may hold different or similar values, these may be ranked differently from one person to another. Schwarz argued that, wherever we are in the world and whatever community or cultural groups we look at, it is possible to identify only ten values: 'self-direction', 'stimulation', 'hedonism', 'achievement', 'power', 'security', 'conformity', 'tradition', 'benevolence' and 'universalism' (Schwartz, 1992). What differs between people, groups, communities or cultures is the meanings and rankings that people assign to values, although they all represent goals that they can pursue.

In some contexts, the expression of these values even be in tension or conflict with each other. For example, it might be challenging to believe that someone should be self-directed or self-determined while strongly adhering to the value of 'conformity', because self-direction requires people to think independently, whereas conformity requires people to do as prescribed. If placed in the same situation with the same ethical dilemma to manage, a person who prioritises the value of self-direction would probably not come to the same decision as someone who prioritises the value of conformity. This is just one example of how our values influence our choices and decisions (Pakizeh et al., 2007), and it is for this reason that they must also be examined carefully as one engages in ethical practice.

Therefore, we encourage readers to remain aware of how their attitudes, experiences, values and social position can all potentially influence their understanding of a given situation, as well as their professional relationships with individuals, groups and communities. What is important to remember is that values and positionalities have an impact on intervention and, ultimately, ethical practice. Whether a Social Worker shares a value or a positionality with service users, groups or a community can have positive or negative impacts. This is why reflecting about positionality while engaging in intervention is fundamental to developing Social Work practice that is ethical; ethical practice, as we have already suggested, is a practice that questions and challenges the assumptions on which a decision is based.

Social Work Values

Although values can differ from one person or group to another, there is one document that proposes a set of values that can be regarded as foundational within the post-war world II: the United Nations Declaration of Human Rights (1948). While it does not explicitly state a set of universal values, it implicitly highlights universal values such as 'freedom', 'dignity', 'equality' and 'rights', which were taken as a basis for articulating the principles that follow in the Universal Declaration. This document is fundamentally important for Social Work because the profession is known to have a special commitment to human rights, which provide the foundation for the Social Work International Code of Ethics. Other important documents in Social Work include the International Convention of the Rights of the Child (United Nations 1989) and other conventions aimed at eliminating discrimination (IFSW, 2018), such as the United Nations Declaration on the Rights of Indigenous Peoples (2007), which are also be discussed in this book.

Although not all Social Work organisations in the world use the same words to articulate Social Work values, the ideas of respect, self-determination, social justice and integrity are often cited as core values of the profession (Banks, 2020). Many of these values are critically analysed in Part II. As for other types of values, professional values can also have different meanings for different people and evoke conflict or tensions. We often talk about these conflicts in value when we refer to an ethical dilemma.

The Regulation of Social Work Practice

In many places where Social Work is practiced around the globe, professional Social Work associations and state regulatory bodies have published Codes of Ethics or Codes of Conduct to support practitioners in their work and help them manage difficult situations. For example, in the United Kingdom, the British Association of Social Workers (BASW, 2021) produces a Code of Ethics for UK Social Work as a whole, while different bodies perform regulation for the profession and uphold the Professional Standards (2019) in England, Wales, Scotland and Northern Ireland. In Canada, the Canadian Association of Social Workers (CASW, 2024) publishes the Code of Ethics and Scope of Practice, but each province, such as Nova Scotia or British Columbia, is responsible for regulating Social Work professionals, although provincial codes of ethics largely echo CASW values and principles. For example, in Ontario, a large province in Eastern Canada, the Ontario College of Social Workers and Social Service Workers (OCSSSW) plays a regulatory role in professional jurisdiction, reflecting a mandate to protect the public from the Government of Ontario. There are different arrangements of this nature both between and within other countries. For example, in the state of South Australia, the title of 'Social Worker' is now protected, which means that professionals cannot use it without being a member of the Social Worker Registration Board and meet minimum requirements set by the organisation, although there are different regulations in other Australian states.

In some places, the title of 'Social Worker' may not be protected, which means that professionals can use it without being registered with a Social Work regulator. Having protection for the title comes with not only some advantages, such as ensuring a minimum level of ethical practice with service users, but also disadvantages, such as creating a financial burden for professionals who must usually pay an association fee and potentially reducing their level of professional autonomy, at the very least (Tangney and et Mendes, 2023). Protecting titles is common in many places, such as Canada, the United States, New Zealand and South Africa. In places where the title of 'Social Worker' is protected, people who are not registered can only use other titles, such as 'social care practitioner', even if they have completed their qualification in Social Work. Before using any title, we encourage readers to check the situation in the jurisdiction where you are studying to clarify this aspect.

The guidelines produced by associations and Social Work regulators, such as *Codes of Ethics*, *Codes of Conduct* or professional *standards*, are important because they provide guidance to Social Workers and help maintain ethical practice. At the same time, they serve other functions, such as protecting and reassuring the public, legitimising Social Workers' claim to professional status and fostering members' allegiance to the profession (Witkin, 2000). All of these codes, whether they are part of a regulatory body such as Social Work England or the Canadian Association of Social Workers Code of Ethics and Scope of Practice, make up part of what we call 'prescriptive ethics' in the earlier part of the introduction.

While a Code of Ethics or Conduct should be used as general guidelines to help Social Workers manage ethical dilemmas, they must be carefully used. Because practice is so varied, unless the code is very broad and general, one Code of Ethics cannot answer the needs of Social Workers who practice using different methods or approaches, let alone in different types of professional social care settings, nor do they always provide a clear answer on how to manage an ethical issue. For example, it is not uncommon to see one statement in a Code of Ethics conflict with another one on a different page. This sort of challenge, which emerges from conflicting principles within the same Code of Practice, was highlighted by Proctor et al. (1993) in a research project in the US, which found that 85% of conflicts mentioned by Social Workers reflected a conflict in principles listed in the US-based National Association Social Workers Code of Ethics (in Harrington and Dolgoff, 2008). Such Social Work Codes of Ethics are important, but they are not a panacea and cannot ensure ethical practice on their own.

Furthermore, Social Work practice sometimes takes place in the context of an unclear social landscape, whereby some norms that were formally accepted in society become increasingly challenged and sometimes rejected by many people, sometimes even a majority. For example, in North America, we have seen a movement to restrict access to reproductive health, although this was more widely accepted in the past. Sometimes, society transforms to the detriment of some groups, which may become marginalised and oppressed. For instance, the anti-immigration sentiments observed over the past few years have led to a decrease in support for immigration in places such as Canada (Robitaille, 2024); this trend has also been seen in the United States, Australia and across Europe.

Sometimes, society takes longer to change, and marginalised groups remain so because of the status quo. For example, while gay, lesbian, bisexual, transgender and queer (LGBTQ) groups have engaged in struggles and legal battles to have their rights legally and socially recognised, it is still illegal in many countries to be gay or transgender or enter into same-sex marriage. In these situations, we need to make a distinction between norms enshrined in the laws of a country and wider questions of ethics. Under apartheid in South Africa, laws which enshrined racial discrimination were ruthlessly enforced; yet, they were anything but ethical. The human rights organisation Amnesty International describes contemporary Israel as having instituted a comparable form of apartheid in which Palestinians are denied rights as citizens (Amnesty International, 2022). In other places, different struggles for recognition have led to changes in law and policy. For example, homosexuality has been decriminalised and transgender people have gained greater recognition of their specific health care needs in many countries. This shows that struggles and conflicts in value can lead to the development of new rights.

In conclusion, we can see that society's values and what is considered socially accepted can change and evolve over time. This may involve a recognition of greater levels of equality and social justice, as seen with the ending of apartheid in South Africa in 1990. However, important social rights can also be taken away, as demonstrated by the quashing of the *Roe v. Wade* judgement in the United States, which allowed different states to determine women's access to abortion rather than the federal government and represented a substantial attack on women's reproductive rights.

It is also important to note that social norms which can influence laws and policies cannot in and of themselves be taken as the ethical basis for Social Work practice. In other words, we need to think about ethics in a more reflexive manner, as described by Clark (2000); that is, we need to question 'taken-for-granted' ideas and the arguments on which social norms are defined. This was echoed by Clifford and Burke (2009) who asserted that, although 'authority' establishes standards, principles and concepts, this does not mean that they must be accepted as 'ethical'. Therefore, Codes of Ethics, Codes of Conduct and even laws should always underpin interventions but never replace critical judgement. To be ethical in your practice, you need to be critical in your reflection while taking into account the legal, organisational and professional context in which a Social Worker's action takes place. In this book, we propose an approach to ethics that considers the person as a professional, professional norms and standards in Social Work and, more broadly, the context in which an intervention takes place. We do this in a way that centres the importance of practical reasoning in the process of ethical deliberation.

Ethics as Practical Reasoning

As noted, it is crucial for Social Workers to engage in critical self-reflection about their social location and values. We argue that, as Social Workers, we must also be aware of the various norms and standards that make up Social Work practice in a given jurisdiction and the basis on which these codes and other moral norms (which are often used as the basis for prescriptive ethics) were developed.

In order to support this process of critical reflection, this book introduces and examines a series of concepts which we consider to make up what we call the 'ethical foundations' of Social Work. These come from social theory and moral philosophy which, when combined, can be very valuable in exploring the kinds of ethical issues that are emerging in Social Work practice.

One of the key themes that we address throughout this book is that 'ethical practice' never exists in a vacuum. What we call 'ethical practice' becomes real through the ways in which practitioners use ethical concepts in concrete situations, and, in a wider sense, these situations are themselves located in particular societies and historical moments. It is in this sense that we see ethics as having a strongly social dimension – that is, they are concerned with the issue of how people relate to each other and how individuals and groups relate to social institutions. Many writers on Social Work ethics (e.g. see Rhodes, 1986; Clark, 2006; Clifford and Burke, 2009; Weinberg, 2018) have seen in this the political dimension of ethics, and we also sought to develop this line of argument by drawing attention to how ethical issues in Social Work are always contextualised and situated within power relationships. For this reason, 'conscious' ethical practice needs to involve questioning assumptions and critically challenging the various forms and structures of oppression encountered in Social Work practice.

This question of 'conscious' ethical practice is a key theme throughout this book, and we draw here from the work of contemporary moral philosopher Alasdair MacIntyre. In his book *Rational Dependent Animals* (1999), Macintyre set out an argument for what he called the 'practical reasoner'. We see this idea as very useful for Social Work and, indeed, something which may become an important paradigm for Social Work practice. MacIntyre suggested that people – in this case, Social Work students and practitioners – need to develop as practical reasoners. He characterised practical reason as a process which involves both reflection and self-knowledge – an enquiry that "provides us with grounds for criticism, revision, or even rejection of many of our judgments, our standards of judgment, our relationships and our institutions" (MacIntyre, 1999, p. 157).

There are a number of reasons why practical reasoning skills are so applicable to Social Work practice. Firstly, becoming a practical reasoner represents a set of understandings and skills which need to be consciously acquired. It requires active engagement rather than passivity, an unquestioning reliance on external guidelines. Being a practical reasoner means developing your own voice rather than simply going along with what is happening around you because it has 'always been done like that'. Secondly, the concept of the practical reasoner situates ethics in a social and relational dimension. When we think of ethical dilemmas, we often think of an isolated individual confronted by a series of difficult choices. However, in reality, the moral dilemmas addressed in Social Work (if not in life in general) are invariably located in relationships with others and particular institutional settings. In this sense, ethical decisions are not simply individual decisions but involve other people, both directly and indirectly. A key implication of this is the critical dimension of ethics, which is not only about an immediate situation but also related to wider questions about what the role of a Social Worker is and who they are meant to be accountable to – another key theme throughout this book.

This concept of Social Workers as practical reasoners is central to how we conceive of ethical practice in this book, and we explore this concept in a range of ways. Like other books on Social Work ethics, our approach is thematic, but the themes take their starting point in theory and are applied to practice, rather than the other way around which is more typical. We adopted this approach because we feel that a 'conscious ethical practitioner' must be able not only to grasp the realities of ethical dilemmas as they present but also understand how ethical theories can help us think differently and better understand the issues within these dilemmas.

It is equally important to state that, because ethics are a practice, they must bring together theoretical understandings and the acquisition of particular skills which are exercised in practice settings; it is in this way that practical reasoning skills are developed. Therefore, it is crucial to locate the process of developing ethical consciousness within the real world of Social Work practice, and it is for this reason that we make extensive use of case studies throughout the book. We draw from case studies not only to illustrate contemporary ethical dilemmas but also to demonstrate the process of analysing the situation, making links between theory and practice and applying a conscious ethical framework to a particular situation. The use of case studies allows readers to conceptualise Social Work practice as a process in which ethical principles can be applied to concrete situations.

Organisation of This Book

This book is divided into three parts, which include two to five chapters each. Part I, 'What Is Social Work?', includes two chapters; it considers the historical evolution of Social Work up to and including contemporary Social Work values and policy perspectives. Rojek et al.'s (1988) pioneering investigation of Social Work's 'received ideas' made the important point that "European Social Work can best face up to the actuality of value questions through a critical examination of its own historical roots and its received ideas in the context of their various discourses" (1988, p. 44).

Chapter 1, 'The Historical Emergence of Social Work', aims to recover the importance of this historic perspective as a means of revisiting the frequently asked question of what Social Work is. It focuses on two divergent conceptions of Social Work: those of the Charity Organisation Society and the Settlement Movements. In the Charity Organisation Society model of Social Work, the 'problems of the poor' were identified as a failure of 'morality' rather than a consequence of the destruction of a pre-existing social fabric, which occurred as a result of the development of industrial capitalism in Britain. Conversely, the Settlement movement, which branched into most of the large industrial centres of Britain, the United States and Australia, constitutes a tradition in which people with appropriate skills and understandings sought to place these at the service of the disenfranchised, working alongside those who suffered the effects of deprivation and advocating on their behalf where necessary.

This examination of the historical development of Social Work leads to Chapter 2, 'Contemporary Social Work: Care or Control?'. It examines the contemporary definition and manifestation of Social Work values and ethics, specifically Social Work practice over the last 30 years and the rise of neoliberalism and new public management. In particular, it looks at the implications of neoliberalism for ethical practice in an era when Social Work has been characterised as dominated by managerial and regulatory frameworks. Chapter 2 concludes by briefly looking at the Social Work value base, as deployed in current Codes of Ethics in Social Work, particularly within the IFSW.

Part II, Ethics and Social Dynamics, further develops the material presented in Part I by examining four key issues in Social Work: (1) power and oppression, (2) 'epistemic justice and injustice', (3) 'empowerment' and (4) radicalisation and the extreme right, and their significance for 'conscious' ethical practice. The chapters in this part lie at the intersection of social theory and ethics and consider the wider factors which frame the practical context in which Social Workers operate.

Chapter 3, 'Power and Oppression', examines different approaches to understanding power, beginning with key issues from classical social theory and moving on to contemporary theorisation. It also looks at their ethical implications for Social Work and considers the relationship between different forms and conceptions of oppression. Notably, Chapter 3 examines a number of key theories of power, Marxist, Weberian and Foucauldian, and considers the ethical dimensions of their work.

Closely linked to the first concept of power and the development of knowledge in Social Work, Chapter 4, 'Epistemic Injustice', examines the work of Miranda Fricker (2007), who described a distinctively *epistemic* genus of injustice in which an individual is specifically wronged in their capacity *as a knower* and therefore wronged in a capacity essential to human value.

In Chapter 5, 'Radicalisation, Social Work and Society', we begin by considering the historical context of the rise of violent authoritarian movements, both violent Islamist groups and Neo-Nazi movements. We examine the similarities between these groups, as well as the many misunderstandings that surround them and the complexity of the processes where people are drawn into them. We conclude by examining how practitioners can work with people whose vulnerabilities are being exploited so as to draw them into the hatred and nihilism of these political movements.

Chapter 6, 'Empowerment' examines different conceptions of of 'empowerment' in social work and how these have been used in the language and practice of Social Work. The chapter looks at the different ways in which this concept can be understood, concluding by looking at the work of Paulo Freire and his conception of 'empowerment' as critical consciousness and democratic practice.

At last, Part III, 'Ethical Perspectives for Social Work', examines core principles of Social Work through a number of ethical theories. We chose to explore five overarching ethical theories and perspectives that have greatly influenced professional ethics in Social Work or are considered increasingly important today. Chapter 7, 'Decolonial Ethics', presents some of the necessary principles for working with Indigenous people and populations. In many places around the globe, Social Workers have intervened in the lives of Indigenous communities in ways that have often reflected deeply held colonial assumptions embodied in law and policy and been detrimental to both Indigenous people and communities. Ioakimidis and Wyllie's (2023) work offers an extensive documentation of how Social Workers have been complicit in the legacy of colonialism and racism. For example, in both Canada and Australia, Social Workers have actively contributed to the implementation and enforcement of colonial policies which saw Indigenous children removed from their families and placed in institutions (Yu, 2019). National professional associations are increasingly recognising their responsibility to do better and not repeat the harm previously committed (Yu et al., 2024). Therefore, Chapter 7 begins Part III discussing Indigenous worldviews before colonisation, illustrates the impact of colonisation and articulates how a decolonial ethics standpoint can help non-Indigenous Social Workers engage with Indigenous people and communities to contribute to reconciliation efforts and, ultimately, decolonisation.

The next two chapters, Chapters 8 and 9, examine principle-based ethics perspectives, which use principles or rules to help define right and wrong actions. Chapter 8, 'Kantian Ethics', proposes an exploration of Social Work's underlying roots in the moral philosophy of the Enlightenment. It looks at the central concepts of self-determination and human dignity through the work of Immanuel Kant. The chapter also outlines the ways in which Kant's work has framed the understanding of these concepts in modern Social Work. Chapter 9, 'Utilitarian and Rawlians' Ethics', examines the idea of social justice though different ethical theories and highlights different ways of understanding the concept. It explores this theme through a discussion of utilitarian theories of ethics from the works of Jeremy Bentham and John Stuart Mill. Principles of distributive justice developed by John Rawls are also examined. The legacy of these frameworks on the contemporary legislative framework of Social Work is also considered.

The last two chapters move away from principle-based ethics and introduce the idea of *character-based and relationship-based ethics. These branches of ethical theory* do not rely on rules to follow but instead focuses on the sort of person who makes the decision and their relationships with others.

Chapter 10, 'Virtue Ethics and Ethics of Care', examines the work of Socrates and Alasdair MacIntyre, alongside the idea of 'ethics of care', an influential development in virtue ethics. Finally, Chapter 11 presents the ethics of recognition. The concept of recognition, as developed by Honneth (1996), draws attention to three areas of social life in which recognition can be produced or is lacking: intimate and personal relationships, the state (laws and rights) and social interactions. This ethical perspective focuses on relationships and can help identify where factors of oppression and resistance may emerge, which allows professionals to think about how a more ethical society – that is, one that produces recognition for everybody – can be fostered through Social Work. We conclude with a discussion of the centrality of ethical practice to Social Work as a whole, which expresses our hope that, in writing this book, we have contributed to keeping alive the idea of Social Work as a project of practical humanitarian social change.

Part One

What Is Social Work?

1 The Historical Emergence of Social Work

When we talk about Social Work, what are we talking about? One of the complications of defining the nature and content of Social Work practice is that it varies considerably according to where it takes place. Sarah Banks has noted that:

> Social work is, therefore, a difficult occupation to encapsulate. It is located within and profoundly affected by diverse cultural, economic, political and policy contexts in different countries of the world. Social work embraces work in a number of sectors (public, private, independent, voluntary) and it takes place in a multiplicity of settings (residential homes, neighbourhood offices, community development projects). Social work practitioners perform a range of tasks (caring, controlling, empowering, campaigning, assessing, managing) and the work has a variety of purposes (redistribution of resources to those in need, social control and rehabilitation of the deviant, prevention or reduction of social problems, and empowerment of oppressed individuals and groups).
>
> (Banks, 2020, pp. 1–2)

There are those Social Workers employed by governments, there are those who work in national voluntary organisations and NGOs, while there are others who work in small, grassroots organisations. Are they all doing Social Work? Can they all call themselves Social Workers? Can we define Social Work independently of its context of practice? Just as the question of what activities actually count as Social Work has had different kinds of answers, so equally we find different definitions of what Social Work is. Consider, for example, the following two definitions of Social Work:

> Social work is 'a profession which promotes social change, problem solving in human relationships and the empowerment and liberation of people to enhance well-being…Principles of Human Rights and social justice are fundamental to social work'.
>
> (The International Federation of Social Work (IFSW) quoted in Horner, 2018, p. 4)

> Social work is 'a very practical job. It is about protecting people and changing their lives, not about being able to give a fluent and theoretical explanation about why they got into difficulties in the first place.'
>
> (Jacqui Smith, former UK Minister of Social Care, quoted in Horner, 2018, p. 4)

DOI: 10.4324/9781003458715-3

When we think about these two definitions, it becomes apparent that the authors of these two definitions are emphasising quite different conceptions of Social Work. The first definition, from the International Federation of Social Work, evokes a concept of the Social Worker as the agent of individual and social change, placing their skills at the service of the excluded and disempowered. The second definition from Jacqui Smith, former UK Minister for Social Care, by contrast, does not talk about social change, empowerment or liberation – instead she emphasises that Social Workers need to be 'practical'. This definition promotes the idea that Social Workers should be 'doers' rather than 'theoreticians'. At first glance, that may sound like a more realistic definition, but what about the way this definition presents action as something which is separate from thought? In the context of this book particularly, if we are concerned with the ethical dimensions of Social Work practice, don't we need to be 'thinkers' as well as 'doers'? Isn't there a danger in putting such emphasis on 'doing' that we fail to consider the ethical basis of the things that we are doing? At a deeper level, aren't all forms of doing connected to thought?

These are the sorts of questions we will be addressing throughout this book, but the key point which will be explored in this chapter is these different definitions are not just about people being confused about what Social Work is. Rather this confusion comes about because the definitions offered reflect different assumptions about the role of Social Workers and what it is they are supposed to be doing. Are Social Workers advocates and campaigners for the people they are working on behalf of, or is their role to support people through the implementation of particular laws and policies? Who are Social Workers supposed to serve – the organisations they work for or the service users they work with? Is the wider purpose of Social Work to serve the 'nation' or to serve the 'citizen'?

In this chapter, we want to suggest that one really good way to understand this is think about the emergence of Social Work historically. There is a tendency in some Social Work text-books to take the context of practice as a given – and then to see the role of the book as explaining to people the best way to do this. However, if we look at the historical emergence of Social Work, including the way it is continuing to develop across the world, we can get a better sense of why there are these different conceptions of what the responsibilities of Social Worker are. This allows us to see that Social Work never was and probably never will be just one thing; there have always been different and even radically opposed conceptions of the role and purpose of Social Work.

Social Work Ethics in History

Philanthropy, which means the process of helping others without expectation of personal gain, is as old as human society itself. Almost all societies have to deal with the fact that there are problems which manifest themselves on an ongoing basis and which will simply become more and more serious if some kind of help, assistance or relief is not provided. In his study of the origins of Social Work, Malcolm Payne noted that as far as back as Ancient Greece and Rome, there were important traditions of charity and philanthropy which have emerged from the need to deal with social problems such as divorce, child abuse, abortion and prostitution (Payne, 2005, p. 13). In Medieval Europe, as well as in China and India, organised religion was not only one of the most powerful forces in society but came to be a focus for charitable work because of the association between religious virtue and assisting the more vulnerable in the community. Throughout history, there have been people who became involved in charitable work and set up organisations which sought to help individuals in difficulty, and Social Work grows out of those traditions.

Payne and Kirk note that

> unlike a number of traditional professions such as medicine, law, teaching, pharmacy and engineering that can be traced to classical Greece and Rome and throughout the medieval period in Europe, the emergence of social work did not take place until the second half of the nineteenth century.
>
> (Parton and Kirk, 2009, p. 24)

This is a significant point which tells us something important about the reasons why Social Work emerged historically. The connection between Social Work and social problems is central to way Social Work emerges as a defined activity. Parton and Kirk (2009) note that the development of 'Social Work' as a defined activity "emerges at times of rapid social change, at the time of war, or when communities break up under pressure from increased market forces and where industrialization and urbanization are rapid". Social work emerged in England and the USA in the second half of the nineteenth century where traditional communities based on kinship and geographical proximity were no longer able either to meet the needs of their members or provide appropriate social order. Similarly, they note that Social Work developed in formerly communist countries in the late twentieth century when the more regulated and compulsory communities forged by the coercive collective inclusionary policies of state communist societies began to collapse under the demands of liberalisation and privatisation in the post-Soviet era (Parton and Kirk, 2009, p. 25). We could extend this argument to understand way that Social Work has now become a global profession concerns the way these profound social processes of urbanisation, industrialisation and changes in the way societies organise their political and economic structures have developed across the world, bringing about the undermining and transformation of community networks based on traditional forms of kinship and ways of life. In terms of understanding Social Work's origins, it is therefore important to examine the specific context in which Social Work has emerged and is continuing to emerge.

Before we begin, it is worth asking why a book on Social Work ethics might begin by talking about the need to have an understanding of the history of Social Work. The reason for this comes back to one of the key arguments we put forward in the introduction; which is that 'ethical practice' in Social Work never exists in a vacuum; ethical choices are always grounded in a particular historical moment, a particular political period and a particular society. Take for example the issue of child labour. The vast majority of people who live in the West would regard this practice as cruel and exploitative – they would believe that children are too young for this type of work and that the right place for these children should be in school. Yet for many decades, across Europe and North America children worked in mines, factories and farms. This related to the way families needed to have as many members of the family as possible working and bringing in an income: and that children just as much as adults were seen as capable of work. Employers themselves had absolutely no problem with the morality of child labour; as a British campaigner against the practice noted in 1908:

> Child labour being regarded by the manufacturers as absolutely essential to the speedy piling up of fortunes, the morality of which no-one questioned, it was

> universally employed in the cotton mills and factories which sprang up in the land. Manchester, specifically the seat of the cotton trade from its earliest days, was a positive employer of child labour...A positive majority of the workers in the cotton mills were young children.
>
> (Dale [1908] in Alexander, 1988, p. 53)

The views expressed above were an example of the language of the political campaigns aimed at eradicating child labour as they developed throughout the early twentieth century in the UK. They are also related to significant changes taking place in society in which attending school became to be seen as more important than working at this particular age. It was in this particular context that child labour came to be seen as 'unethical'. However, in much of the world today, particularly sub-Saharan Africa and South Asia, child labour is practised for much the same reasons as it was in Europe and North America last century; poverty is widespread, there is little or no enforced regulation governing employment practices, and education is seen as the preserve of children from wealthy families. That is not to say that child labour cannot be considered unethical in all societies; and there are people all over the world campaigning on this basis. However, the point we are trying to make here is that the basis of what we regard as an 'ethical issue' is an expression of particular assumptions and expectations people have of the way they will live their lives. In that sense, our conception of what is an ethical issue is always grounded in a particular context, and framed by particular understandings related to that context. This is the value of having a historical understanding, as it allows us to look beyond our own immediate situation and values and situate those within a wider context.

Reflection Break: Are Ethical Issues Universal or Relative?

One of the big debates in the field of ethics is the question of whether issues are universal, that is applicable in all situations, or relative, which means specific to particular contexts. In terms of this debate consider the following:

1 Child Labour is now outlawed in most European countries, but does that mean that Child Labour was and is always wrong from the perspective of social justice? What is it about child labour that makes is morally objectionable?
2 Many religious organisations object to women who have unwanted pregnancies obtaining abortions on the basis that they consider this to be the 'taking of life', a major offence in the eyes of their religion. Consider a situation where group-based social housing for young people seeking to overcome drug problems is being provided by such a religious organisation. If the funding for this housing provision comes from the government, should the religious groups providing the housing be allowed to refuse to carry literature or information which gives young women advice about obtaining a termination? Would you consider the refusal to carry this information a legitimate expression of faith, or should the state, as funder, insist that women from all communities should have access to this information about the termination of a pregnancy if they require this? Finally, what are the mechanisms or principles we would use to decide on an issue like this?

This chapter is not attempting to offer a full history of the development of Social Work, and readers who are interested in this may want to look at Mark Hendrickson's book on *The Origins of Social Care and Social Work* (2022) for a more detailed account of this. We have chosen to focus on instances from of Social Work practice in different contexts to allow us to explore the question of what Social Work practice involves as well as the ethical questions that may emerge from them. We have chosen to focus on these because they highlight not only the contextual but also the inherently political nature of ethical dilemmas in Social Work.

This chapter begins with a discussion of the way Social Work in its current form emerged as a strategy for dealing with the consequences of social deprivation in Britain and the United States at the end of the nineteenth century. The second part of the chapter considers Social Work practices in the Global South, looking particularly at the Social Work with homeless people in cities in India.

Social Work as a 'Product of Modernity'

As already noted, the motivation which some people feel to help and assist those in distress is something which is universal to all societies, and probably to human existence itself. However Social Work's arrival on the historical stage in the particular form which it now takes is a product of a particular history, and having a historical perspective allows us to grasp the way in which Social Work's existence is related to the emergence and persistence of particular kinds of social problems. It is in this sense that Social Work can be thought of as a 'product of Modernity'. We can think of Modernity as a set of historical experiences based on capitalism as an economic system, industrial production, urbanisation and particular ideas about the political rights of 'citizens', which themselves emerged from the Enlightenment and the French Revolution in the Eighteenth century.

What Is Modernity?

Austen Harrington notes that the word Modernity derives from the Latin word modus, meaning 'of our time'; here and now, as opposed to the past. It is this meaning that we evoke when we refer to something as 'very modern'.

However, the term can also be used to refer to a particular period, as we do here, where it refers to the influence of the Industrial Revolution, and the spread of the ideas from the French Revolution and of 'Age of Enlightenment'.

(Harrington, 2005, p. 17)

Prior to the emergence of modern urban societies of the sort we now see across the economically developed world, the vast majority of the population survived through subsistence farming and people lived in small communities rather than in large cities. In Medieval Europe, people would not even have much of a sense of 'society' and Peter Knapp and Alan Spector argue that this idea is itself a central feature of modernity. This is because what we think of as 'modern' was defined in relation to the traditional subsistence economies which modernity was displacing. Hence it only became possible to "conceive of 'society'...when different kinds of social structure can be observed". These different structures were represented by the conflict between "two kinds of social system – one feudal, agrarian, monarchical, religious, aristocratic, traditional and rural, and the other capitalist, industrial, more democratic, secular, dynamic and urban" (2011, p. 53). Karl Polanyi's book *The Great Transformation*, which traces the history of the emergence of capitalism in Europe, gives an interesting example of this. He demonstrates that 'the poor' first became visible as a social problem in the sixteenth century as a consequence of the emergence of a group of people who were "unattached to the manor 'or any feudal superior'" (Polanyi, 2001, p. 109). In other words, while the vast majority of people in medieval society lived in what we would consider today grinding poverty, the problem of 'the poor' only came to be seen as a problem when groups of people who were not incorporated within traditional social bonds became noticeable.

For the development of capitalism to take place, firstly farming had to be industrialised, as it was through the introduction of machinery, and much land had to be 'enclosed'. This meant the peasants who had for generations worked that land had to be removed from it, and this happened through brute force in many instances. It was through this process a labour force for modern industry was created. What we call modernity thus arrived in people's lives through the destruction of centuries-old ways of life, as former peasants left the land, or were forcibly removed from it, and emigrated into new urban centres like, in England, the cities of London, Manchester and Birmingham. It is the momentous nature of these social changes which Karl Marx was seeking to understand when he wrote his now famous book *The Communist Manifesto*. He noted that:

> The bourgeoisie, wherever it has got the upper hand, has put an end to all feudal, patriarchal, idyllic relations. It has pitilessly torn asunder the motley feudal ties that bound man to his "natural superiors", and has left remaining no other nexus between man and man than naked self-interest, than callous "cash payment". (...) All fixed, fast-frozen relations, with their train of ancient and venerable prejudices and opinions, are swept away, all new-formed ones become antiquated before they can ossify. All that is solid melts into air, all that is holy is profaned, and man is at last compelled to face with sober senses his real conditions of life, and his relations with his kind.
>
> (Marx [1848], 2012, pp. 37–38)

The key point we want to remember from Marx here is that the way capitalism, a system he sees as driven by a new class of entrepreneurs he calls the bourgeoisie, needs to be understood as a radically different sort of economic system. In order to establish itself, it had to destroy the feudal world, and the 'ancient and venerable' social bonds associated with that, which brought about social dislocation, poverty and squalor on a scale never previously witnessed. As a commercial, and then an industrial society emerged throughout the eighteenth and nineteenth centuries in Britain, as Polyani puts it "sporadic destitution had grown into a torrent of misery" (Polanyi, 2001, p. 113). While the new factories producing goods that were now being sold across the British Empire created great wealth for this emerging class of factory owners, the vast majority of workers lived in unsanitary and impoverished conditions which were rife with disease and destitution. While rural communities had worked on a seasonal basis, the new factory work involved long hours and constant work. The older traditional communities had absorbed the disabled, the elderly and the frail within the structure of the family; however, the need to care for those not able to work within the new system exacerbated problems of deprivation. We would argue that it was concern around the problems associated with the development

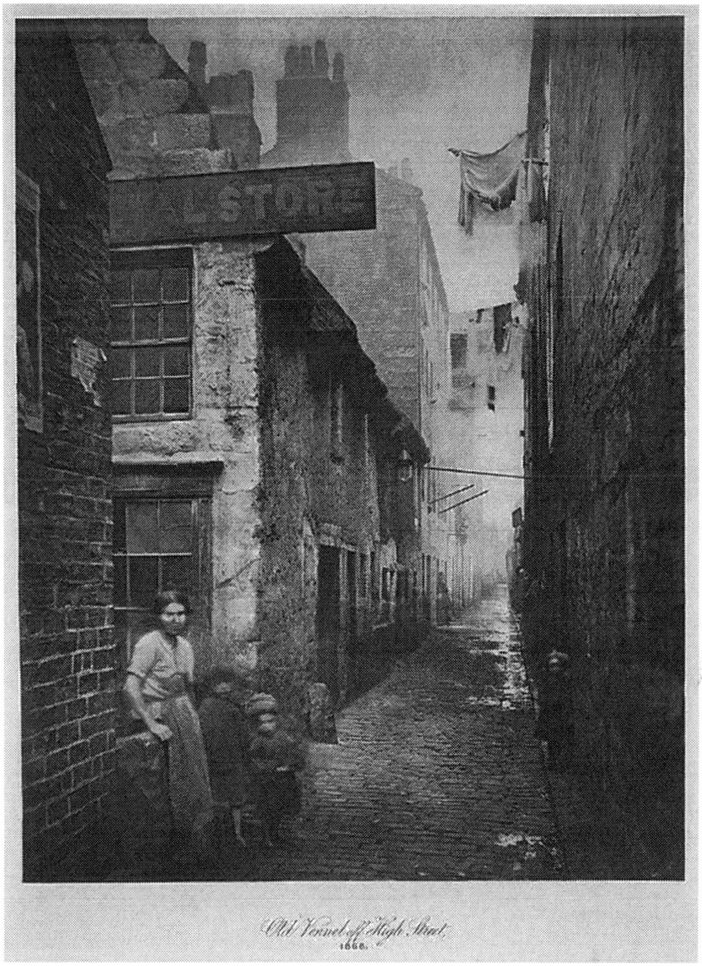

Figure 1.1 A mother and her children in London's East End during the Victorian era, depicting daily life and social conditions of the time

Source: http://www.makingthemodernworld.org.uk/stories/the_industrial_town/06.ST.02/?scene=6&tv=true

of industrial urban capitalist societies that initiated the basis for modern Social Work (Figure 1.1).

In places like the United States, Europe and Australia, Social Work is a paid profession; however, as Social Work is now across much of the developing world and Global South, activities associated with the Social Work role are often organised by charitable groups. Throughout the eighteenth and nineteenth centuries, in the UK and North America, a range of charities and philanthropic individuals expressed concern with the conditions of the poor. One of the most famous examples of this was a book put together by the British social investigator and journalist Henry Mayhew, which published in 1851 with the title *London Labour and the London Poor*. In this book, Mayhew and his team of researchers documented the impact which unemployment, substandard housing and rampant disease were having on the conditions of the working classes in London. The work of Charles Booth in the late 1900s developed this still further with the development of 'poverty maps', where social inequality indicators were mapped onto particular geographical areas. While charity and philanthropic work developed during the nineteenth century in relation to the questions of poverty and what needed to be done to address it, these forms of social investigation took place in a context in which the dominant view of political leaders and established opinion saw the problem not so much concerned in terms of the suffering caused by poverty and the need for the authorities to understand and do something about it, as the problem of the lack of moral behaviour of the poor themselves – so the problems of poverty were seen as problems of personal 'character', which were related to the frequency with which the poor engaged in drunkenness, 'idleness' and various other forms of 'vice'; in more strictly economic terms, 'unproductive labour' (Jones, 2014). The poor thus presented to the governing classes as both an object of concern and a threat, both potential and actual, to the dominant order. This is significant for Social Work's emergence since the justification for Social Work activities is related to both of these concerns.

Many of the voluntary activities which were the forerunners of contemporary Social Work were forms of self-help which emerged from working class communities themselves. Throughout the nineteenth century, Friendly Societies, Building Societies and Co-operatives where working class people pooled their resources to make payments during periods of sickness or unemployment were formed (Payne, 2005, pp. 33–34). These developments in working-class self-help were closely related to the growing influence of Trade Unions and the increasing belief that working class organisations needed their own political party, which lead to founding of the Labour Party in Britain in the early years of the twentieth century. These forms of grass roots Social Work point to the way Social Work's legacy is also connected to the history of Socialism in places such as the UK, Australia and the United States (Payne, 2005; Crocker, 1992).

Charities by contrast were generally set up by philanthropists from the middle classes, often with religious motivations. The nineteenth century saw a substantial growth in charitable organisations, which were often set up within the major churches, but which were also partially separate from them. Typical of this was an organisation such as that set up by Thomas Barnado, a mission preacher who had initially planned to work in China, but who, upon witnessing the destitution of orphaned and abandoned children in the East End of London, decided that his charitable energies were more needed in his own country. He set up a 'ragged school' where children could obtain a basic education in 1867, and his first home for orphaned boys in 1870. Barnardo's entrepreneurial and fundraising skills allowed this grow into a nationwide network, and the organisation he founded continues to this day (Payne, 2005, pp. 29–30). Middle-class women were also often prominently involved in organised charitable work, and practices which developed out of this period were 'social visiting', where volunteers from charities would visit the houses of the poor, offering them advice on family life, budgeting etc. The origins of Social Work casework lie in this method of observation and recording (Jones, 2002). There were thus a range of different forms of provision which emerged with substantially different approaches – and this itself depended on the underlying philosophy of the organisation. This is significant because the different forms of provision which emerged in this period have all in their different ways, fed into what Social Work became when its work was primarily organised by the state. In terms of bringing this out, we want to focus on two different organisations whose legacy to modern Social Work is fundamental in terms of the different ways in which they sought to provide assistance to the urban poor – these are the Charity Organisation Society (COS) on the one hand and the Settlement Movement on the other.

The Charity Organisation Society

The COS was founded in 1869 with the explicit aim of co-ordinating charitable giving. From the outset, the organisation sought to providing key principles under which charitable giving was seen as desirable and beneficial. These principles were as follows:

1. Full investigation into the circumstances of the applicant to be undertaken in every case.
2. No relief to be given that is not adequate, that cannot hope to render the person or family relieved self-supporting.
3. No relief to be given to cases that are so 'bad' in point of character or so chronic in their need as to be incapable of permanent restoration.
4. All 'hopeless' cases, however deserving, to be handed over to the poor law.

(Townsend [1911] in Alexander, 1998, p. 183)

As the principles above imply, the COS model of welfare was based on the idea that the poor had to demonstrate particular qualities – such as patience, cleanliness, thrift, sobriety, and in particular the ability to become 'self-supporting' – in order to be seen as worthy of receiving help. The family was assessed through the process of 'social visiting', where middle class mostly female volunteers would visit the houses of the poor, offering what was seen as appropriate advice, and most importantly assess them for whether the family was deemed to be worthy or unworthy of receiving charity. The influential secretary of the organisation, Loch, argued that unless this process of assessing families was undertaken, charitable giving was "as husks, flung before the poor as if they were without common humanity" (in Payne, 2005, p. 35). This reflects the underlying fear within large sections of the political establishment that while charitable giving was 'worthy', there was also the danger that it would simply encourage dependency and 'idleness' from the working classes.

As well as contributing the casework method and the model of home visiting to modern Social Work, the COS model instituted the process of allocating support based on a distinction between the 'deserving' and 'undeserving'. Underlying this was an idea central to attitudes to poverty in Victorian England, which was that it was not a problem of the structure of society, but a problem of the 'character' of the poor themselves. In this the role of Social Work was to reforming this 'character'. Bernard Bosanquet, one of the founding members of the COS, expressed this as follows:

> Here then we find the true meaning of Social Work. Whenever it may start its goal is the same; to bring the mind into order; into harmony with itself. Social disintegration is the outward and visible form of moral and intellectual disintegration.
>
> (in Jones, 1998, p. 36)

The COS model of Social Work was an individualist model which placed the responsibility onto the applicant for charity to demonstrate they had the capacity to 'raise themselves up' beyond the difficulties caused by poverty, unemployment and destitution. This implies that difficulties experienced were essentially individual misfortunes rather than structural features of the wider society and economy, and the despair and demoralisation resulting from these were seen as 'moral failings', rather than understandable responses to feelings of powerlessness and isolation. While this attitude to poverty as a product of character rather than circumstances would appear crude and patronising to contemporary Social Work, Chris Jones has argued that this conception of Social Work has had a profound influence:

> Despite the many changes in language and knowledge based of Social Work since the end of the nineteenth century, Social Work has remained an activity that is not only class specific but has also continued to practice as if the primary causes of clients' problems are located in their own behaviour, morality and deficient family relationships. Mainstream Social Work, despite its immersion in poverty and amongst the least powerful sections of the population, has rarely ventured to seek explanations for these difficulties beyond family and interpersonal relationships and dynamics.
>
> (Jones, 1998, p. 37)

As well as raising questions about how Social Workers understand and make sense of the experiences of service users, Jones is also raising the question about how the organisational context of Social Work influences the ethical decision making which Social Workers undertake, an issue which will be picked up in other chapters in the book. Jones point is also significant as he is suggesting that the legacy of the COS model of Social Work is far more influential than is generally acknowledged.

Reflection Break: How Much Do Social Workers Acknowledge Poverty as a Factor in Their Assessments of Service Users?

There is considerable evidence to demonstrate the fact that contemporary Children and Families Social Work intervention is almost entirely experienced by the poorest and most socially marginalised families in society. Discuss the following questions:

1. Why do you think it is that the poverty is such a consistent factor in families seen by Children and Families Social Workers?
2. What impact might this have on the way these families experience Social Work intervention?
3. Are there things that Social Workers can do about this? What are they?

The Settlement Movement

This conception of poverty as caused by the 'moral weakness' of the poor, while being the dominant view within the COS, was not universally accepted. For example, one local branch secretary noted in the records of her local branch that "human beings cannot be treated as simple units… – the man with his character such as his temperament and surroundings have made it, can only act within the limits of the community of which he is a fraction" (Woodroofe, 1962, p. 60). This comment points to the idea that the choices, which people made were not simply shaped by their individual moral character but were also significantly influenced by their wider situation in which they were living. It was these sorts of understandings that led to the development of different conception of the role of Social Work Social Work: the Settlement Movement. Settlements were a significant social reform initiative which consisted of students and well-educated groups moving into deprived areas and using their skills to facilitate a greater level of education, dignity and quality of life for working class communities. The original Settlement in the UK was Toynbee Hall in Whitechapel in East London, which was established by Canon Samuel Barnett in 1884. Clement Attlee, one of the architects of British Welfare state, was closely involved in Toynbee Hall as a young man. Toynbee Hall was visited by the North American social reformer Jane Addams; after seeing the work that went on there, she went back to her home town of Chicago and founded the first Settlement in the United States, Hull House, in Chicago. In her autobiography, Jane Addams describes an incident which was pivotal in demonstrating what was wrong with the charity model of Social Work, with its central distinction between the deserving and the undeserving, and which went on to shape the direction in which she took Social Work at Hull House Settlement. Describing her early involvement in charity work, she explains that she was given the task of assisting a man who had lost his job as a shipping clerk:

> I told him of an opportunity for work on the drainage canal and intimated that if any employment were available, he ought to exhaust that possibility before asking for help. The man replied that he had always worked indoors and that he could not endure outside work during the winter. I am grateful to remember that I was too uncertain to be severe, but that I held to my instructions. He did not come again for relief, but worked for two days on the canal, where he contracted pneumonia and died a week later. I have never lost trace of the two little children he left behind him, although I cannot see them without a bitter consciousness that it was at their expense I learned that life cannot be administered by definite rules and regulations; that wisdom to deal with a man's [sic] difficulties comes only through knowledge of his life and habits as a whole, and that to treat an isolated episode is almost sure to invite blundering.
>
> (in Conway, 1992, pp. 518–519)

Settlements in this sense emerged out of a critique of the individualistic nature of the dominant Victorian charity model. Beatrice Webb, a committed Socialist who was involved in numerous disputes with Bernard Bosenquet of the COS in the UK, argued for the need to understand poverty as a structural problem, and it was this that was central to the philosophy of the Settlements (Figure 1.2).

While the Settlement movement was, like most forms of nineteenth-century Social Work, inspired by Christianity, the philosophy of Settlements tended towards a more radical reading of the Gospels than the COS and other church-based charities. As W. Moore Ede explains, the philosophy of the Settlements was not about conversion of those seen to be suffering from deficiencies of 'character' – those living in deprived areas:

> (…) will not be converted by missionaries and tracts sent by dwellers in the West End. The dwellers in the West End must go to the dwellers in the East themselves, share with the East those pleasures which give interest and delight to the dwellers in the West, and make up the fullness of their lives.
>
> (in Woodroofe, 1962, p. 65)

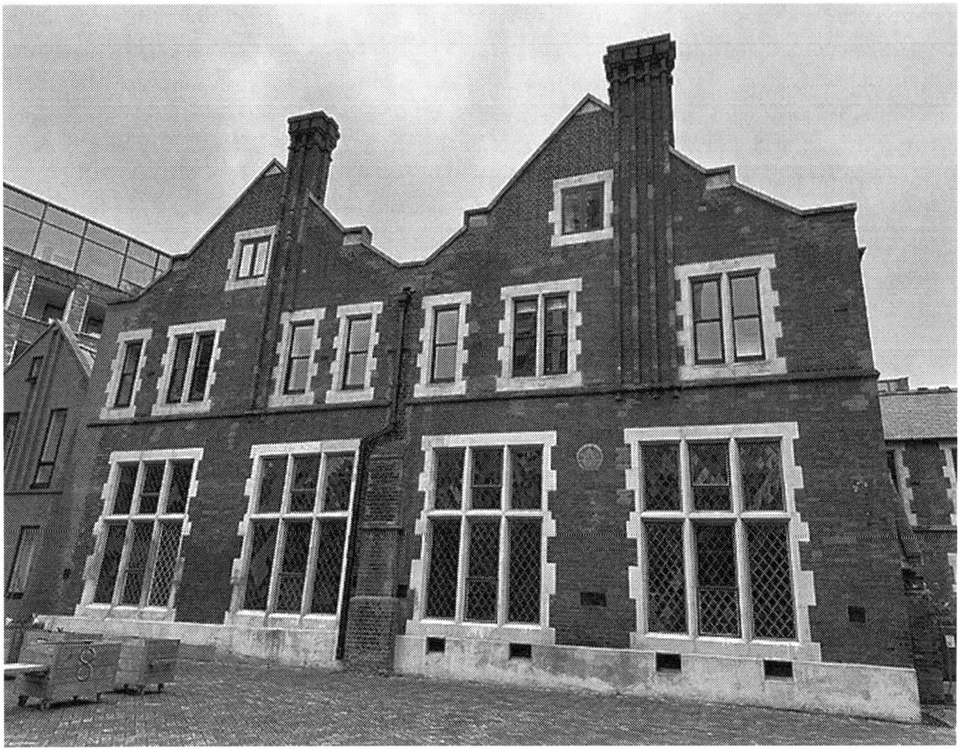

Figure 1.2 Toynbee Hall, in Whitechapel, London

Active participation in the lives of people living in deprived areas was therefore central to the ethos of the Settlement movement, reflecting the idea that in order to change the degraded conditions in which communities were living in, you first needed to understand through first-hand experience the kinds of pressures and difficulties which they faced. Unlike the COS approach in which the individual was assessed according to strictly defined rules, the Settlement movement involved a more collaborative relationship between helper and helped, emphasising the value of allowing the helper and the helped to learn from each other.

The Two Souls of Social Work

One of the founders of the Social Sciences was a Frenchman named August Comte (1798–1813), and he argued that one of the most important things that people in modern societies had to learn was the capacity for altruism – which he defined as "living for others" (Dixon, 2008). This kind of idea is crucial to the development of Social Work, and interestingly enough we can see it as something which animates and motivates both the Settlement Movement and the COS, as well as being an ethical concept which is still central to contemporary Social Work. While both conceptions of Social Work were based on the idea of "living for others", the interpretations of what this meant were profoundly different. The COS volunteers and leaders certainly saw themselves as 'living for others' and they were motivated by concerns about the appalling conditions in which poor people lived in Britain's industrial cities. However they did not question the dominant order and saw the helping role of Social Work in terms of a moral crusade to change the individual character of the poor and oppressed. While the COS was a charitable organisation, its central concerns was that the poor needed to show their willingness to become 'self-supporting'; that is to go out to work. In this sense, the COS shared the fears, which we have noted were dominant with the political establishment of the time, that charitable giving could potentially encourage 'idleness' amongst the poor. Work was understood by the COS volunteers as an expression of religious virtue; by helping people to become 'self-supporting' they were helping people to be 'better people'. What this leaves out of the picture is the experience described by Jane Addams – the unsafe, unsanitary and exploitative conditions in which work was frequently undertaken. By overlooking this, charities such as the COS were promoting a conception of Social Work as the promotion of 'individual independence' rather than thinking about the underlying causes of poverty and deprivation. As Mrs Townsend, a Fabian critic of the COS commented at the time: "They stuck to the theory of individual independence…in a world where man-made laws were enabling the rich to grind the faces of the poor" (in Alexander, 1998, p. 184).

The Settlement movement by contrast sought to work around practical problems from the perspective of, in the words of Jane Addams 'knowledge of the lives and habits' of the community as a whole. Rather than seeing the problems of poverty and destitution as problems of individual character, they promoted a concept of Social Work based on campaigning, advocacy alongside practical measures to improve the lives of people. We see the two approaches to social problems embodied in these two movements as representing what we would call 'the two souls of Social Work'; one representing a vision of Social Work based on the reform of individual character and support for the 'deserving poor', the other representing an attempt to understand the circumstances of communities which experience poverty as a whole, and working collaboratively with those communities. They also represent Social Work's two souls because the different assumptions and values embodied have both become incorporated into what Social Work became once it was formally institutionalised within the State in Britain. In concrete terms, how much in Social Work practice in countries like the UK today do we see problems such as the neglect of children purely in terms of action, or inaction, by 'bad parents'? How are problems such as parental mental health or alcohol abuse understood in the context of the profound level of stress caused by poverty and social exclusion? How significant are issues such as low level of social benefits, the low wages and lack of job security which characterises the lives of many families working with Social Workers seen as factors which shape the kinds of relationships which people have? And how do we incorporate our understanding of the impact of these experiences within our practice?

The Emergence of State Social Work in the Global North

As already noted, these different conceptions of Social Work derived from a time when Social Work was a voluntary activity, and governmental involvement in the arena of welfare provision was minimal. It was the experience of the Great Depression in the 1930s, followed by the Second World War that substantially changed the political landscape in Europe and North America leading to the institutionalisation of Social Welfare within the state. In the context of Britain specifically the historian Richard Titmuss has argued that the essential precondition for this related to the way "the circumstances of the war created an unprecedented sense of social solidarity among the British people [and] made them willing to accept a great increase of egalitarian policies and collective state intervention" (in Thane, 1982, p. 223). In Britain, it was the Beveridge Report in 1942 which acted as the founding document for development of the welfare state, proposing a blueprint for fighting against the five 'evils' of the modern world: Want, Disease, Ignorance, Squalor and Idleness. The report's solution to this was a free, universal and comprehensive provision of service from 'the cradle to the grave' in the spheres of both social care and health, with the creation of the National Health Service (Payne, 2005). Following the election of the Labour government led by Clement Atlee in 1945, which implemented these major changes, the Welfare State slowly began to take shape in the form of a universal system, aimed at providing services to everyone in need in of health and social assistance. It was during this period that Social Work came to be institutionalised as one of the key professions within the welfare state, and it is this change that meant Social Work moved from being a voluntary activity to a public service with legally defined roles and responsibilities. Throughout the subsequent decades of the 1950s, 1960s and 1970s in Britain the responsibilities of Social Workers grew and developed, extending into completely new areas such as mental health and 'juvenile delinquency'. The framework of statutory responsibilities for Social Work also developed, encompassing such crucial issues such as Childcare and Mental Health. The most significant reorganisation of Social Work took place in the wake of the Seebohm Report in 1968, and this sought to rationalise and simplify access to services, leading to the development of Social Services Departments within Local Authorities. The report sought to recommend the creation of "a new local authority department, providing a community based and family-oriented service, which will be available to all" (Seebohm Report, cited in Harris, 1999, p. 919). John Harris notes that the Seebohm Report

> represented the consolidation of Social Work's position as part of the post-war social democratic welfare state...The period has been described as the 'high tide of Social Work' coming at the tail-end of the commitment of 1960s social democracy to tackling the problems of society through expertise located in the state and to promoting citizenship through solidarity.
>
> (1999, p. 920)

Alongside the growth of Social Work provision in Local Authorities, Social Work education in colleges and universities also became formalised during the early 1960s. State-based Social Work was never intended to eliminate the need for voluntary activity, and this period also witnessed the growth of the 'voluntary sector', which was itself increasingly professionalised, though its name was a reminder of its earlier history. These same processes took place across the economically developed world in the post-war period, as welfare states developed in different forms and to different degrees in Scandinavia, Canada, Australia as well as in Southern Europe. This same dynamic also impacted newly independent countries such as India, which gained its independence from Britain in 1947. Within the Constitution of India, Article 38, Part 4 states that:

1 The State shall strive to promote the welfare of the people by securing and protecting as effectively as it may a social order in which justice, social, economic and political, shall inform all the institutions of the national life.
2 The State shall, in particular, strive to minimise the inequalities in income, and endeavour to eliminate inequalities in status, facilities and opportunities, not only amongst individuals but also amongst groups of people residing in different areas or engaged in different vocations.

While the application and enforcement of these principles has not been as extensive as in the Global North, it is important to note the extent of adoption of these sorts of principles concerning the role of the state in having responsibility for the welfare of the people.

Social Work as a Global Profession

The story we have told so far has emphasised the growth of Social work in places such as the UK and the USA in the second half of the nineteenth century as part of a wider social process where traditional communities based on kinship and geographical proximity were no longer able either to meet the needs of their members or provide appropriate social order (Parton and Kirk, 2009, p. 25). However we have also noted the extent to which social welfare embodied in a wider sense of the state having responsibility for well-being of the population as a whole was part of the post-war world. In terms of the development of Social Work practice, we can also understand its global development as part of the same dynamic as processes of industrialisation and urbanisation as these have spread across the world. While Social Work has become institutionalised within the state in the Global North, Social Work has and is developing in its own distinctive way in Global South, though usually without state recognition or support, and sometimes often in opposition to the some of the processes within the state itself. Here we want to look at how Social Workers have become involved in addressing the problem of homelessness in some of India's large cities as an example. In seeking to understand this problem, Nambiar and Mathew's research on the problems of homeless people in India notes that:

> Another key feature of the past few decades is urbanisation, which has been largely unregulated and unplanned, occurring in the broader context of neoliberalisation in many parts of the world, including in India. In the domain of health, there was an expanded role of private sector in healthcare, and a reduction in finances of Urban Local Bodies (ULBs) over time, leading to weakened state-led governance. Insufficient investment in cities has resulted in substandard delivery of public services. The urban poor have meagre access to basic amenities such as sanitation and water and are more likely to live in hazardous environments, leading to greater vulnerability to diseases.
>
> (Nambiar and Mathew, 2022, p. 1)

In their work, they also note that what they call Civil Society Organisations, which are groups such as doctors, Social Workers and other professional groupings, have come to play an important role in supporting and mobilising marginalised groups such as the homeless. The aim of these Civil Society Organisations is to both offer direct practical support to the homeless and place pressure on the authorities to recognise the needs of these people and act on the responsibilities they have towards them, such as those outlined within the Indian Constitution. The work of these groups around homelessness involves activities such as organising housing shelters, and once people are in these, to address the many other issues and difficulties they have also need to be addressed, such as support with health care needs and problems with alcohol and substance abuse (Nambiar and Mayhew, 2022). Social Workers are an important component within these Civil Society Organisations, and alongside the practical support they offer, they are also involved in campaigning for authorities to recognise and then address the problems of the homeless. While the Indian State does have responsibilities for social welfare, there are also those elements within the political class unwilling to acknowledge this responsibility, and they have sought to treat homeless people as though they are a public nuisance. Here, we see Social Workers operating in a contested space where questions about the responsibility for social problems are being raised, which at the same time raise important questions about the ethical and political questions about the role of Social Work.

We can gain insight into how these issues play out on the ground by listening to accounts of the work Social Workers undertake here. Swati Singh is a Social Work researcher and practitioner who has worked in both India and Finland around this issue of homelessness, and in the writings below, she describes her experiences of Social Work practice in New Delhi:

> As part of the field work, I went to Pul Mithai near Old Delhi Railway Station in the year 2010. The visit was in regard to the forceful eviction of the homeless families living under the railway bridge. The government law itself suggests that if the poor and the homeless people have to be evicted, there should be one-month prior notice so that they have a certain time to vacate the place. I went to capture the narratives of the homeless people living there as a testimony to prove the violation of the rights of the homeless people. They were evicted without prior notice. It was a forceful eviction followed by exploitation. I saw demolished shanties which seem like a pile of garbage thrown in a place. Children crying, older members of the homeless families narrating the incident which took place, some of the homeless people were injured, severely injured among them were a ten-year-old girl. Police had lathi-charged which caused severe injury and she was hospitalized. Looking at this situation, I collected three testimonies which narrated their experience on the day of forceful eviction. I also read the Indian Railway Affidavit which conducted the forceful eviction in the name of service of the railway tracks. The affidavit also blamed the homeless people for creating a nuisance on the urban place. The three testimonies were then submitted to the Hon'ble High Court of Delhi on 4th June, 2010. Even though the testimonies were submitted, it was also important to gather more information about the history of the place and people. It was also an effort to understand why and how the homeless people were settled here [we] (...) conducted a Participatory Rural Appraisal (PRA) with (...) groups of women, men, and children. I also facilitated the process and it was conducted on 10th June, 2010. One of the methods of the PRA was used; Community Mapping with each group was facilitated to make Venn Diagrams. The whole process was documented and prepared final brief documentation which can become a base for both applying Social Action Method in the field and also as evidence in court.
>
> (Singh, 2020)

At the start of this chapter we noted that one of the complications involved in defining Social Work was that it involved such a diverse range of activities. The example above demonstrates this in that it shows a very different kind of practice between a country like India and the kinds of institutionalised Social Work we would expect to encounter in the Global North, where practice is more highly regulated by law and policy, but at the same time more recognised professionally. We also noted earlier that there is a tendency of Social Work textbooks to treat practice as a given. Here we've tried to problematise this by pointing to the way Social Work as a profession emerges in relation to specific sorts of social issues which we can think of as the specific problems of industrial, urban, capitalist societies. These are problems that emerge historically; and the way in which those societies seek to address or resolve those problems will depend on all sorts of factors; things such as the kinds of government that is in power in a particular place, the kinds of political ideologies which will define the way the government understands its responsibilities towards the citizenry, the extent to which people are able to express a range of views openly about what is happening in society and the extent and level of the presenting problems. It is these sorts of issues that form the essential context of Social Work practice, and as we noted earlier, these are practical activities, but activities which always bring ethical questions to the fore. Hugh McLaughlin has addressed this same point:

> Social work is not a neutral activity. Social work can lead to a positive outcome for the service user or the social worker or it may lead to a negative outcome for one or both of them. To this end it is imperative for social workers to be in a continuous reflective relationship with their practice seeking to find evidence and answers that help them to identify whether their intervention is effective or mere interference.
>
> (2012, p. 1)

It is precisely because Social Work is not a 'neutral activity' that ethical questions are central to Social Work practice, and these are connected to the methods and interventions we adopt, which are themselves related to the research and evidence base which underlies those. One of the issues which is raised very powerfully by the example of Social Work practice described above in India is the way the people Social Workers are working with are very often people who have no voice in society. Comparing the attitude to homelessness in Finland to that in India, Swati Singh notes that while provision is Finland is much better than that in India,

> the attitude towards the issue of homelessness remains same in Finland and in India. The expression seems to echo "Not in my neighbourhood". Even though homelessness is seen as the structural issue still individuals are blamed for being homeless. This is reflected in the derogatory language used in reference to the homelessness. In our meeting with Tampere City Housing Services, it was narrated that the negative connotation was used towards homeless people. The word used was 'pummi' which refers as 'human trash' although it was publicly criticized in Finland. In the same way, in India the negative connotations have been criticized but there are certain sections of people who are of the opinion that the homeless people are beggars, drunkards, mentally ill and thieves etc.
>
> (2020)

Again this points to the need for Social Workers to be aware of the language, attitudes and underlying assumptions made about the people we work with, as these are ethical questions. While the context of Social Work practice can vary greatly when comparing the Global North and Global South, the attitudes to homelessness Swati Singh is describing in comparing India and Finland also points the continuities in attitudes towards people who are socially marginalised. Just as there is commonality in the way these people are blamed for their situations, so there is an important continuity in the ethical challenges this creates within the Social Work response. This raises the question of whether in talking about Social Work as a global profession, we can think of the ethical approaches we adopt to the people we work as embodying the same approach. The approach adopted by the Social Worker Vidhya Biju, who was awarded the 2017 'Social Worker of the Year' prize in the UK, is interesting in this respect. Vidhya Biju has also worked with the homeless in New Delhi, as well as in children's and adults' services in Birmingham and Walsall in the UK. She insists that the values which guide her understanding of the problems she has worked and her ethical response to those problems are the same in both contexts:

> To me, Social Work is about changing lives for the better for vulnerable people, who believe you can turn things around for them when their world appears upside down… My grass roots experience of working in the deprived areas of the city slums of New Delhi helped me to understand the effects of oppression, poverty, disability, isolation and loneliness on human lives. This understanding always maintains and ignites my passion and commitment to the most vulnerable individuals and apply the values of social justice, social inclusion, equality and empowerment in my everyday practice.
> (in Dennis, 2018)

Conclusion

This chapter has considered aspects of the historical development of Social Work, looking initially at the Victorian Charity and the Settlement Movements as two of the most important streams which lead to the formation of Social Work in the UK and USA. We characterised the tensions between these two traditions as a something which was carried over into State Social Work, when it ceased to be a voluntary activity and became a recognised part of the welfare state after the Second World War in Britain, Europe and North America. The bottom-up tradition of the Settlements, which has largely been forgotten about in the UK and USA, has important continuities with the way Social Work is being undertaken in India today, as the example of Social Work practice amongst homeless people in New Delhi demonstrates. While we have noted significant differences to these contexts, there are also important ways in which they are connected, and this is what we sought to capture in the quote from Harriet Beecher Stowe at the beginning of the chapter; "the past, the present and the future are really one".

We would note by way of conclusion that the argument throughout this book is that Social Work's role in 'mediating the social' is as necessary and important now as it has ever been. Social Work practice, whether it is located inside or outside of the state, continues to be a space which contains real possibilities for improving the lives of individuals and communities, and the further chapters in this book will seek to set out ways in which the challenges facing the present generation of Social Work practitioners can be thought about and engaged with. However, it is always going to be the case that Social Work practice and what it is able to achieve is contextualised within the political, social and economic environment in which it is operating. With the rise of neoliberalism globally, we have seen not only huge reductions to the provision of welfare but also a reframing of social problems away from governmental responsibility for social well-being to the way contemporary social policy has been re-made through the lens of 'individual responsibilization' (Liebenberg et al., 2015). In this context, the problems which people have are seen as the consequences of their own 'bad choices'. This individualistic approach frays the fabric of civil society and democratic life, and it also creates a culture of blame for people who are the victims of structural problems, such as homelessness. In this sense, the argument central to this book, which is that Social Workers need to be 'consciously ethical', is more important than ever. In the next chapter of this book, we expand this argument by looking at what ethics and ethical framework are and how they work in Social Work practice.

2 Contemporary Social Work

Care or Control?

In the first chapter, we discussed the social dynamics which gave rise to Social Work as a defined area of activity, and how these kinds of activities took different forms related to the contexts in which Social Workers were acting. In the West, we noted that one of the key changes in post-World War II period was the development of Social Work as a paid profession which existed primarily within the state. This chapter develops this discussion by thinking about the organisational changes within Social Work in those parts of the world where it has been a state-based profession. As this chapter is focused on the role of Social Work within the state, and is part of the state bureaucracy, we have situated this discussion within sociological approaches to the understanding of bureaucracy. We begin by talking about Max Weber's ideas on bureaucracy, thinking about how relevant this theory is for the contemporary challenges that face Social Work practice. We then think about the impact which the rise of neoliberalism and New Public Management have had on the organisation of Social Work. What are the implications for ethical practice in an era where Social Work decision making is dominated by managerial expectations and by reporting requirements (Pascoe et al., 2023)? How are neoliberal structures that are in place changing the way we think about social welfare, and what can we do about this as Social Work practitioners seeking to honour the Social Work value base in our practice. We conclude with a discussion of values and why these remain so central in defining the uniqueness of Social Work.

Social Workers: Prisoners of Bureaucracy?

In 2021–2022, the British Association of Social Workers (BASW), the professional body for Social Work in the UK, carried out research to look the pressures on Social Work practice. Some key findings of this work were:

- Seventy-two per cent were unable to complete their workload within their contracted hours. Among this group, 24% were working at least 10 hours extra per week on average.
- The three biggest challenges in their roles that respondents cited were administrative demands and adequacy of staffing levels (both 51%) and workload demand (47%).
- The three biggest challenges for the profession were a failure to fund social care adequately (67%), cuts to local services (61%) and having not enough time with people who use services (35%).

DOI: 10.4324/9781003458715-4

- The three things respondents felt were most rewarding about their role were having a positive impact on people's wellbeing (50%), enabling them to have more choice and control (44%) and promoting social justice and anti-oppressive practice.

This survey of BASW members shows that around three quarters of those interviewed could only complete their work by doing unpaid hours outside of works. This survey highlights the intense time pressure Social Workers are under. This pressure is related to the imposition of austerity policies on social services budgets, which, as well as significantly increasing workloads, has also reduced the resources Social Workers have available to support the individuals and families they are working with. It also points to the extent to which those practitioners believe in the Social Work role and the positive work that can be done within that.

In 2023, Pascoe, Waterhouse-Bradley and McGinn published a major literature review on *Social Workers' Experiences of Bureaucracy*. Surveying a huge body of work on this topic, they concluded that Social Work was experiencing a huge resurgence of the 'bureaucratic method', arguing that:

> An environment of regulation and control has expanded across social services in western and westernised countries through the rise of managerialism. Driven by New Public Management reforms which sought to transform the public sector through implementing private sector performance criteria and practices in the pursuit of efficiency and economy, managerialism focuses on risk management, control, fragmentation of services and accountability, consequently increasing demands for paperwork and procedure compliance from street-level bureaucrats (SLBs). The nature of this resurgence warrants attention to question the impact on service delivery and public servants.
>
> (2023, p. 514)

This research points even more sharply to the pressures on Social Work practice in the current environment and the tension practitioners experience between the part of the job where they feel they are really helping people and the part of the job where they feel they are serving the bureaucracy. In a recent personal account of Children and Families, Social Worker noted that:

> Child protection social work in particular has become so bureaucratic and paper-laden that 80% of a practitioner's time is spent form-filling rather than supporting service users. The less time you spend with the person that you are supposed to be supporting, the less you understand their needs and wishes and the less likely you are to advocate for them effectively. And because you are unable to build up a strong professional relationship, a breeding ground for resentment is created when service users feel big decisions are being made for them, rather than with them.
>
> (Novell, 2014)

While the tension between the 'bureaucracy' and the 'actually helping people' dimensions of Social Work has been around as long as Social Work itself, the form which this tension is taking may be becoming more acute at the moment for very particular reasons. It is these issues which form the focus of this chapter on Bureaucracy and Social Work.

We begin this chapter by trying to define bureaucracy, and our starting point here is the sociological writings of Max Weber. Weber's work remains a crucial landmark in thinking about the significance of bureaucracy in modern industrial capitalist societies, and for this reason, it is important to understand his contribution. After outlining his ideas, we then turn to one of the key ambiguities in his arguments, which concern the question of who the bureaucracy is responsible to. This is a question which impinges directly on Social Work, and in particular, the issue, which has been discussed previously, of who Social Work is 'answerable' to, both in a practical organisational sense, as well as ethically.

This leads us to the question of how much Social Workers are controlled by the bureaucracy, or how much space the professional role gives Social Workers to themselves define what their role and tasks actually are. We approach this by considering the arguments of two different schools of thought, which we broadly categorise as pessimistic and optimistic. Firstly, we consider the arguments put forward by Margaret Rhodes in her book Ethical Dilemmas in Social Work Practice (1991). We class these as pessimistic in the sense they she sees an inherent contradiction between the needs of the bureaucracy itself, and the needs of those whom it is supposed to serve, which she argues are almost always resolved in favour of the former. For Rhodes, the demands of the bureaucracy are what undermines Social Work as an ethical enterprise. The other side of this story, what can be characterised as optimistic arguments, follows the work of Michael Lipsky in his book *Street Level Bureaucracy: Dilemmas of the Individual in the* Public Services (1980). Lipsky's distinctive argument is that while policy makers and managers never stop seeking to define and control what frontline professionals actually do, the very nature of the frontline role means that they can never fully achieve this. Lipsky can be characterised as an optimist in the sense he sees discretion as ever present in the work of frontline professionals, who are forever in the business of inventing, improvising and working in, through, around and even against the substantive policy objectives of those higher up in the bureaucratic food chain.

The next part of our discussion brings us right up to the present and concerns the issue of whether contemporary Social Work is now subject to new types of bureaucratic control. These have been characterised by Clake, Gewirtz and McLaughlin as 'Managerialism' and concern "the forms of organisational control and direction, and the relations between leaders, staff and customers involved in the production and delivery of welfare outcomes" (Clarke et al., 2000, p. 1). Clarke links the rise of Managerialism with the impact of neoliberalism on state policy, and this continues the discussion of the significance of neoliberalism's impact on Social Work from the previous chapter. We conclude by asking whether these new forms of bureaucratic control are a key issue in the often-voiced dissatisfaction and frustration of Social Workers about what the way they feel recent changes are so detrimental to the job, as exemplified at the beginning of the chapter.

Defining Bureaucracy

What is a bureaucracy? The sociologist Max Weber is hugely significant for being one of the first social theorists to talk about why bureaucracy has become such a pervasive feature of modern society as well as to define its central operating principles. Writing at the end of the nineteenth and beginning of the twentieth centuries, Weber was seeking to understand the phenomenon of bureaucracy; what it was and why it was that they had become so important. His key argument was that the rise of the bureaucracy needed to be understood as a consequence of the rational, calculating spirit of capitalism, which was leading to the emergence of new kinds of social organisations which were called upon to deal efficiently and equitably with large numbers of people. Bureaucracy was for Weber the most typical organisational form to develop out of a society based on what he called 'legal-rational principles' which he saw as characterising the modern state. This was because unlike 'traditional' or 'charismatic' forms of power, where power was seen to reside in the person themselves, bureaucratic authority is understood as vested not in the person but in the rules. Frank Parkin explains that for Weber:

> The hallmark of bureaucratic domination is its studied impartiality. Its officials act without prejudice or passion, applying the same rules to all irrespective of rank or condition. The bureaucrat moreover is not the ultimate fount of the rule. Unlike the traditional or charismatic leader, the official in the modern state are themselves a servant of a higher political authority – typically an elected government and its ministers.
>
> (Parkin, 2002, p. 88)

Weber on Bureaucracy

Weber defined the features of the bureaucracy as follows:

1. That it was a continuous organisation bound by rules.
2. That each individual in the bureaucracy occupied a specified sphere of competence.
3. That the organisation of offices follows a principle of hierarchy.
4. That the conduct of an office is based on the acquisition of technical skills.
5. That in the rational type of organisation it is a matter of principle that the people who administer the bureaucracy must be separated from ownership of the means of production.
6. That the administrators of the bureaucracy cannot appropriate their official positions.
7. That administrative acts, decisions and rules are recorded in writing.

(From Craib, I *Classical Social Theory* (1990, pp. 139–140)

While the centrality of impartial rules was crucial to Weber's view of the bureaucracy, he also saw the role of the bureaucrat in a large organisation as representing a particular way of working. In his 1914 work *Economy and Society*, Weber characterised this as follows:

> The individual bureaucrat cannot squirm out of the apparatus into which he [sic] has been harnessed (...) In the great majority of cases he [sic] is only a small cog in a ceaselessly moving mechanism which prescribes to him [sic] an essential fixed route of march. The individual bureaucrat is, above all, forged to the common interest of all the functionaries in the perpetuation of the apparatus and the persistence of its rationally exercised domination.

> The ruled, for their part, cannot dispense with or replace the bureaucratic apparatus once it exists, for it rests upon expert training, a functional specialisation of work, and an attitude set on habitual virtuosity in the mastery of a single yet methodologically integrated function. If the apparatus stops working, or if its work is interrupted by force, chaos results, which is difficult to master by improvised replacements from among the governed...Increasingly the material fate of the masses depends on the continuous and correct functioning of the ever more bureaucratic organisations of private capitalism, and the idea of eliminating them becomes more and more utopian.
>
> (in Kalberg, 2005, pp. 214–215)

Weber notes that a key feature of the bureaucracy is that it is based on the acquisition of technical expertise, and Social Work is just one of many examples of this. The point Weber is making here is that as a hierarchically structured organisation, bureaucracies define not just the remit and activities but also the thinking, of those who work within them. It is important to note Weber's aim in discussing bureaucracy here was not to criticise them or to object to their existence; rather his objective was to argue that given the development of large-scale societies which had to process huge numbers of individuals, alongside the demands for rationality and efficiency in these dealings, the development of the bureaucracy was inevitable. Indeed, when people complain about 'bureaucracy' and 'red tape', often what they are complaining about is not bureaucracy as such, but about bureaucracies which do their job badly or incompetently. For Weber, these complaints only point to the extent to which we all rely on them, and in that sense, Weber argued that the technical mastery of the bureaucratic office was invaluable to the functioning of society. As the quote above demonstrates, he thoroughly rejected the idea that a complex modern society could ever do without bureaucracy, however frustrating we may find our dealings with them.

After setting out these arguments mid-way throughout his career, towards the end of his life, Weber came to see the development of the bureaucracy in a less positive light. While he never shifted from his view that they were an inevitable feature of modern societies, he used the memorable phrase "the iron cage of bureaucracy" as means of expressing his concern about the vast impersonality of the bureaucratic organisation. He was particularly concerned with the way a mechanistic loyalty to rules and impersonal specialisation could act to stifle individual creativity, independence and initiative. He was also concerned about the way they had grown and argued that bureaucracy was absorbing an increasing range of activities within society – religion, music, art, war, law, education and family life had all entered the 'iron cage'. These concerns are significant in the light of how much bureaucracy has expanded since his death, particularly the bureaucracy associated with monitoring and surveillance. However, this image of the 'iron cage' remains significant for the way it expresses a particular view of the modern rational world, dominated by a ceaseless search for efficiency. Weber saw this as a world in which charm, wonder and awe had disappeared, and he concluded his work on bureaucracy by noting that:

> So much more terrible is the idea that the world should be filled with nothing but those cogs who cling to a little post and strive for a greater one....The central and further question is not how we further and accelerate it but what we have to set against this machinery, in order to preserve a remnant of humanity from this parcelling-out of the soul, and from this exclusive rule of bureaucratic life-ideals.
>
> (in Pampel, p. 111)

It should be apparent from this brief account of his ideas that Weber has bequeathed us a somewhat ambiguous view of the bureaucracy. On the one hand, he argued that complex modern urban societies have no alternative to bureaucratic forms of organisation, which were central to the way the state organised its responsibilities in the context of complex, large-scale urbanised societies. However, the comments he made about the stifling impact these could have both on individuals and on society as a whole suggest that though they may be inevitable, this did not make them a particularly positive feature of modern society. The sociologist Bryan Turner has noted that another key ambivalence in Weber's work concerns the legitimacy of the norms which being followed by those bureaucracies. Turner argues that is one thing for Weber to insist on the inevitability of bureaucracy as a means by which modern societies need to organise, but it is another thing to say what the rationale of this bureaucracy is or should be (1996, p. 358). This is a question with substantial implications for Social Work, since Social Work agencies have legal powers which allow them to intervene in the lives of the individuals and families we work with. Social Work Children and Families teams have the ability to remove a child from the child's parents and this is a rationale which seeks to ensure particular standards about parenting and how children need to be treated. At the same time, there is good research evidence which demonstrates a strong connection between poverty and child neglect. According to Skinner, Bywaters and Kennedy, who have researched this area:

> Poverty was found to be consistently and strongly associated with maltreatment, be that in terms of familial or community-level poverty, or in terms of economic security. Findings demonstrated that both the type and the quantity of economic insecurities impacted child maltreatment. Certain economic insecurities – income losses, cumulative material hardship and housing hardship – reliably predicted future child maltreatment. Likewise, as families experienced more material hardship, the risk for maltreatment intensified.
>
> (2022)

It is one thing to say that we as a society vest responsibility in the Social Work profession to protect vulnerable children – but it is another thing to state that there is political consensus about the underlying causes of child maltreatment and also about the forms of intervention Social Work bureaucracies undertake in addressing this concern. How much are factors like poverty and insecurity central to how Social Workers, or for that matter government policy, a key part of how we think about child maltreatment? These things are important because they form the context of the way people encounter the state bureaucracy, and this is an important ethical question for us as Social Workers. This leads us to the question of how we make sense of and conceptualise the actual day-to-day operation of policy and procedures for Social Work in the context of bureaucratic organisations, and it is to these issues that we now turn.

Understanding Life in the Bureaucracy: Pessimists and Optimists

While most books on Social Work ethics contain extensive discussions of different ethical theories, there is, by comparison, much less discussion of what we could think of as 'real world' of ethical decision making, which is invariably located in the context of the bureaucratic agencies within which most Social Workers are employed in the West. Margaret Rhodes book *Ethical Dilemmas in Social Work Practice* published in 1991 is significant for the way she offers an extremely forthright discussion of bureaucracy which can be regarded as one of the most distinctive contributions to this debate within the Social Work literature. Whilst she published this book some time ago, the questions she addresses are still, in our opinion, very relevant. In the opening pages of her chapter on bureaucracy, Rhodes argues that in a world in which public bureaucracies increasingly shape Social Work practice "individual workers often seen caught up by organisational forces beyond their control", finding their work "determined more by institutional rules than by client needs". She argues that in spite of the attempts by well-meaning people to improve the functioning of bureaucracy, the frontline Social Worker "must continue to make her decisions despite inadequate resources, case overloads, excessive paper work, and a labyrinth of rules, all of which contribute to a sense of helplessness and hopelessness" (1991, pp. 133–134). While these sentiments are ones that many Social Workers would agree with, the key question for our purposes here is to ask why this is. According to Rhodes, the fundamental problem is that

> bureaucracies, by virtue of the kind of decisions they promote, undermine our ordinary concepts of morality. In particular, human service organisations undermine our moral concepts, because of their contradictory nature; their stated goal is to help clients, yet their actual operation serves the interest of preserving the bureaucracy. When this conflict is not recognised, workers often function as if their day to day decisions do not have ethical dimensions.
>
> (1991, p. 134)

Hence, for Rhodes, the key issue is that there is an inherent contradiction between the ethical impulse of the Social Work professional as an individual, and the demands of the bureaucracy upon that individual.

Rhodes returns to Weber as part of her discussion of the basis of bureaucracy, and while she deploys the same categories for describing the bureaucracy as he does, she fundamentally rejects the idea that his description of the bureaucracy could simply be an objective description. The very features which Weber sees as those which allow the bureaucracy to work effectively, Rhodes characterises as the key factors which undermine ethical decision making in Social Work. To take for example the question of impartial decision making. While Weber sees as a central feature of bureaucracy, Rhodes argues that this brings about a 'double standard' in that rules allow people to be 'freed from the demands of their personal moralities'. Consider an instance a situation where a Social Worker may personally believe that a particular service user is in need of support, but is also aware that the agency's eligibility criteria specify this at a particular level which that service user does not meet. Because the rules predominate over 'personal morality', the Social Worker dealing with this situation will feel that it is morally legitimate to not offer any further service to that service user because they do not meet the criteria for this support. The Social Worker, Rhodes argues, is able to see this decision as morally legitimate because they:

> (...) do not hold [themselves] personally responsible for the action, because the choice is made impersonally by the organisation. The result of this split between personal and organisational morality is that an employee can dismiss general ethical considerations from evaluation of job performance.
>
> (1991, p. 137)

At the core of Rhodes' argument is a powerfully expressed view that bureaucracies through being bureaucracies undermine an ethically based approach, as they are inherently based on a split between personal moralities and the rules and procedures of the agency concerned.

Another of the features of the bureaucracy outlined by Weber is the specialisation of particular roles. Rhodes also sees this as undermining an ethically based approach in Social Work as it allows workers to only see themselves as responsible for the one part of the process which is their particular role, and in doing so they fail to consider the impact of different interventions on service users overall: "Workers and agencies may spend considerable energy denying responsibility for a case...with the result that no-one will take primary responsibility" (1991, p. 141). An example of this could be a person with Learning Disabilities and additional Mental Health issues which neither a Social Services Mental Health or Learning Disabilities team is willing to take responsibility for. While some might argue that the way to deal with this is to generate guidelines which specify what those agencies should do to avoid this happening, Rhodes argues that this is to miss the point about the way these forms of behaviour are inherent in bureaucracy. She concludes her indictment of the bureaucracy stating that:

> It may be argued that the failings of human service organisations do not result from bureaucratic structure, but from inadequate resources combined with increased demand. Certainly in this decade of new cutbacks to social programmes and higher caseloads, characteristics like impersonality of work and objectification of the client are magnified. These bureaucratic features, however, characterise human services whatever the political climate and are basic to bureaucracies as they are currently structured.
> (1991, p. 144)

It is on the basis of this account that we have classified Rhodes approach to the role of bureaucracy in Social Work as pessimistic. It is important to note, based on her concluding statement, that she is not just criticising particular procedures, which may be seen as unfair or discriminatory, or particular organisations, which may do their job badly or treat service users oppressively. Her account locates the problem as inherent in bureaucracy itself. There is no doubt that many of the examples Rhodes gives will resonate with many Social Workers; but the question we need to think about here is whether these issues are inherent in bureaucracy itself, or are consequences of bureaucracies which function badly, or treat people badly because they are shaped by powerful forces external to the bureaucracy. We want to now examine Rhodes' central arguments that the core of what is wrong with bureaucracy is this split between personal morality and bureaucratic rules through a case study.

Patience's Placement

Patience is a Social Work student who has been living in the UK for six years after arriving from Zimbabwe as an Asylum Seeker and having now obtained the right to remain in the UK. She worked as a teacher before leaving Zimbabwe, and was inspired to train as a Social Worker after being helped by Social Workers in an Asylum Team. Prior to coming on the Social Work course Patience worked for several years in a residential home for older people, and she has also been involved in assisting other Zimbabweans who had recently arrived in the UK with practical and emotional support issues in work that she organised through her church.

For her first Social Work placement, she joins a fostering team, and while she is very happy to have this placement, she is deeply shocked to realise not just that the team she works with places children with gay or lesbian couples, but that she may be herself expected to work with these people. The situation becomes clear to her after she undertakes a visit to a gay male couple with her Practice Assessor, Neelam. The couple whom she meets, Don and Warren, have done some short-term fostering with the Local Authority, which has gone extremely well. They are now interested in being assessed as potential adoptive parents. For Patience, the visit to their house was extremely challenging in itself, and while she feels nothing personally against Don and Warren, the visit has raised a series of issues she needs desperately to discuss with Neelam.

At their next supervision Patience explains to Neelam that 'as a Christian' she feels it is "morally wrong to place innocent children with a homosexual couple". While she has nothing against the men personally, their practices are 'against God's laws'. Neelam responds by saying she can understand where Patience is coming from, but as a Social Worker in training, she needs to think about Social Work values in relation to her own personal values. Neelam, who is from a Hindu background herself, says she felt similarly to Patience when she first trained as a Social Worker, but has since worked with several gay and lesbian couples, and now has absolutely no concern about it and indeed has come to champion the rights of gay and lesbian foster carers and adoptees as part of a wider campaign on issues of justice with her the Local Authority. She says she feels proud that the Local Authority, having previously changed many of their policies on areas of 'race', have also now acknowledged the rights of gay and lesbian couples, many of whom are amongst their team's best foster placements. She offers Patience Social Work literature which explains these issues in more detail, as well as giving her a copy of the Local Authority's policy guidelines for Fostering and Adoption, pointing out that it is Authority's policy to welcome Foster Carers and Adoptees from all sections of the community.

Questions:

1 In a case such as this, should personal morality be allowed to predominate over organisational objectives? Why?
2 Consider this case in the light of Margaret Rhodes argument that problem with bureaucracy is that it undermines 'personal morality'. What does this case suggest about that view?
3 Finally, consider the following outcome from this situation. After thinking long and hard about all the issues involved in this situation, Patience decides that in order to be successful on the Social Work course, she needs to accept that she has to work within the Local Authority guidelines. However she cannot but feel that her own personal values have been compromised, and she explains this to Neelam. This leaves Neelam with the dilemma of whether to pass the case which they previously visited to Patience, as she was hoping to do. What do you think Neelam should do here?

We noted earlier that a key assumption in Margaret Rhodes' argument about the relationship between Social Work and bureaucracy is that individual morality represents a superior form of morality than agency policy and procedure. While this may be true in many instances, it is not universally true. This assumption, which is central to Rhodes' arguments, has been explicitly challenged by the sociologist Paul Du Gay in his book *In Praise of* Bureaucracy (2000). Du Gay characterises the position taken up by Margaret Rhodes as expressive of

> a thoroughly romantic belief that the principle of a full and free exercise of personal capacities is akin to a moral absolute for human conduct...[Within such a view] the specialisations of function and conduct attendant upon bureaucratic organisation are represented as introducing a violent 'split' into individual subjective and social being. The instrumental 'spirit of bureaucracy' makes fragmented (...) that which should be organic and 'whole'. It is because bureaucracy fosters only rational and instrumental human faculties...that it must be seen as a fatally flawed vehicle for the realisation of a moral personality.
>
> (2000, p. 3)

Du Gay is arguing here that it is simply romantic to propose that instead of a bureaucratic structure for Social Work, Social Workers should be able to allocate resources to all service users on the basis of what they as individuals feel is appropriate – how would such an organisation function? Du Gay is suggesting, following Weber, that one of the great advantages of regulation is that it ensures consistency, and without this we would lack criteria for establishing what we considered was fair towards service users. He is also questioning the assumption that it is inherently unethical to take a decision which deploys one set of values in one setting and to use another set of values in another. Rather than this something of an absolute distinction between ethical versus unethical decision making, as Rhodes suggests, Du Gay is suggesting that it depends on the context.

In terms of our Case Study above, imagine that after some time Patience came to accept that in terms of her role as a Social Worker, she did need to be able to consider the qualities of foster carers and adopters regardless of sexual orientation. While such a shift would involve something of a split between her role as a Social Worker and her life outside of Social Work, is it right to characterise this as being based on an abandonment of personal responsibility or a rejection of ethical practice within Social Work (which would be the implication of Rhodes arguments)? Du Gay is suggesting that because we live in a world which has "different socio-ethical comportments", meaning that different things are expected of us in different situations, that the recognition of this is not the same as a distinction between ethical versus unethical behaviour. Neither can it be simply understood as a 'split' between a concept of personal responsibility versus an acceptance of purely technical rationality (2000, p. 3). In other words, he is saying that it in a complex and diverse world, it is commonplace that we make ethical decisions using particular criteria in a particular situations and these may be different from other criteria we may use in other situations, but that doing this does not necessarily make our decision making inherently unethical – again that would depend on the situation we were in.

Indeed Du Gay takes this argument about bureaucracy and ethics one stage further and suggests that rather than being dominated by a technical rationality and thereby devoid of ethics, that bureaucracy needs to be understood as an ethical domain in its own right:

> The ethical attributes of the 'good' bureaucrat – adherence of sub- and superordination, commitment to the purposes of the office and so forth – do not represent an

> incompetent subtraction from a 'complete' or 'all-round' conception of personhood. Rather they should be represented as a positive moral and ethical achievement in their own right. They represent the product of particular ethical techniques and practices through which individuals develop the disposition and capacity to conduct themselves according to the ethos of the bureaucratic office.
>
> (2000, p. 4)

To put this point into the context of our previous example, one of the most important things which Patience needs to learn as a Social Work student is precisely the question of how to operate within the bureaucratic office environment – the things she needs to do immediately and the things she can leave to do later, the things which are irrelevant and the things which must be followed up and pursued, the people she needs to develop a relationship with in order to get a particular process happening, the distinction between those procedures which must be followed to the letter and those where there is a certain room to manoeuvre. Du Gay is arguing that it is entirely mistaken to see the acquisition of these skills as involving a diminution of our own personal moralities – instead he argues, we need to see the acquisition of these as crucial 'moral and ethical achievements' which will allow Patience to achieve what she has come into Social Work to do – help people.

So far, we have set out what we have called the pessimistic view of the bureaucracy through looking at the work of Margaret Rhodes, as well as considering a critique of that, looking at the work of Paul Du Gay. Now we want to look at what could be called the optimistic accounts of bureaucracy. As noted above, these accounts are optimistic not in the sense that they suggest that everything that happens within bureaucracies is good – it is rather that they suggest that people within bureaucracies cannot be thought of as simply controlled by those organisations – but rather that people often have a certain room to manoeuvre. The key work which looks at this is Michael Lipsky's book Street Level Bureaucracy: Dilemmas of the Individual in Public Services (1980). Lipsky's work grew out of research which he carried out with frontline public service employees in the United States – people such as teachers, police officers, Social Workers, public lawyers, whose role is to "grant access to government programmes and provide services within them" (1980, p. 3). It is through this research that he has developed a distinctive account of role of practitioners within the bureaucracy. Rather than seeing, as Rhodes does, that public policy determines the role of frontline practitioners, Lipsky emphasises the element of active agency exercised by frontline practitioners, arguing that it is their actions which in essence make that policy. He characterises frontline professionals as 'street level bureaucrats', and argues that:

> Most citizens encounter government (if they encounter it at all) not through letters to [their political representatives] or by attendance at school board meetings, but through their teachers and their children's teachers and the policeman on the corner or in the patrol car (...)

In other words, we experience the state bureaucracy not through grand statements of purpose and intent, or through the vast amounts of policy documents published by government departments, but through particular kinds of everyday interactions we have with state employees – teachers, health workers, Social Workers and police. These people are significant for the way they form the interface between the public on one hand and politicians and policy makers on the other. The argument of his which is most suggestive in the context of our discussion here is the idea that each one of these everyday interactions between the public and frontline practitioners

> represents an instance of policy delivery (...) Although [frontline practitioners] are normally regarded as low-level employees, the actions of most public service workers actually constitute the services 'delivered' by government. Moreover when taken together the individual decisions of these workers become, or add up to, agency policy.
>
> (1980, p. 3)

It follows from Lipsky's argument that one of the reasons why frontline professionals such as police, Social Workers, teachers and health professionals are so often controversial figures, often in the news, often singled out for either criticism or praise by politicians and other commentators, is that the decisions they make, frequently in situations of considerable stress, can have a massive impact on the people on the receiving end. As Lipsky notes:

> (...) in delivering policy, street level bureaucrats made decisions about people that affect their life chances. To designate or treat someone as a welfare recipient, a juvenile delinquent, or a high achiever affects the relationships of others to that person and also affects the person's self evaluation (...) A defining feature of the working environment of street level bureaucrats is that they must deal with client's personal reactions to their decisions...[and this means that] the reality of the work of street level bureaucrats could hardly be farther from the bureaucratic ideal of impersonal detachment in decision making.
>
> (1980, p. 9)

Lipsky is emphasising that is rather than seeing street-level bureaucrats as defined by the rules and procedures they work within, as both Weber and Margaret Rhodes argue, it makes more sense to see them as intermediaries between policy guidelines and the public. In the context of Social Work, one of the most significant skills the Social Worker has to acquire is how to carry out this mediating role between the wider bureaucracy, to which they are formally accountable, and to the service user, to whom they are also accountable. This accountability is both formal – in the sense that an agency employs a Social Worker and could terminate this employment if the employee's behaviour was seen to be inappropriate – and ethical in that the Social Worker is likely to feel a sense of responsibility to both the agency and to the service user. The way the Social Worker and their agency may experience this sense of duty may vary significantly from person to person and agency to agency; however, the point being made here is that frontline professionals are not simply automatons who exist simply to carry out the will of policy makers and managers. The way a Social Worker manages accountability to service users may not be the same as the way they deal with accountability to the agency, and links with Du Gay's discussion regarding different 'ethical domains'.

Lipsky's focus on the mediating role of frontline professionals is significant because it points to one of the issues which he sees as central to the role of street level bureaucrats, which is the way they exercise discretion:

> Unlike lower-level workers in most organisations, street level bureaucrats have considerable discretion in determining the nature, amount and quality of benefits and sanctions provided by their agencies...That is not to say that street level bureaucrats

> are unrestrained by rules, regulations and directives from above, or by the norms and standards of their occupational group. On the contrary the major dimensions of public policy – levels of benefits, categories of eligibility, nature of rules, regulations and services – are shaped by policy elites and political and administrative officials...[At the same time] even public employees who do not have claims to professional status exercise considerable discretion.
>
> (1980, p. 14)

This discretion comes about for a number of reasons. Firstly, the range of situations which street-level bureaucrats encounter are too broad and too complex to be easily fitted into a single series of rules – there are never enough rules to cover the range of situations which frontline workers will find themselves in. Secondly, part of the expectation of the professional role which Social Workers have is not simply to respond mechanistically to what is in front of them, but to read the human and relational dimensions of a situation and devise a response accordingly. The 2011 Munro Review of Child Protection into Children and Families Social Work in the UK reinforced exactly this point in its recommendations, a key one of which was that:

> Good social work practice requires forming a relationship with the child and family and using professional reasoning to judge how best to work with parents. The nature of this close engagement means that supervision, which provides the space for critical reflection, is essential for reducing the risk of errors in professionals' reasoning.
>
> (2011, pp. 11–12)

The significance of this recommendation is that while Children and Families Social Workers are expected to work within policy and guidelines and the legal framework for intervention, Professor Munro is saying that the exercise of discretion where there is scope to do so, is equally crucial to their work.

Lipsky is therefore arguing that while the major parameters of policy and practice are fixed at the top level of the state, that within street level bureaucracies, much frontline practice is conducted in this more indeterminate realm. It is in situations where policy and legislation offer only partial and sometimes even contradictory guidance, that discretion, and the issues of ethical judgement which accompany this, come most to the fore. The following case study considers the way two Social Work students exercise discretion in differing ways.

The Case of John Garson

John Garson is a young British man who has come to the attention of Social Services after contacting the Duty team of a Physical Disability Social Work team requesting help with an application for financial support from a charity which helps members of the Armed Forces. John is 23 years old and grew up in Local Authority care. After leaving school with few qualifications, he worked in a series of factory jobs, and frustrated with the lack of any direction or security offered by these, he decided to join the Army. John liked life in the Army well enough, though he found the tension of aspects of life on tours of duty in Afghanistan got to him at times, and to deal with this, he started using opiate-based painkillers, which were available from army medics, as a means of relaxing. These were widely used amongst soldiers and John would not have considered his use of these to be any sort of problem. On his third tour of duty, John was severely wounded by a roadside bomb, and it was only through the quick thinking of his fellow soldiers in getting him quickly to a field hospital that he survived at all. John is now severely disabled and due to injuries in his legs and spine is confined to a wheelchair for the rest of his life. He has been back in the UK for just over two years now, and while he has had very good Occupational Therapy and Physiotherapy, he was not offered any psychological support or counselling, and neither would he have felt able to ask for this sort of help. In addition John has become very isolated from his social networks; his former girlfriend is now in another relationship with another man with whom she has just had a child, he only ever had intermittent contact with his mother and was never close to her, and with the passage of time, his former comrades in the army have stopped visiting him. John is seriously depressed and after coming off painkillers for his injuries has started drinking heavily.

John is in receipt of an army pension and disability benefits, but has got into financial problems largely though bills he left unpaid and rent arrears he failed to deal with. He was able to deal with some of the rent arrears with assistance from a charity for injured service people around six months previously, and was supported in this by a Social Work Student who was working with the Physical Disability Team who helped him complete the relevant paperwork and helped him obtain the necessary independent verification of his financial difficulties. He has now come back to the same service following being threatened with court proceedings by a debt collectors following non-payment of his utility bills. Unfortunately, the charity he applied to successfully previously only allows a single application every two years unless there is a substantial deterioration in the individual's condition. Secondly, while John was vague about the reasons for getting into debt in the first place with the first student Social Worker, when John is visited this time around, he takes the opportunity to talk about his difficulties, in terms of his drinking, his debts and his isolation. John makes this disclosure because he is concerned about the way his life seems to be slipping out of his control.

Reflection Break: Exercising Discretion

The purpose of this exercise is to think about the way two different practitioners exercise discretion in different ways. Read through the two scenarios and consider them as alternative ways of dealing with this situation.

Scenario 1: John is visited by Susan, a Social Work student. She is 23 and came onto the Social Work course with a background in working with street homeless men. On visiting John, she is extremely concerned about his isolation, his drinking, as well as his financial problems. She sees the sorting out of his finances as the beginning of a much wider programme of support for John, including support around his alcohol dependence and psychological support. While she recognises that on a strict interpretation of the criteria for the charity application he is technically ineligible, she feels they are also open to interpretation such that John could be considered again. She also sees it as significant that John has opened up to her about his wider problems and in her work with him expresses the view that clearing his debts is only the beginning of the support she feels he needs.

Scenario 2: John is visited by Wayne, a Social Work student. He is 32 and came onto the Social Work course with a background working with older people.

On visiting John, he is extremely concerned about his isolation, drinking and the general chaos of his life. On looking at the charity application form, he informs John straight away that he is ineligible to obtain further support from them; the question of whether the rules are open to interpretation is not something he would not see as acceptable. Wayne's approach is to try to help John deal with his debts by obtaining a low interest loan to clear the debt. He feels this will help John to take back responsibility for his life, rather than just clearing the debts through 'another handout'. Alongside this, he puts in place support for John around his alcohol dependence as well as psychological support.

1 Discuss the ethical rationales and strengths/weaknesses of these two approaches.
2 Which Social Work Student do you think is 'more ethical', and why?
3 Think about the scope for exercising discretion that you have in your own work/ placements. How do you exercise this yourself?

In summary, the question of how we understand the way a bureaucracy actually works is more complex than it may appear at first sight. What we have tried to demonstrate here is that there are a range of different approaches. We characterised Margaret Rhodes as a pessimist, since her emphasis is consistently on way Social Workers are determined, and almost entirely negatively in her view, by the structure of the bureaucracy. Lipsky on the other hand could be seen as an optimist, since he emphasises the discretionary and improvisational element, noting that this exercise sometimes exists to the point of being able to work in ways that are entirely different to the intentions of those who drafted the legislation or policy. However, rather than seeing this optimistic and pessimistic positions as alternatives to each other, it may be useful to think of them applying to different situations along a kind of 'discretion continuum' – at the one end of the spectrum are Social Work situations in which staff have very little room to manoeuvre, while the at other end are situations in which front-line workers have considerable opportunity to do so. As well as different situations, Social Workers are also people who have different experiences which have shaped the way they understand the issues within Social Work practice – exemplified by the Social Work students Wayne and Susan in the case above. This is a question that concerns not only values but also what sociologists call 'agency', meaning the things people feel they are able to do in a particular situation. So in this situation, agency refers to the things people are prepared to do to make the values they believe in a reality; this combination of values and agency could be seen to come together in the form of a person's understanding of what the professional role means to them in Social Work. To use our above example, we could see Wayne as someone feels the 'handout mentality' is not just unhelpful for John, but bad for society in general. In John's case, he would see this as something which is preventing him from becoming independent and taking control of his situation. For him, the charity guidelines are a 'given' and they are not something he would see it as appropriate to question or challenge. Susan, on the other hand, looks upon John as someone who has already sacrificed a huge amount, having served his country as a soldier and ended up being severely and permanently disabled in the process. As she sees it, John should be entitled to much greater support than he has received so far and would see the fact that he has to rely on charity applications as something of an indictment of the way he has been treated by society. From her perspective, the charity application is the least of what John should be entitled to.

Hence it is the different conceptual understandings of the presenting problem, which shapes those different values and informs the question of what these two students are prepared to do for the service user. This demonstrates the way professional discretion has an important ethical dimension, and this brings us back to the question of the scope for discretion within bureaucratic structures. How has the nature and scope for professional discretion been impacted by the shift towards neoliberalism and New Public Management? This is the focus of the next part of our discussion.

Neoliberalism, Managerialism and Professional Discretion in Social Work

We began this chapter with a discussion of the 2021–2022 BASW Members Report and with Pascoe et al.'s research into Social Workers' experiences of bureaucracy. We want to argue here that we cannot understand the kinds of things these Social Workers are reporting or what Pascoe et al.'s research is saying without understanding the significance of neoliberalism and the impact that it has had on Social Work practice. David Harvey defines neoliberalism as:

> a theory of political economic practices that proposes that human well-being can best be advanced by liberating individual entrepreneurial freedoms and skills within an institutional framework characterized by strong private property rights, free markets and free trade. The role of the state is to create and preserve an institutional framework appropriate to such practices.
>
> (2010, p. 2)

This points to the way neoliberalism has fundamentally sought to change the relationship between the citizenry and the state. *The Social Policy* writer John Clarke has argued that there are two key strands within neoliberalism: an anti-welfarist strand and an anti-statist strand. For the anti-welfarist strand, welfare spending is seen as both unproductive, in the sense that it is 'a drain on the real economy', and undesirable, in the sense of that is produces 'welfare dependency' and a 'handout mentality'. For the anti-statist element within neoliberal thinking, the problem is excessive state involvement in what should rightly be the role of the free market, seen as the most appropriate mechanism for allocating resources, goods and services (Clarke et al., 2000, pp. 2–3). Neoliberal policies were introduced by in the world by the government of Margaret Thatcher in the UK and Ronald Reagan in the US, as part of the rejection of the post-war settlement described in the first chapter, which led to Social Work becoming a state-based profession, and in which the state accepted responsibilities for the economic welfare for society as a whole. What we have also seen throughout the twenty-first century across the world is that while these neoliberal policies have often been unpopular, they have become a dominant common-sense amongst political elites, including amongst Labour and Social Democratic parties which had previously stood for an alternative to this. The extent to which the state accepts responsibility for the overall welfare of its citizens, and the way in which governments understand the role of the state in social provision, has shifted fundamentally. Neoliberalism is not just a project which has simply sought to reduce state expenditure on welfare, it is also, as John Clarke has noted, sought to change "the meaning of welfare" (Clarke et al., 2000, p. 3). This has real implications for how the problems of vulnerable populations – such as people living in poverty, or people living with mental health problems or long-term support needs such as people with learning disabilities – are understood within state policy.

In terms of understanding the remaking of the role of the state, and in looking at the impact this has on Social Work, it is important to note the way these different strands converge. On the one hand, Social Services agencies have been reduced in size, and on the other, as an organisation, Social Work agencies, and the government bureaucracy as a whole, are now required to model themselves on the practices of private sector organisations with their claims of 'greater efficiency'. This was hugely facilitated by the privatisation and outsourcing of large areas of Adult Social Care, where those areas of provision once run by the state have now been taken over by private sector companies. The logic of this privatisation of former state-run agencies gave a huge boost to the values and attitudes embodied under managerialism, and provided further justification for the managerial revolution of changing the way people were "expected to think and behave" within bureaucratic structures. (Clarke et al., 2000, p. 9). This has particular significance for Social Work as managerialism has sought to displace the professionally based ethos which had previously been dominant in Social Work bureaucracies. Clarke et al. note that:

> Managerialism – like professionalism – defines a set of expectations, values and beliefs. It is a normative system concerning what counts as valuable knowledge, who knows it and who is empowered to act in what ways as a consequence. Indeed a central issue in the managerialisation of public services has been to displace or subordinate the claims of professionals. It can no longer be assumed that 'professionals know best', rather we are invited to accept that managers 'do the right thing'...Public service organisations have [thus] come to 'think' managerially about themselves, their 'business' and their relationships with others.
>
> (2000, p. 9)

Macalpine and Marsh have described the use of New Public Management as 'management which increased both direct and indirect methods of control, in order to enhance productivity, increase profit and/or reduce costs' (Macalpine and Marsh, 2008). Spolander et al. have noted that whilst the state aim of these is to increase efficiency and accountability, this is accompanied by the way what might be considered core values of Social Work, such as equality, equity and participation, are de-emphasised. They note that we are now living in a time in which 'the state sector has been increasingly criticized for being the cause of social problems such as crime and poverty, with the Social Work profession who are integral to the welfare state also experiencing a reduction in status'. The profession has become vulnerable in its response to this criticism, its efforts to lift itself out of this predicament especially through adopting neoliberal ideas such as risk management, promoting the use of markets through individual budgets and the erosion of universal Social Work services (Spolander et al., 2014, pp. 305–306). Cowden and Singh have made further observations about the shift represented by neoliberalism when then discussed the changes in language which is now used. Where Social Work terminology once referred to 'clients' and 'citizens', services now describe their users as in the language of 'customers' and 'consumers', reflecting the way the purpose of public organisations has been remoulded as replicas of the business world (Cowden and Singh, 2007).

As the logic of 'markets' becomes increasingly embedded across society, the values associated with this become internalised in people's thinking, and these policy changes impact on people in their social and personal lives. The policy of personalisation for people with learning disabilities is an example of this. Here we have seen a shift away from universal state-based provision, represented by services such as Day Centres for people with learning disabilities, towards policies like Personalisation, which represent a form of provision where the service user is seen as a consumer who is purchasing services tailored around their individual needs. While the old Day Centres could be very limited in what they offered to people with learning disabilities, they also created a context for people with learning disabilities to interact with the wider community, as well as offering respite for their unpaid carers. When these Day Centres were closed, as most were following the introduction of the Personalisation policy in the UK, these became the focus of protest for people with learning disabilities and their families (Pitt, 2010). Emily Holzhausen, director of policy and public affairs at Carers UK, has noted that closures of Day Centres has often left carers with the primary responsibility for looking after family members, and has stated that:

> In some areas, closing a day centre will have been a false economy. If you turn to a more fragmented care package and a family can't work as a result, you leave people in poverty, both short and long term.

She also notes that social isolation of both people with learning disabilities and their carers is another problem that has followed day centre closures (Pitt, 2010). Within the language of neoliberal social policy, the development of initiatives such as Personalisation are not presented simply as the withdrawal of services; rather this policy is represented as a 'modernisation' of services, offering an enhancement of people's personal freedom.

But has this been realised? What impact has this shift had on the lives of people with learning disabilities? The research of Power et al. (2022) explores the impact of Personalisation by looking in detail about the changing nature support services as they have been experienced by a small group of adults with learning disabilities in England and Scotland who are the focus of their work. They are seeking to find out the extent to which Personalisation has facilitated the process of these people 'building a life' for themselves. In discussing the origins of the policy of Personalisation, they note:

> This principle emerged from demands in the 1990s by the disability rights movement for a redistribution of power, more choice over community-based support, and crucially control of the funding that went with it. For people with learning disabilities, person-centred support emerged as a parallel agenda based around a care and support plan to enable individuals to exercise more choice and control in their lives and recognition of inclusion and empowerment as the foundations of support provision.
>
> (2022, p. 221)

This is important because it notes the way policies such as Personalisation represented a response to the state to the demand for greater control by people with learning disabilities over the kind of support provision which they wanted. However, it is important to be aware that the implementation of this demand has taken place 'in the context of reduced welfare provision that has unfolded in many nations advancing personalisation' with the consequence that 'the policy has manifested itself [as]... an expectation for people to self-build a life as individual consumers within a care market' (2022, p. 221).

After discussing the experiences of their research respondents and looking in detail at what their daily lives are like, they offer the following conclusion:

> Firstly building lives is a relational process; it requires relational agency (as opposed to solely individualised autonomy). Secondly building lives...is about developing and expanding one's learning and networks and not primarily about consuming or participating in sets of activities. As such, building lives relationally can be transformative...Thirdly, building lives requires an environment that is conducive to creativity and gives people the tools to both challenge negative and fearful attitudes and bolster more encouraging ones... [However] by channeling funding only to these individuals, personalisation policy holds them responsible for outcomes they cannot control – that depend on factors within their social networks and local area, and on wider social structures, policies and attitudes. In this way, policy fails to recognise adequately the socially shared dimension of care and support.
>
> (2022, p. 224)

What it points to is the gap between the positive aspirations represented by the idea of giving people with learning disabilities more control and choice in how they 'build' their lives, but that the language of Personalisation reflects the neoliberal focus on individual autonomy which completely misses the centrality of relationships in the process. In a discussion of the social philosophy of neoliberalism, Stuart Hall has noted that 'neoliberalism is grounded in the 'free, possessive individual', with the state cast as tyrannical and oppressive (Hall, 2011, pp. 10–11).

We see this manifested in the language and approach of the Personalisation where individual choices are presented in opposition to the 'one-size-fits-all' policies of the state, as well as the way society is understood as a collection of autonomous individuals. Power et al.'s research, however, points to the how flawed this understanding is: their research demonstrates that we live in a 'relational world', that is our lives are built not as autonomous individuals but rather through our relationships with other people. This is true for everyone, but it is particularly so for vulnerable groups such as people with learning disabilities, who do not have access to the networks of relationships many neuro-typical people have. They do not have the same opportunities to develop friendship networks, and they are usually excluded from the experiences of education, work and careers through which many neuro-typical people build the networks of important people in their lives. It is in this sense that Power et al. argue that:

> personalisation has failed on the terms under which it has operated, because the policy and ideology which underpins it do not recognise and value the relational (rather than individualistic) actions and responses of people, social groupings and organisations. We propose that social care policy needs to challenge the way personalisation has manifested itself and recognise the relational ways in which people build their lives. In doing so, perhaps it can reclaim one of the fundamental principles of person-centred support; to achieve people's aspirations and become more included within their communities.

This research offers similar findings to other work which demonstrates that in spite of the many inadequacies with the Welfare State as it once was, the introduction of market forces into social care has largely failed to realise the improvements into the welfare provision which were offered. Malcolm Carey notes the impact of the shift from public to private provision of care homes:

> Within the private sector dominated market of residential and nursing home care, complex and convoluted rituals of mergers, take-overs, sales and closures have continued...As a consequence such markets have helped to generate unstable (and therefore potentially unsafe) living and 'support' environments for many residents. For example, recent research has highlighted how many private sector providers have failed to meet basic standards of care...Also recent plans by the Commission for Social Care Inspection to reduce the number of care home inspectors, including children's homes, suggests that presently unacceptable standards may fall even further.
> (2008a, p. 923)

Most of the evidence for Carey's conclusions comes from government's own reports, and material such as this makes depressing reading when thinking about the ways in which bureaucratic structures limit the scope for ethical agency by Social Workers. In an overall sense, the response to the dominance of managerialism within the Social Work profession has been one of frustration and disorientation at the changes that have come about. This sense of fragmentation is exacerbated also by the way large sections of the Social Care direct provision has further declined in quality through privatisation, particularly where work is undertaken by lowly paid, lowly skilled or untrained staff. As Carey notes, "key sectors of social care are now dominated by business interests, many of which, in principle, seek to gain profits" (2008a, p. 919), and he goes on to note that:

> the consequences for Social Work practitioners have been many and have included adherence to numerous (and typically convoluted) administrative procedures and protocols, the rationalisation of Social Work practice, which has led to intense deskilling, and the virtual removal of therapeutic interventions and service provision.
> (2008a, p. 919)

In a related piece of research, where Malcolm Carey has asked frontline practitioners to describe the nature of the changes in their jobs which have brought about by managerial practices, similar issues emerged. One Social Worker, Linda, expresses these in terms of how different the job is compared to her expectation of what it would be like:

> It's just such a routine job now, and quite tedious. There's no real freedom in what you do, and everyone seems pretty fed up most of the time...It's just all this paper work and there's no money for services...I do feel terrible completing those assessment forms knowing there's no budget for anything...We are always hearing about new policies – 'best value' is the most recent (...) but I've seen little evidence [of positive change] (...) Nobody cares about Social Work.
> (Carey, 2008b, p. 349)

In the same article, Carey interviews another worker Tony, who expresses a more optimistic picture of his work:

> There's too much bureaucracy in the job, that's the main problem. However you can find a way around [the bureaucracy], and make time for carers and clients (...)

> I enjoy the work (...) There's little money about [for support services for clients] but you can still change things for some people (...) I've counselled people during assessments, and also done a bit of group work with families, especially [informal] carers (...) You have to believe in something (...).
>
> (2008b, p. 351)

These accounts tally with the 2023 BASW report discussed at the beginning of the chapter, which builds a picture of a disjuncture between the priorities of people running Social Services and the issues faced by Social Workers on the frontline. The sociologist Pierre Bourdieu has argued that it is this which constitutes the "profoundly contradictory basis of the mission" of Social Work under present conditions:

> Social Workers must fight unceasingly on two fronts; against those they want to help and who are too demoralised to take a hand in their own interests, let alone the interests of the collectivity; on the other hand, against administrations and bureaucrats divided and enclosed in separate universes.
>
> (2002, p. 190)

Conclusion

The question which has been addressed throughout this chapter concerns the issue of Bureaucracy and Ethical or Moral Agency – how much do bureaucratic structures suppress, undermine, facilitate or encourage ethical practice within Social Work. The answer is not entirely straightforward. Certain kinds of bureaucracy and bureaucratic roles undoubtedly do undermine moral agency, though it would be a mistake to see this as an inherent quality of bureaucracies. We note here the value of Paul du Gay's arguments about bureaucracy and ethics for Social Work, in that one of the most important ways ethical attributes may be experienced in Social Work, by service users at the very least, is about the way practitioners behave within a bureaucracy. To be a good bureaucrat in this sense is not about a coldly technical rationality, but rather is about an awareness of the needs of the people relying on you (2000, p. 4). It is in this way that Du Gay could be seen as linking the issue of behaviour within the bureaucracy with an ethics of public duty. However, it is in this sense of a focus on ethics that we can return to the point made by Bryan Turner on Weber; that is, it is one thing to argue for the inevitability of bureaucracy as a means of organising society, and another to endorse the rationales of the bureaucracy at any given point in time (1996, p. 358). This point becomes all the more pertinent in a world where the state is continuing to privatise what were once functions controlled by the state, leaving those practitioners working for the state with reduced leverage to effect the positive changes which are the very rationale for Social Work itself. Are Social Workers therefore destined then to remain prisoners of this particular form of neoliberal form of bureaucracy? Pierre Bourdieu makes an insightful point when he argues that:

> Paradoxically, the rigidity of bureaucratic institutions is such that, despite what Max Weber said about them, they can only function (...) thanks to the initiative, the inventiveness, if not the charisma of those who are the least imprisoned in their function (...) And it is undoubtedly these contradictions emanating from bureaucratic divisions that open up a margin of manoeuvre, initiative and freedom which

> can be used by those whom, in breaking with bureaucratic routines and regulations, defend bureaucracy against itself.
>
> (2002, p. 191)

Amongst Social Workers, there will always be some of us who feel 'the weight of the world' more than others. But what Bourdieu offers here is the idea that bureaucratic rules can be so dysfunctional, that they create the conditions for people to have find ways around them, in order to help the people we want to help. In this sense, our ethical duty may be best served by refusing to allow ourselves to become mentally, psychologically and practically imprisoned by the 'iron cage', and in doing so, we can come to realise that its bars are not as fixed as we are told they are. It is important to realise in this sense that Social Work only became a profession out of a form of imagined social solidarity which the Welfare State represented. The dominance of neoliberalism has frayed these forms of solidarity and in some cases undermined these altogether. The research of Power et al. into the lives of people with learning disabilities fully embodies the wider critique that has been made throughout this chapter – that the world of 'autonomous individuality' described by neoliberalism is a false and deeply flawed description of how most people live their lives. It is precisely because of the gap between neoliberal ideology and the reality Social Workers encounter when seeking to support vulnerable individuals and families that we need to hold onto a different sense of what is important. As long as people continue to believe in and articulate a conception of the social where it is people and their real needs that are what is most important, the system which we have to work within is far from invulnerable to challenge. As Spolander et al. note:

> by working together, developing collaborative research methodologies and collectives we can work, lead and promote the role of social work at a global level. If we think that as individuals we have no power, then as an old African proverb may tell you, you have never spent a night in a closed room with a mosquito.
>
> (2009, p. 309)

In other words, it in this process of challenge that new forms of solidarity will emerge and Social Work's ethical mission will again be fought over and reconstructed. It is in this context that questions about the value base of Social Work values are so significant, and it is to this issue that we turn in the final part of this chapter.

Part Two

Ethics in Social Dynamics

3 Power in Social Work

This book so far has discussed issues concerning the evolution of Social Work as well considering the ethical significance of the way it is organised. In this chapter, we turn to the question of power in Social Work practice. As Roger Smith notes in his book *Social Work and Power*:

> Social Work is not just concerned with direct interactions between service users, practitioners and their agencies, but is closely implicated in the conflicts and inequalities that characterise the contexts of their interventions, including those that reflect the wider forms of oppression and discrimination.
>
> (2008, p. 7)

It is the way Social Work is implicated in questions of power, at the many different levels in which this is expressed and manifested, which we want to explore in this chapter. By using the work 'implicated', we are wanting to suggest something more than the idea that Social Workers exercise power or have it exercised over them; rather we want to point to the way it is both of these, and often at the same time. As Smith (2008) has noted:

> [Social Workers] are at one and the same time, acutely aware of their own relative powerlessness in an organisational and structural sense, and yet concerned as to how to manage their own authority over service users.
>
> (2008, p. 17)

Smith is pointing here to the ambivalence of Social Work's relationship with power, and this is an issue which we see as important to think about in considering ethical issues within practice. Ambivalence refers to the feeling of being simultaneously pulled in opposing directions, and this a feature of many Social Work interventions. In Chapter 1, we discussed the way Social Work arises historically as a response to the persistency of problems which are essentially about power, powerlessness, questions of 'social order' as well as questions about what is acceptable in terms of how people live in society. People who have become involved in Social Work are motivated by the desire to act as a 'power for good', to be an individual who can, as is said, 'make a difference' to these problems. Almost all people who want to become involved in Social Work are seeking in some way to help people experiencing difficulties and distress. But a key issue within that desire to make change is the question of how Social Workers understand and work with the problems they are presented with. The book so far has

DOI: 10.4324/9781003458715-6

offered different ways of thinking about this. The Social Work with homeless people in India described in the first chapter could be described as a 'bottom-up' intervention where Social Workers are seeking to 'give voice' to people whose needs are being disregarded and in fact being trampled on by more powerful groups and interests. For these Social Workers, it is not homeless people themselves who are the problem, but rather, the fact that they are homeless is a manifestation of another problem – most likely the lack of housing which is available and affordable to those people. In understanding the issue in this way, Social Workers are seeking to articulate the needs and interests of the homeless against more powerful forces, such as the government and landowners. The example of the different ways the two British Social Workers in Chapter 2 understood the needs and issues in working with the former soldier illustrates this same phenomenon; that the different ways through which the difficulties faced by individuals are understood are related to questions of power. Social Workers all over the world are concerned with assessing and responding to need, but because the question of how we understand and address that is very much bound up with "wider forms of oppression and discrimination" (Smith, 2008, p. 8), questions of power are always present. The last chapter discussed the way in which Social Workers' professional discretion and sense of what a family or individual needs can at times be circumscribed by organisational imperatives. How much time are Social Workers able to give people they are working with? How much are Social Work interventions shaped by what they see as the key issues and how much are they determined by predominance of a particular approach which becomes dominant within the organisation they are working for? These are questions about how Social Work is organised, as we discussed in the last chapter, but they are also questions of power. In this sense, issues of power interact closely with Social Work's ethical framework. This is not least because the actions taken, or in some instances not taken, by Social Workers can have far-reaching implications in the lives of service users and their families. As Hugh McLaughlin (2012) has noted:

> Social Work is not a neutral activity. Social Work can lead to a positive outcome for the service user or the Social Worker or it may lead to a negative outcome for one or both of them. To this end it is imperative for Social Workers to be in a continuous reflective relationship with their practice seeking to find evidence and answers that help them to identify whether their intervention is effective or mere interference.
>
> (2012, p. 1)

This process of finding evidence and seeking answers that McLaughlin (2012) refers to here is very much concerned with the exercise of power in Social Work. Power and ethics can be thought of as inseparable twins in a constant process of interaction, as the tensions between Social Work's idealistic 'helping' mission, the process by which service users' 'problems' are conceptualised, and the organisational and political context in which Social Workers are operating are played out. Because Social Work is 'not a neutral activity', questions of ethical practice within Social Work are always contextualised within power relations. In this chapter, we begin by looking at how power has been defined, moving to a historical discussion which looks at where our present conceptions of power come from. The chapter concludes with a Social Work example in which we try to exemplify the different conceptions of power discussed.

What Is 'Power'

What Is Power?

Power is a word we use all the time, but the definition of it is not straightforward. The Oxford English dictionary for example lists no less than 15 different senses in which the word can be used. The most commonly understood meaning of the power is "the ability to control people or things", and this is one of the most widely used definitions. However when moving into a deeper discussion of power, this definition is really just a starting point for a longer discussion.

In an interesting discussion on the question of Social Work and power, Arnon Bar-On (2002) argues that "if Social Workers are to help their clients, then they must master the discourse of power and use it effectively" (2002, p. 998). This writer is pointing to the centrality of power within Social Work practice. But before we can think about whether we agree with this statement, it is important to ask ourselves, what do we mean when we are talking about 'power'?

The Sociologist and Philosopher Steven Lukes has spent much of his life writing about the nature of power. In a recent discussion of his, he noted that:

> The topic of power is inexhaustible. One reason is that it raises a series of uniquely hard questions from various, related points of view: ontological, epistemological, methodological and normative. Another reason is that it is a topic that arises at every level and in every sphere of social life, from the most intimate to the most macro-geopolitical settings – from hidden power within marriage, to gender-related and racial subordination, to war and diplomacy between states and governance across the international political economy.
>
> (2021, p. 97)

Power is pervasive in our lives. It can touch our everyday experience very directly through people we are in direct personal contact with – think of your relationship with your line manager at work. But we can also be profoundly affected by decisions which are made many thousands of miles away – consider, for example, the impact of trade agreements between countries. While these agreements are made in London, Paris or Washington, this can have a profound effect on things such as the availability of work in the countries of Latin America and the income people gain or lose as a result of tariff agreements in North Africa. Another example is the issue of climate change. Decisions made by fossil fuel companies based in Europe or the United States can decide whether people who live on islands in the South Pacific have to abandon the land they have lived on for centuries due to rising sea waters. Because its impact can both be so near and so far, power can be hard to define. Lukes tried to do this when in 1974 he wrote an influential book entitled *Power: A Radical View*. The book became such an influential text that Lukes rewrote the book in two subsequent editions, which included the original discussion alongside additional chapters. Here we want to think about some of the issues Lukes advanced in his original work. His starting point is no such thing as a neutral definition of power – the process of defining this is "ineradicably value-dependent" (2005, p. 30). When we talk about power, are we talking about the power to achieve a particular end, or does it also involve the power to define legitimate courses of action? Does people's apparent acceptance of a situation which might be considered unfair suggest that that this might not all be that bad for the people affected, and they are in effect giving their consent to this, or might it suggest that those victims of unfairness go along with their treatment because, for a whole range of reasons, they cannot see any alternative to the unfair situation they are in? Why do people support the actions of more powerful people who appear to be acting against what we might think of as their 'best interests'? This brings us to the question of how we can define and understand questions of people's 'interests'. Lukes (2005) notes that rather than being self-evident, 'the notion of 'interests' is an irreducibly evaluative notion. If I say that something is in your interest, I imply that you have a prima facie claim to it, and if I say that 'policy x is in A's interest' this constitutes a prima facie justification for that policy. In general, talk of interests provides a licence for the making of normative judgments of a moral and political character. So, it is not surprising that different conceptions of what interests are, are associated with different moral and political positions' (Lukes, 2005, p. 37). In his book, Lukes (2005) is trying to develop what he calls a 'three dimensional view of power' in which instead of seeing it primarily as the capacity to undertake a particular course of action which embodies something a person wants, considers that these wants "may themselves be a product of a system which works against their interests, and, in such cases, relates the latter to what they would want and prefer, were they able to make the choice" (2005, p. 37). The terrain of power is one that can give voice to a particular person or group, as well as being that which silences, and this is a topic we develop further in the next chapter on 'Epistemic Injustice'. Power includes within it the power to name particular experiences, and this is important as Social Work is a profession which has played an important role in making visible issues that are known about, but which are not able to be talked about in public; Child Sexual Abuse is an example of this. Having been named, this is now an issue which fully exists in the domains of law, public policy and professional practice.

Lukes (2005) argues for a conception of power that includes power as persuasion, power as influence and power as coercion. This is useful as all these different manifestations of power are present in Social Work. For example, consider a Social Worker working with a young person suffering with severe anxiety. In the first instance, the Social Worker can try to work therapeutically with the young person so that they develop different strategies of dealing with their anxiety, or they could encourage them join a support group which has been set up for people to address these sorts of concerns. These are instances of persuasive power, but they also morph into questions of power as influence in that while we are seeking to persuade the young person that doing these things is in their best interest. Our capacity for influence also extends to a Social Worker's ability to involve other professionals, such as Psychologists or Psychiatric Nurses, into the care of this young person. This might lead to a Community Psychiatric Nurse prescribing medication which the young person is expected to take. Imagine that none of these strategies work and the young person's anxiety becomes so severe that they are perceived to be 'a risk to themselves and others'; a Social Worker in this situation has the power to deprive the person of their liberty and compel them to enter a psychiatric hospital for a defined period of time.

This example points to the different ways in which power is exercised in Social Work, and Roger Smith (2008) echoes this observation when he notes that this often makes it difficult to "identify consistent underlying precepts which guide interventions" (2008, p. 2).

Part of the difficulty with this can be seen to lie in the fact that power has these different manifestations in Social Work, and the movement from one into the other can be at times subtle. A key issue within this concerns the authority Social Workers possess – and this is an issue which cuts across the three manifestations of power which Steven Lukes (2005) talks about – whether one is talking about power as persuasion, influence or coercion, all are reliant on an underlying sense of authority. The German sociologist Max Weber was one of the first of many sociologists who have been interested in the many forms of professional power in the specific context of modern societies. Weber was significant for the way he tried to understand the nature of power as authority in societies.

Power as Authority

Max Weber (1864–1920) was one of the first sociologists to argue that we need to understand the issue of power through its exercise in the form of authority. He set out three different forms of authority: Traditional, Charismatic and Rational-legal (see Craib, 1997, pp. 133–141 for a longer discussion of this). Traditional authority is vested in an individual on the basis of tradition and custom; the British Monarchy or the Roman Catholic Pope are good examples of this. Charismatic authority is also vested in an individual, but this is exercised by virtue of their personality; think of African-American leaders like Malcolm X or Martin Luther King, whose soaring oratory and incisive analysis inspired people to join the political movements they developed. However the key form of authority held in modern societies Weber called 'rational-legal' authority. This form of authority is not a possession of an individual, but is invested in a person on the basis of their being the holder of a particular office. This is the form of authority which is exercised by social care and health professionals in modern societies, which was additionally maintained through specialist training (Weber, 2005, p. 214). Rational-legal authority, backed up by Social Work's recognised specialist role, is manifest throughout almost all Social Work interventions.

Understanding Power Historically: The Enlightenment and its Critics

We have begun by setting out some of the complexities in defining power, which derive from the way the word can be used to describe many different things at one time. A useful way of understanding this is to think about the way different thinkers have tried to define the nature of power as it has emerged historically, particularly looking at the development of modern forms of power. Having a historical understanding of these issues is valuable because the operation of power, however much we talk about it abstractly, is always situated in relationships between people, and between people and institutions, within particular societies. These relationships and the way they have been understood have changed considerably over time across different historical periods.

Medieval Power and the European Enlightenment

In Medieval Europe, power was vested in the figure of the Sovereign, and the Kings and Queens and members of the nobility who ruled Europe and believed completely and genuinely that they occupied their place as part of a divinely ordained social hierarchy. This is the archetypal example of what Max Weber called 'traditional authority'. In this period, deference to authority and to the power of tradition was synonymous with obedience to the will of God. The sociologist Barry Hindess (1996) has noted "in this view we are all born subjects" (1996, p. 13); in other words rather than seeing ourselves as being born free, but then having power taken away from us in different ways, as people in modern societies generally do, the starting point in the medieval world was that we were born into a particular role in society, and for better or worse, it was that role that defined how our life would be lived. In this sense, people saw themselves as 'subject' to power as a consequence of the circumstances of their birth. The idea of someone's status in a social hierarchy changing – say a very clever or hardworking peasant working his way up to becoming a member of the nobility – would have been seen as outlandish to people in this period as the social strata in which you were born was seen to define your place in life almost entirely.

It was during the period known as the Enlightenment in Europe, which began in France and Scotland during the 1700s, that these ideas about a fixed and divinely ordained set of social relationships were fundamentally challenged. This was not the first time in which thinking like this took place, but it was something that emerged in a significant period of history. The people involved in this thinking represented a new grouping of journalists, writers, philosophers and activists. One of their most influential spokespersons was Immanuel Kant (1724–1804), whose writings on moral philosophy have had a huge influence and whose main contributions and influence on Social Work ethics is discussed more fully in Chapter 8 of this book. Here we want to discuss him in the context of the significance of these new ideas of power which developed in the Enlightenment. In a famous essay written in 1784 called 'What is Enlightenment', Kant argued that the Enlightenment represented "man's [*sic*] emergence from his self-incurred immaturity" (cited in Porter, 1990, p. 1). Kant's work shook the intellectual foundations of the medieval world, as he set out an entirely new basis on which morality and authority should be established. He argued that people needed to stop passively following tradition and established authority, but instead needed to see their lives and the choices they made as things in which they should be actively involved in. Central to this shift was the idea that human beings were defined by the capacity to reason. Kant's key arguments regarding the importance of reason emphasised that it was the ability to possess and exercise reason which gave human beings the capacity to exercise free-will. This was a crucial issue for all the Enlightenment philosophers, and the historian Roy Porter (1990) has characterised them as a movement which was:

> (…) aiming to put human intelligence to use as an engine for understanding human nature, for analysing man [sic] as a sociable being, and the natural environment in which he [sic] lived. Upon such understanding the foundations for a better world would be laid.
>
> (1990, p. 3)

The advocates of the Enlightenment called themselves 'philosophers', but far from being locked in ivory towers as we often think of philosophers, they saw themselves as a kind of intellectual political activist. Denis Diderot (1713–1784), another of their leading members, defined the 'philosopher' as a person intent on "trampling on prejudice, tradition, universal consent, authority, in a word, all that enslaves most minds" (cited in Porter, 1990, p. 3). In other words, while the Enlightenment philosophers were very concerned with ideas, they wanted not just to share these ideas, but to change the societies in which they lived for the better by implementing these ideas. Another book which had a huge impact within the Enlightenment period was Jean Jacques Rousseau's (1712–1778) *The Social Contract*, which was published in 1762. This book opened with the now famous words: "Man [sic] is born free, and everywhere he [sic] is in chains" (1998 [1762], p. 5). This statement sums up one of the most powerful themes within the Enlightenment, which was about challenging the medieval concept that existing power relations were simply a given, and that to question these was in some way sacrilegious. By emphasising the idea that every person had the potentiality to think and reason for themselves, and to act accordingly on the basis of that, the Enlightenment philosophers laid the basis for our modern views of morality and ethics.

Reflection Break: Do you see yourself as the 'subject' or 'object' of Power?

1 Think about your own life, and some key decisions you have made up to this point. Do you feel as though those decisions were made by you, or do you feel they were made for you?
2 Do you think of yourself as someone who has had a degree of control over how you have lived your life, or do you see yourself as someone whose life has been governed by other people's expectations of you and your role. Are you happy with this?
3 The fact that most of us will relate to these kinds of questions is a testament to the ongoing influence of the Enlightenment and its emphasis on 'free-will'. What are some of the things that prevent people exercising 'free-will'?

Rousseau's (1762) arguments sought to challenge not just the medieval world's conception of morality, he also took the argument one step further and claimed that because people had this capacity for reason, the state itself should be organised on the basis of this recognition. In this way, the Enlightenment set the stage for a radically different means of understanding the relationship between the individual and the State. In opposition to the Absolute Monarchy of France, where the king saw himself as being placed on the throne by God himself, Rousseau argued that the only form of legitimate State order was one which was directly elected and accountable to "the general will" (Rousseau, 1998); anything other than this represented a fraud by the powerful upon ordinary people. It was the combination of these radically democratic ideas and the yawning gap between the opulence of the lives lived by the aristocracy and the poverty of ordinary people which laid the basis for the French Revolution of 1789. In the course of this revolution, the aristocratic order which had dominated France for centuries was overthrown, and this event sent shock waves across the world. The aristocratic families that had controlled the reins of political power in Europe for centuries were challenged by revolts and insurrections from the newly emerging social groupings, as the ideas of the Enlightenment began to change the way people thought about political participation and power. The ideals of the French revolution had a major impact not only on the American War of Independence (1775–1783) but also on lesser-known historical events such as the anti-colonial rebellion in Ireland led by Robert Emmet (1803), and first successful slave revolt in Haiti, which began in 1791, in which slaves claimed their right to be treated as free human beings (James, 1963).

Georg Hegel (1770–1831), a German philosopher highly influenced by the Enlightenment and the French Revolution, took this concept of the centrality of the active rational subject still further in a book called *Elements of the Philosophy of Right* (1821). Hegel (1821) argued that every person simply by virtue of their humanity inherently possessed "Abstract rights" (Houlgate, 2005, p. 186). This could be seen as the origin of our present concept of 'Human Rights'. However, Hegel (1821) did not just want to philosophise about rights – he argued that these rights needed to be made a reality through being enshrined by that state in a written constitution, and one which specifically sought to balance between individual needs and desires and more universal needs. Political liberty was the theme of another influential English philosopher, John Stuart Mill (1806–1873). In a famous essay entitled 'On Liberty', he argued that "the only purpose for which power can be rightfully exercised over any member of a civilised community, against his will, is to prevent harm to others" (1989, p. 223). The work of John Stuart Mill and other related thinkers known as 'Utilitarians' was another important development for ethics in Social Work, and this legacy is explored further in Chapter 9 of this book.

New Understandings of Power: Karl Marx

The political world of the period after the Enlightenment was a turbulent world in which aristocratic monarchies crumbled in the face of popular revolt and new ideas of democracy and popular participation came to the fore. It was a period in which, as Andrew Bowie (2003) has noted, "the tensions inherent in modern philosophy…became increasingly manifest as concrete problems in the socio-political world" (2003, p. 118). Nowhere was this concern about the nature of the relationship between the world of ideas and the world itself manifest more strongly than in the work of Karl Marx. Marx's philosophical manifesto could be seen to be expressed in the words of his famous 11th Thesis on Feuerbach: "The philosophers have only interpreted the world in various ways; the point is to change it" (Marx, 2004). In other words, the validity of philosophy was not just at the level of philosophy itself, but in the way these ideas moved out of the pages of books in libraries and into the real world of people's lives. This expresses one of Marx's key ideas about the way ideas, what is called theory, are realised through informing action in the world. The term for this is 'praxis', which means the unity of theory and practice, and this term was one Marx revived from the Greek philosopher Aristotle.

Marx is important in any discussion of the history of the concept of power, since he was both a product of the Enlightenment, as well as one of its major critics. His work is both hugely influenced by the Enlightenment, but he also marks out a new understanding of power which went beyond the aspirations of the Enlightenment philosophers. The distinctiveness of Marx's views can be seen by comparing the way he looked at Christianity with the views of the main Enlightenment philosophers. Like all the Enlightenment philosophers, Marx was strongly critical of the Christian Church as an institution. However, while the Enlightenment philosophers tended to dismiss Christianity as an 'illusion' which would disappear once people become more 'enlightened', Marx argued that you could only understand the influence it had amongst ordinary people by grasping the sense in which it spoke to their actual situation:

> Religious suffering is at one time the expression of real suffering and a protest against real suffering. Religion is the sigh of an oppressed creature, the heart of a heartless world and the soul of soulless conditions. It is the opium of the people.
>
> (Marx, 1975, p. 244)

Marx's (1975) description of religion as the 'opium of the people' has often been misunderstood to mean that he was simply dismissive of religion. Rather, he saw it an analogous to an opiate, in that it dulled the pain and struggle of people's lives, making carrying on a little more bearable. While the Enlightenment philosophers believed their devastating critiques of religious ideas and clarion calls for free-thinking would finish off the Church as a force in society, Marx (1975) argued that instead you need to look at the real conditions of people in society, and it was only through this that you could understand the appeal of religion. He argued that "the abolition of religion as the illusory happiness of the people is the demand for their real happiness" (Marx, 1975, p. 244); in other words, the problem with religion was not simply that is was an illusion, but rather its illusions were the veiled expression of a truth about power and exploitation which was painful and difficult to apprehend, but which at the same time needed to be understood if this suffering was ever to be alleviated or ended. An example like this demonstrates the way Marx built on the insights of the Enlightenment, but by grounding these insights in relation to the lives of ordinary people, came to offer a much more radical understanding of the way power operates.

Marx looked at the Enlightenment theme of 'free will' in much the same way. In a well-known quote, he commented that people do 'make their own history, but they do not make it just as they please; they do not make it under circumstances chosen by themselves, but under circumstances directly encountered, given and transmitted from the past' (Marx, n.d.). So, while Marx saw that people certainly had the capacity to change the direction of society, this wasn't an abstract capacity – it was a capacity rooted in specific concrete circumstances. Marx's importance here in understanding power lies in the fact that he both drew on the ideas and values of the Enlightenment, but always sought to locate apparently abstract questions in a world of real power relations. It was this which led Marx to conclude that the freedom of the property-owning classes was actually that which guaranteed the unfreedom of the working class – the class with nothing to sell but its labour, hence the need for workers to collectively discover their power as workers, and remake society so it was organised in the interests of the majority of people. These insights have acted as a major inspiration for the development of socialist, communist and trade union movements, including the Settlement movement, discussed in Chapter 1. Marx's major contribution to our understanding of power, and an aspect highly relevant for Social Work, is that it is always embodied materially, that it always exists in social relationships, and for him the central issues was the relationships between classes.

Who Is a 'Rational Subject': Issues of Gender and 'Race'

The Enlightenment philosophers saw Freedom and Equality as Natural Rights, but as Marx pointed out, for most workers, they were trapped within coercive economic relations which meant that those rights could only become a reality if workers challenged and resisted those relations. If we think about the Enlightenment in relation to Gender and colonisation the same issue is present. The working class, women and people from countries colonised by European powers have all had to fight bitter political struggles in order to gain even limited access to Enlightenment ideals. Why was this? It has been argued that a key explanation for this lay in the way the concept of reason came to be interpreted. As noted earlier, Immanuel Kant characterised the European Enlightenment as part of the process of "man [sic] coming to maturity" (Kant, 1784 cited in Porter,

1990, p. 1); maturity in this context meaning the ability to use 'reason'. As Ramazanoglu and Holland (2002) point out:

> The dominance of reason put the reasoning mind in a position of mastery. The 'knowing subject'– the conscious self who reasons – could master the 'object of its knowledge' – the matter to be known. The natural scientist, the man of culture, could unlock the secrets of nature in order to master her. One consequence of this logic was to conclude that the rational, civilized, cultured man, with his access to certainties, could master the savage, primitive or barbarian, who was subject only to passion or a childlike mind.
>
> (2002, p. 28)

Within this view, the civilised mind came to be associated with the male members of the European educated classes, and uneducated workers, and 'natives' in colonised countries were seen as 'uncivilised' or 'barbarian', lacking the intelligence or refinement to understand or use reason. Women too, with their 'emotionally driven' natures, were equally seen as incapable of exercising reason. Stefan Johnsson (2010) has similarly noted the paradox of the way Enlightenment ideas were claimed as universal, but that the expression of this universality historically:

> (...) reflected the specific values and interests of those persons through whom it is articulated. With few exceptions universal subjectivity had been articulated by white men of upper-class background, and resulting body of thought had been shaped according: a mixture of humanist ideals and patriarchal values, universalism and racism, knowledge and bourgeois ideology.
>
> (2010, p. 116)

This tension between universal values and the lived experience of most women during the years of the Enlightenment is revealing in this respect. The lives of most women at this time were lives of unceasing labour, both within and without the home. The ideas of the Enlightenment did influence the educational opportunities available to women of the middle and upper classes; however, as Richard Hooker (1996) has noted, the serious disciplines of science and philosophy were seen as reserved for men. For women, education was about developing the 'accomplishments', which meant various skills that contributed "to the moral development and the 'display' quality of a wife: music, drawing, singing, painting, and so on" (Hooker, 1996). The famous novel *Pride and Prejudice* (1813) by Jane Austen demonstrates these dynamics through the story's focus on what constitutes a 'good marriage' for women of the propertied classes. Hence, while the Enlightenment emphasis on education greatly increased the numbers of people who were learning the new sciences and philosophies, the presumption was that women were not able to cope with these more serious disciplines and that they were unsuited for life beyond the domestic sphere. While men could master their passions through the use of 'superior reason', women were by definition located with the world of emotion and it was 'dangerous' to allow them to move out of that. Educated women did of course challenge these ideas, and one of the most notable examples of this was Mary Wollstonecraft's feminist manifesto *A Vindication of the Rights of Woman* published in 1792. This document, still relevant today, makes a passionate appeal for women to be given access to education in particular, in order to end their marginalisation within the domestic world. Feminism emerged as a political movement in the mid-1800s, and one of the milestones of this was the Women's Rights Convention held in Seneca Falls, New York, in 1848. One of the central demands of this movement was the Right to Vote, and the bitterness of the political battle over the extending voting rights to women indicated how powerful the idea that women belonged in the domestic sphere, rather than the wider public sphere, was. New Zealand was the first country where women were granted the right to vote in 1893, and in the UK, women's voting rights were not made equal to men's until 1928. One of the most powerful accounts of the oppression of women was a book by the French philosopher Simone De Beauvoir, called *The Second Sex*, and first published in 1949. Her central argument is expressed in the memorable phrase that "One is not born, but rather becomes, a woman" (1972, p. 267), and she argued that this process of becoming involves the internalisation of the idea that she is an object, forever defined as the 'other' in relation to a male 'subject':

> Humanity is male and man defines woman not in herself but as relative to him; she is not regarded as an autonomous being...Man can think of himself without woman. She cannot think of herself without man...With man there is no break between public and private life: the more he confirms his grasp on the world in action and in work, the more virile he seems to be, human and vital values are combined in him. Whereas woman's independent successes are in contradiction with her femininity, since the true woman is required to make herself object, to be the Other.
>
> (De Beauvoir, 1972, p. 262)

This work became something of a manifesto for the second wave of global feminist activism which developed from the late 1960s onwards, and even though women have gone on to gain considerable numbers of political rights in wake of this, assumptions that women remain responsible for children and for the home, the 'other' to the male with his focus on the external world of work, remain strong, even though large numbers of women now are working as many hours as the men they are living with (Hochschild, 1989). It is in this, as well as many other ways that the question of gender remains central to discussions of power, and this is particularly the case in Social Work. A contemporary example of this will be looked at the end of this chapter.

As we noted earlier, the fact that the pinnacle of 'reason' came to be seen as the white male from the bourgeois classes was also significant from the perspective of the politics of 'race' as well, since colonised peoples were similarly defined by ideas of immaturity, superstition and backwardness. Writers such as Frantz Fanon (1925–1961) and Edward Said (1935–2003) have famously characterised the way in which colonised peoples were never seen to be capable of representing themselves but could only manage in the modern world by being spoken for and directed by whites. In his 1952 book *Black Skins, White Masks*, Fanon spoke of the way colonisation created a situation in which black people were socialised into deferring to an image of themselves as inherently inferior to the white coloniser based on a process of only being able to look at themselves through the eyes of the coloniser. It was in this way that Fanon pointed to the psychic dimensions of colonialism. *Black Skin, White Masks* (1952) was groundbreaking for the way Fanon understood that the processes of racialised objectification on which colonialism was based were not just about the political economy of colonialism; they were, at the same time, embedded in the psyche of the colonised:

> If the black man is overcome by to such a degree by the desire to be white, it is because he lives in a society that makes his inferiority complex possible (...) it is to

> the extent that society creates his difficulties that he finds himself positioned in a neurotic situation
>
> (Fanon, 2008 [1961], p. 80)

These ideas were developed further in his later book *The Wretched of the* Earth (1961) which was deeply influenced by Fanon's experience of working as a psychiatrist in the psychiatric hospitals in northern Africa, particularly the hospital at Blida-Joinville in Algeria. As someone working within the psychiatric system, Fanon became intensely aware of the way the psychiatric treatments which were used in the hospitals medicalised and individualised the psychic distress of Algerian patients, while failing to grasp the way colonialism itself was a direct cause of these people's psychological distress. He described the colonial world in Algeria as one that was:

> (...) cut in two. The dividing line, the frontiers are shown by barracks and police stations. In the colonies it is the policeman and the soldier who are the official, instituted go-betweens, the spokesmen of the settler and his rule of oppression. (...) It is obvious here that the agents of government speak the language of pure force [bringing] violence into the home and into the mind of the native.
>
> (Fanon, 2004 [1961], p. 38)

In this quote, it is clear that Fanon (1961) understood colonial violence not just as simultaneously shaping the physical organisation of social space but also the psychic space. In this Manichean world, the natives were seen as incapable of ethical thought or action, compared to white settlers, who embodied 'civilization' and 'goodness' at the same time as relentlessly asserting their superiority and the inferiority of the colonised. These social tensions forced the colonised person to live psychically "in a state of permanent tension" (2008, p. 41). David Macey (2012) has noted that "Fanon always stresses the sociogenic aspects of symptomatology: symptoms did not, in his view, originate from the person's unconsciousness or repressed sexual impulse as much as from (...) the internalisation of social conflicts" (Macey, 2012, p. 320).

Edward Said has addressed similar issues in his 1978 book *Orientalism*, which is concerned with the way people from 'the East' come to be defined and categorised by 'the West' as fundamentally alien to the West. The knowledge produced about the Orient, which is what he called 'Orientalism', is thus a "western style for dominating, restructuring and having authority over the Orient" (Said, 1978, p. 3). The key point which Said (1978) drew attention to was the fact that the context of the colonised subject coming be 'known' by the West is the context of colonisation, where the Indigenous people of those countries were economically exploited and in some cases enslaved – and to be a slave was literally to be an object, a non-person. While most former colonies now have their independence, it is a mistake to think that the social relations which developed during the period of colonisation have gone away and do not continue to frame and shape our understandings of these issues. The restrictive immigration laws which have been introduced by most European countries over the last two decades, disproportionately target people from the Global South, and laws about immigration either implicitly or explicitly address the relationship between 'race' and nation. An example of this is the UK's 'Windrush Scandal'. In 2017, after it emerged that hundreds of Commonwealth citizens, many of whom migrated to the UK from the Caribbean in the 1950s and 1960s, had been illegally detained, deported and denied legal rights. An important report into this issue noted that: "There was widespread shock and outrage at the fact that so many Black Britons had had their lives devastated by Britain's deeply flawed and discriminatory immigration system" (The Joint Council for the Welfare of Immigrants, 2024). Just as women were categorised as lacking the capacity to reason on the basis of their inherent 'emotionality', racist ideas originate in this process of classifying people from colonised countries as inherently different and inferior, in short denying their capacity to think for themselves and exercise moral agency.

The Enlightenment in this sense offers us both an extremely important, but at the same time contradictory legacy. It was only after a series of long and bitter struggles by the working classes that they gained basic political rights. There were equally arduous, and sometimes bloody struggles fought by colonised peoples before their demands for self-government and self-determination were accepted by European colonial powers. Women also had to engage in bitter political struggles to gain the right to vote, access to education, to equal pay and to be able to enter the professions. In each of these cases, the dominant image of the working classes and colonised peoples was as 'savage' and 'uncivilised', just as the image of women was split between 'angels of the hearth', an idealised version of domestic life, or as 'hysterically emotional'. This relates to the legacy of the Enlightenment in the sense that savagery and hysteria were characterised as the opposite of reason, and therefore used to justify the denial of political rights. Nonetheless, because of the underlying universality of enlightenment ideals, those same arguments came to be used by anti-colonial and feminist movements, when they demanded recognition of their rights as people and to argue for an end to colonial and patriarchal rule on the basis that these forms of oppression were against the spirit of the Enlightenment. In the earlier chapters of this book we posed the question of whether ethical issues were 'universal' or 'particular'. Stefan Johnsson (2010) is interesting for his suggestion that rather than being thought of as polar opposites to each other, as either/or, we need to think of these two as having a more interactive or both/and relationship. He argues that:

> If there is today a global canon of universalism, it consists of documentary traces of past struggles in which oppression was resisted in the name of universal values. Like all canons, that universalism is selective and easily turned into a new instrument of oppression. Inevitably, every coding of universality is a particular representation.
>
> (Johnsson, 2010, p. 118)

The point Johnsson (2010) is making here is that universalism is a double-edged sword, and the dangers of an uncritical use of this can result in a high-minded ideal becoming used to justify oppressive practices. Nonetheless, it would be equally wrong to throw the universalist baby out with the bathwater. Universality remains important, and not least for Social Work, because it implies the idea that as humans, we have something in common. We all have the same needs for food, water, shelter, and safety. Psychologists are increasingly talking about a universal need for 'relatedness'; for a need to feel connected to others around you and the need to feel that those others care about you. The fact is that our concept of what these universal needs are is not fixed permanently across time and space but is something that is revealed to us as our knowledge grows and develops is also important.

Michel Foucault's Theories of Power

It is implicit throughout our discussion so far that modern ideas about power, upon which a profession like Social Work is based, derive from the European Enlightenment and its intellectual and political legacy. It is for this reason that we have devoted later chapters to looking at the work of Kant, the Utilitarians and others, precisely because, whether we are aware of it or not, the ideas developed here have formed a significant foundation for the ethical frameworks which are used in Social Work. For a long time, there was an assumption that while the practice of this was uneven, that the ideas themselves represented progress. The French Philosopher Michel Foucault (1926–1984) is significant for the way he sought to overturn these assumptions and it is important to understand the nature of this challenge, its importance as well as its limitations. Foucault's first work of major significance was a historical examination of 'madness', entitled *Madness and Civilisation*, which was published in English in 1967. In this book, he looks at the way that in the period after the Enlightenment, a 'Great Confinement' of 'the mad' within large psychiatric institutions took place. The placing of people with psychiatric problems in hospitals where they were treated by doctors has generally been seen as a step towards a more rational and 'enlightened' society, even if it is now acknowledged that many abuses of power took place within those institutions. However, Foucault (1967) challenged this assumption, and argued that the rationale to exclude and confine 'the mad' was not only extremely oppressive, but in addition to this, grew out of the Enlightenment's focus on reason as that which defined our humanity. Because 'madness' represented the polar opposite of reason, 'the mad', who were seen as those who had abandoned or lost the capacity to reason, were seen as less than human. In that sense, the degrading treatment they received was not accidental, but was rather central to the way madness was conceptualised and understood as the opposite of reason.

Foucault's (1967) book came to be situated within a wider literature which developed in the 1960s and 1970s, from former doctors and former inmates of psychiatric hospitals, as well as other commentators, concerned with the dehumanising impact of the large psychiatric hospitals and the abuses of power that took place within them. The work of the Scottish Psychologist R.D. Laing and the US Sociologist Irving Goffman's highly influential book *Asylums*, published in 1961, were amongst the most significant writings within this. While Foucault (1967) did broadly belong in this camp, his concern was not just with madness, but with the power which was involved in placing someone in the category of 'mad'. In order to characterise this, he used the phrase 'power-knowledge'.

What Is 'Power-Knowledge'

This is a complex idea which is more than just the idea that 'knowledge is power'. What Foucault is trying to suggest is that knowledge, rather than being neutral, has an intimate relationship with power, and in particular acquires its status of 'truth' as a consequence of its use within power relations. The relationship between power and knowledge is thus a reciprocal relationship, in which power makes use of knowledge, which in turn reinforces the status of this knowledge. To take the example of madness; the knowledge produced in disciplines like psychology and psychiatry, while being presented as objective knowledge, is a form of knowledge which develops within the power relations of hospital settings and is itself an exercise of power over the patients of those institutions.

In a later book on prisons, called *Discipline and Punish* (1977), Foucault argued that the mechanisms for control and surveillance, which are used in institutions like prisons, were not just incidental to our experience of power. The use of surveillance as a means of creating compliance in populations groups usually began amongst marginalised groups who were not well regarded by the rest of the society, such as prisoners or people with psychiatric problems, but were then extended to more and more areas of social life and government. This form of power which he called 'disciplinary power' was, he argued, amongst the most important ways in which power in manifested in contemporary societies. In a lecture he gave in 1976, Foucault argued:

> The judicial systems have enabled sovereignty to be democratised through the constitution of a public right articulated upon collective sovereignty, while at the same time this sovereignty was fundamentally determined and grounded in mechanisms of disciplinary coercion.
>
> (1977, p. 105)

In other words, 'disciplinary power', a power which creates conformity and compliance through surveillance, represents a kind of hidden accompaniment to the Enlightenment philosophy of Rights and Equality. This represents a significant argument about the nature of power in modern society, and one which has become very influential in contemporary social theory, including within Social Work. However, in evaluating the significance of this argument, it is important that we look concretely at the practical implications of Foucault's rejection of the universalist legacy of the Enlightenment. If we consider contemporary psychiatric care, it can be argued that while Psychiatry was undoubtedly implicated in the abusive treatment of patients for much of the twentieth century, it was also able to respond to Anti-Psychiatry arguments which emerged in the 1960s and the growth of the Patients' Rights movement which accompanied this, and to develop forms of practice which did recognise patients' rights and which have been able to position them as active agents in their recovery. As Dunne (2009) noted of contemporary psychiatric practice in the UK, it now seeks to adopt

> a holistic approach to the patient, taking social and cultural backgrounds into account, as well as the general medical status. Treatment may thus involve medication, various forms of psychotherapy, or both, in addition to practical measures such as help with family problems, debts, housing, residential placements and so forth. In recent years, particularly in the UK, there has been a much greater emphasis on psychological treatments and social interventions. The 'medical' approach has taken a definitive back seat.
>
> (p. 59)

While the problems associated with overly medicalised forms of provision towards mental illness have not gone away, it can also be argued here that changes such as this do represent progress and that Foucault's arguments which characterise Psychiatry as inherently oppressive denies the differences that clearly exist between the Psychiatric Hospitals of Victorian England and those in the UK today. This is significant because it suggests that Foucault's argument which positions Enlightenment Reason as the root of the problem is an oversimplification of the issues in terms of how we have understood mental health and illness. The philosopher Miranda Fricker has developed this point in her own critique of Foucault. She argues that:

> Suspicion of the category of reason per se and the tendency to reduce it to an operation of power actually pre-empt the very questions one needs to ask about how power is affecting our functioning as rational subjects; for it eradicates, or at least obscures, the distinction between what we have a reason to think and what mere relations of power are doing to our thinking. If one has an interest in how questions of justice might present themselves (...) then [the approach taken by Foucault] obscures essential distinctions between, say, rejecting someone's word for good reason and rejecting it out of mere prejudice.
>
> (Fricker, 2007, p. 3)

So to go back to our example of mental health, the way in which Foucault has presented the problem of the abusive and stigmatised treatment of mental illness as an essential product about the operation of Reason, we lose the capacity to distinguish between forms of psychiatric treatments which do unjustly abuse the rights of patients and those which see the recognition of those rights as an important part of the process of recovery. This is important for Social Workers working in the area of mental health conceptualise and understand the work they are doing.

A further problem associated with the ongoing influence of Foucault's ideas is the rejection of the category of 'the Universal'. The complexity of the how universality has been defined has been discussed throughout this chapter, but just as Fricker has questioned the wholesale rejection of the concept of Reason in the work of Foucault and his followers, so we can equally point to the problems associated with the wholesale rejection of the category of Universality. These issues are demonstrated in the work of Judith Butler, an influential contemporary sociologist who was a student of Foucault and whose work has significantly developed his ideas. In her book *Gender Trouble: Feminism and the Subversion of Identity* (1990), Butler argues that there is no such thing as a 'pre-discursive' natural body; in other words conceptions of 'woman' are entirely social and cultural constructions which are constituted 'performatively' rather than biologically. She goes on to argue that the category of 'Woman' rather than being connected in any way to the female body is rather an 'effect of discourse', that is the meaning of being a woman is entirely created by language and social practices. The consequence of this argument is that there are no inherent qualities which one can ascribe to all women, and that to do so would be excluding, reductive and 'essentialist'. However, in similar terms to Fricker's critique of Foucault above, the philosopher Alison Assiter (2021) has argued that there is universal significance to the physical materiality of the female body, even if the meaning given to this is socially and culturally specific. Assiter argues that we need to 'remember our biological bodies, since it is in virtue of these that we all share a concern for the natural world on which we all depend and from which we have all emerged' (Assiter, 2021, p. 76). In other words, we can hold onto a conception of the materiality of the biologically defined body without having to see the meaning associated with this body as fixed and timeless. In similar terms we can acknowledge the fundamental importance of biological knowledge, while at the same time accepting that the development of biology as a discipline is and has been culturally and socially situated. So while Assiter (2021) rejects the idea that conceptions of woman should be entirely defined by the physicality of the body, at the same time, she wants to retain the importance of the physical reality as a universal quality of womanhood, even if the meaning of 'womanhood' itself is a category which has many different and evolving meanings. In their critique of Foucault's work, both Fricker (2007) and Assiter (2021) are making the same point in different ways – that postmodern constructivism has thrown the baby out with the bathwater. By creating an either/or position about Reason and about the category of the Universal, this obscures the different ways these concepts have been and which continue to be utilised in social practice. Assiter goes on to argue that a category of universal womanhood, while not being fixed and unchanging, continues to constitute the basis for women's political struggles against violence and inequality: 'if we are to act as women to ameliorate domestic violence against women, to fight against the rape of women, we need the universal category of woman' (Assiter, 2021, p. 78).

Conclusion

What we've tried to do in this chapter is to explore different conceptions of power. The point of this to demonstrate how pervasive a phenomenon this is, but also how complex it has been to characterise it, and how contested this process continues to be. In looking at the ways different thinkers have tried to characterise power, it is clear that they are emphasising very different things. In a discussion of this issue, Keith Dowding noted that as a concept, 'power is essentially contestable' [and this is because] what is essentially contested [are] different views about the way society ought to be governed (2012, p. 121). This is a key issue for Social Work, as the very existence of Social Work as a profession is directly bound up the question of how the social problems of modern societies are defined and addressed. In other words, Social Work is closely connected with the nature of governance in society. It is for this reason that, as we noted at the beginning of the chapter, questions about the definition of power are so bound up with ethical questions. This includes both the way power is exercised upon Social Workers and the ways in which Social Workers exercise the power they have. It also points to the way that Social Work as an 'ethical profession' has a crucial investment in questions of how society is governed and particularly in the role of democratic forms of governance that emphasise social equality. These are themes we develop in the following two chapters. Chapter 4 develops the discussion in this chapter on the relationship between power and ethics still further, while Chapter 5, develops the connection between Social Work practice and wider political governance.

4 Epistemic Injustice and Social Work

With the Collaboration of Barbara Neale

In the previous chapter, we discussed different conceptions of Power, and this chapter builds on this, introducing a dimension of power which is both conceptual and practical. The sociologist Barry Hindess noted that when we think about power, there is always a tendency to explain it as 'the generalised capacity to act'. He suggests we need to see power as involving "not only a capacity but also a right to act, with both capacity and right being seen to rest on the consent of over whom the power is exercised" (1996, p. 1). However, when we talk about right to act, we are also implying something else, which concerns the process where that right is heard and accepted as a legitimate form of expression. In real-life situations, there are some forms of testimony which are readily seen as needing to be listened to, while others are ignored, and others still are actively dismissed. The assumption in democratic liberal pluralist societies which recognise forms of legal equality is that while the existence of inequality is acknowledged, that all citizens possess a legitimate capacity to act within the law, even if that is not the same capacity. But what happens when a person's attempt to describe or seek redress for an experience of injustice is not seen as credible in the first instance? How does it happen that a situation of someone making a claim about unfair treatment results in them being seen as the problem, rather than the problem they are describing? It is these sorts of questions which are the focus of this chapter, which is concerned with what has been called 'Epistemic Injustice'. In this chapter, we begin by outlining the meaning of this term and explaining why it is significant when thinking about the understanding of and ethical use of power in Social Work. The term 'Epistemic Injustice' is important because ethical questions are not just about the distinction between right and wrong, but also about how we come to recognise the expression of that distinction between right and wrong. In other words, 'Epistemic Injustice' is a concept which seeks to connect ethical questions with questions of 'knowing'. We see the concept of 'epistemic injustice' as useful for Social Work as it offers is a theoretical lens which allows for a deeper examination of the operations of power, prejudice and social justice in Social Work, building the core knowledge and skill base that underpin and reflect the professional identity of Social Work.

What Is Epistemic Injustice?

The concept of epistemic injustice is associated with the work of the philosopher Miranda Fricker (2007), and even though the idea which has articulated certainly existed prior to her work, it has been her work which has brought the concept to prominence. In her work on *Epistemic Injustice* (2007), Fricker puts forward a distinctively epistemic genus of injustice where a person is wronged specifically in their capacity as a knower, and

DOI: 10.4324/9781003458715-7

thus wronged in a capacity which is essential to human value. The branch of philosophy concerned with knowledge is known as 'epistemology' and this is concerned with the question of 'how we know what we know'. The term epistemology has been defined as 'concerned with providing a philosophical ground for deciding what kinds of knowledge are possible and how we can ensure they are both adequate and legitimate' (in Crotty, 1998, p. 8). Fricker was inspired to develop her work in this area through being initially trained in philosophy, but then feeling that the branch of philosophy concerned with epistemology was seeing these issues in overly abstract terms and so failing to engage with the way questions of 'knowing' were closely connected with real experiences of just and unjust treatment in everyday life ("Epistemic Injustice", 2021).

Consider the following situation: A woman has just taken her car to the garage for a service. Following the service, on her way back home, she feels that there is something about the steering that does not feel right. She has been driving this car for a long time and knows what it feels like to drive, so she goes back to the garage and describes her sense that something isn't right with the steering. The mechanic listens and then tells her that when new parts have been put into, the car often take a while to 'bed in'. She continues to try and explain to him how she feels when driving, but she is finding it hard to convey the sense that something is not right. He continues to assert that it should sort itself out, and in the end, she accepts his reassurance. However, on driving the car the next day, she finds the problem to be even worse. She speaks to her husband about this and after driving the car himself, he immediately agrees with her that something is not right. As he has time available the next day, he takes the car back to the garage, and when he does this the mechanic agrees to look at the car immediately. The garage subsequently calls him apologising for the situation – the garage had fitted this new part incorrectly and a serious problem could have resulted had this not been addressed.

One response to this situation is that it could be described simply as the sexism which is often manifested in the 'male' world of cars and mechanics. However, what Fricker wants to get us to think about here is the way questions of how we are treated in public life are connected to the validity of testimony. What the incident above illustrates in terms of epistemic injustice is that the woman's expression of her experience carried less weight than that of her husband. This situation illustrates Epistemic Injustice because it is in her capacity as a knower that the woman's account of her situation carries less credibility in the perception of the mechanic.

Reflection Break

Do you recognise this situation?
Have you ever been in a situation like this or a similar to this one?
Why do you think the man in the situation was believed more readily than the woman?

'The Grindr Killer'

This situation might seem like a relatively minor example on which to build the case for a concept which is focus of a chapter of a book on Social Work ethics, so let us think about a more serious example. Here we want to discuss the case of a serial killer who was known as 'the Grindr Killer' due to the way he used the gay dating app 'Grindr' as a means of making contact with the young men who became his victims. Between June 2014 and September 2015, four young gay men were found dead in the East London suburb of Barking, UK. There was a pattern of similarities to these deaths with all four bodies found in a small geographic area. The body of the first victim, 23-year-old student Anthony Walgate, was found outside a block of flats with the subsequent three bodies found by members of the public in a same churchyard, itself only a couple of 100 metres from the location of the first body. All four young men died in exactly the same way, as a result of ingesting excessive amounts of the 'party drug' gamma-hydroxybutyric acid (GHB). During the period in which the later three deaths took place, the UK LGBT newspaper *PinkNews* ran a series of stories warning gay men in the East London area to be aware of men they were meeting on 'Grindr' and other gay dating apps.

While concern was developing about possible connections between the deaths, the police investigations of the deaths continued to treat them as entirely unconnected, being characterised as 'unexplained' or 'non-suspicious' (De Simone, 2021). Even after the death of the fourth victim, Jack Taylor, and in a situation where many of the detectives attending the scene had been present at the earlier deaths, the police investigation continued to see each death as unrelated from the others. Indeed, the police only began to consider that that might be a pattern of connections between the deaths following pressure from the two sisters of the final victim Jack Taylor. Jack Taylor's sisters were so frustrated with the inconsistences in the account of their brother's death offered by the police – in particular the fact that their brother never took drugs and was very opposed to drug use – that they began carrying out their own investigation. It was this amateur detective work, combined with concerns expressed in the media, which pressurised the police into widening the scope of their investigation. This led the police very quickly to a man called Stephen Port, who was then arrested. When the case eventually came to the court, he was not only convicted of all four murders, but what became devastatingly clear how much evidence the police investigation had disregarded, with the killer Stephen Port 'hiding in plain view'. A BBC documentary into the catalogue of errors in this investigation noted that friends and families of the dead men had consistently questioned and challenged the police's explanations for the deaths, but all of this evidence had been dismissed by the police (How Police Missed the Grindr Killer, 2017). The evidence that the police had particularly disregarded was that of other gay men who were the ex-partners and friends of the victims – which was rejected on the basis that these people were "not next of kin". Family members of the victims later alleged that the London Metropolitan Police 'made false assumptions about their loved ones, with homophobia playing a role in the flawed decision-making' (BBC, 2021) As the full extent of the failures, incompetence and missed opportunities to have caught Stephen Port in the early stages of his serial killing emerged, Assistant Police Commissioner Helen Ball responded saying:

> I don't think the Met is an institutionally homophobic organisation. I do think that we need to make a great deal of change to our investigative practices. We have done that – and people need to be reassured that we have done that.
>
> (De Simone, 2021)

What Is 'Identity Power'?

The concept of Epistemic Injustice concerns situations of injustice which take place because some forms of testimony carry more weight than others. Miranda Fricker develops this idea in her work, arguing that the expression of power in society is not simply about practical co-ordination between different agencies. Alongside this practical coordination of social power, there are also:

> operations of power which are dependent upon agents having shared conceptions of social identity—conceptions alive in the collective social imagination that govern, for instance, what it is or means to be a woman or a man, or what it is or means to be gay or straight, young or old, and so on. Whenever there is an operation of power that depends in some significant degree upon such shared imaginative conceptions of social identity, then *identity power* is at work.
>
> (2007, p. 14)

Fricker uses this concept of 'identity power' to describe interactions which work both passively and actively when a shared imaginative conception of what is a group or individual is 'really like' comes to shape the understanding of people's actions and behaviour.

How might the concept of Epistemic Injustice help us understand this situation? Here we want to introduce the concept of 'Identity Power'.

Here we want to suggest that this concept of 'Identity Power' offers one way of understanding the apparent inability of the police to connect what subsequently appeared be clearly connected phenomena in this case. While there was extensive criticism of the police investigation once the full details of this case and the extensive catalogue of errors emerged, much of this pointed towards individual faults and examples of incompetency, and on poor information sharing between different branches within the London Metropolitan Police. But does this, in itself, explain the reasons for why the police saw the four deaths as both 'non-suspicious' and as unconnected to each other for such a long time? If we think about the issue of 'identity power' in this instance, Fricker's argument concerns the harms which this enacts through the way identity prejudices are invoked in such a way that hearers deny or withhold credibility to or from speakers as members of a certain "social type" (2007, p. 4). Evidence to this effect emerged most clearly during the inquest into the trial of Stephen Port, held in 2021, which showed the way that the prejudices of the police shaped the investigation. John Pape, a friend of one of the victims, noted that while the Inquest had exposed underfunding as a factor in the police investigation that

> consequently, they 'prioritised' in ways that exposed their prejudice. It led to incompetence and unequal treatment (…) What disturbs me now, is knowing how the Met actively shut down anything that challenged their incorrect assumption, that the victims willingly took a date rape drug.
>
> (Davies, 2021)

At the centre of the Metropolitan Police's conceptualisation of the murder victims were that they were promiscuous gay men who met others like them through dating apps and who used illegal drugs to enhance their sexual experiences. The 2021 Inquest evidenced the notes of the one of the police family liaison officers who recorded Port's first three victims as "all gay and they were using dating websites to meet men and also attending parties that had been organised where it appeared there were drugs actively being used and sexual activity happened" (Davies, 2021). What this demonstrates is the way in which the police saw the victims as young men were all seen as freely choosing to place themselves in situations which were inherently risky, and which sadly went wrong for them. The fact that these encounters had ended tragically for these four was unfortunate, but this was seen to be in the nature of the kind of deviant sexual encounters which promiscuous homosexuals were known to seek out. This latter point was demonstrated by an email from a police Duty Inspector who described the churchyard where three of the victims' bodies were dumped as a "haven for gay sex (even dogging) and rough sleepers" (Davies, 2021). Hence, it was the police's conceptualisation of the behaviour of the four victims that was central to the way they carried out their investigation. Much of the evidence which contradicted this came from other gay men who knew the victims. However, these accounts of the victims from other gay men carried little credibility within the police; one of the victim's partners of four year described himself as dismissed "in every single way" by police "because we were a gay, unmarried couple" (Davies, 2021). Does this mean that every police officer who was involved with this case was consciously homophobic? Fricker argues that 'identity power' is not just about consciously held beliefs; rather "the primary modus operandi of identity power is at the level of the collective social imagination. Consequently, it can control our actions even despite our beliefs" (2007, p. 15).

If we think about the way this situation played out, we can see that police's actions were not simply incompetent and negligent, though they were that. We can also understand the police's actions as an instance of the concept of Epistemic Injustice; particularly in the way forms of testimony which were fundamental to discovery of the murderer were disregarded by the London Metropolitan Police. The concept of identity power makes the point that when we encounter social institutions, we do not just encounter them as abstract citizens; we encounter them through the lens of collectively held beliefs about the nature of particular sorts of identities. It was this collectively held conception of identity which governed the actions on which the police investigation was based, and which explains why they continued to see the similarities between the deaths as related to the deviant sexual behaviour of the victims, rather than other possible explanations; which in hindsight were staring them in the face. This situation demonstrates 'epistemic injustice' because it shows that ethical questions of justice and injustice are closely connected to the way people bring collectively held beliefs and presumptions to the process of making ethical judgements. 'Knowing' in that sense is not just an individual action but reflects social beliefs and frameworks which are used to evaluate meaning and the significance of events.

Fricker's conception of epistemic injustice connects here with a growing body of scientific evidence, from cognitive psychology in particular, supporting the notion of 'unconscious bias'. This is concerned with the way our unconscious preferences can shape the way we engage with others and make decisions about them, particularly when we are under pressure to make a decision and there is a considerable amount of information to process (Suveren, 2022). This work demonstrates the way our brains are wired to involuntarily categorise people based not only on a host of visible and salient criteria but also on invisible and apparent labels such as gender, age, skin colour, sexual orientation, job title, accent, education and professional status. Culture is about values, but it is also made up of the innumerable engagements between people which take place every day. Within these interactions, we are all the time unconsciously assigning qualities and characteristics to the other people we interact with and encounter. This may remind you about the idea of social location we covered in the introduction of this book, and the importance of reflecting on it as we engage in Social Work intervention. The evidence around this shows that we are more likely to attribute positive characteristics and therefore have better relationships with those who appear to be like us and appear to share the same values. This bias might not involve consciously held beliefs or considered ideological attitudes, and indeed these situations can occur when people consider themselves not to be prejudiced.

Reflection Break

Reflecting on your own life and work:

- Can you identify a time when you personally experienced a situation where your testimony was not validated in an encounter with a social institution?
- Can you think of any experience you have had in Social Work practice where the testimony of a particular service user was invalidated in a way you were unhappy with?
- Do you think the concept of identity power is valid way of understanding these?
- If those situations were to arise again, what do you feel you could do differently in terms of addressing this situation?

Is this concept also relevant in Social Work? We would argue it is very significant because Social Workers are always called upon to evaluate and assess the needs and concerns of different groups of people in the community. The way we understand the accounts of the people we encounter can impact on issues such as quality of care different groups of people might receive, decisions made about the entitlement to support for people we assess and the process through which we recognise the validity of people's needs. In the 'Grindr Killer' situation, conceptions of identity power acted to close down the 'professional curiosity' we would expect the police to show in investigating a murder case. There is comparable evidence in Social Work regarding child deaths where subsequent investigations into the circumstances of the families have revealed a lack of professional curiosity that could have kept a child safe (see below for further discussion of this). In assessing people we work with as Social Workers, what are the explanations for people's behaviour that we consider? How much do we hold the possibility for different explanations in our minds when we are listening to people? Is Fricker's conception of identity power useful for understanding the way people can be treated differently in their capacities as knowers regarding questions of gender, disability, sexuality, class background, ethnicity and 'race', and the connection of these to images of "sincerity and inferiority, lack of breeding, lack of moral fibre" (Fricker, 2007, p. 32)?

Testimonial and Hermeneutical Injustice

Having set out the broad definition of Epistemic Injustice and its relationship to the concept of 'Identity Power', Fricker goes on to define two distinct sub-sections of this concept; 'Testimonial Injustice' and 'Hermeneutical Injustice':

> Testimonial injustice occurs when prejudice causes a hearer to give a deflated level of credibility to a speaker's word; hermeneutical injustice occurs at a prior stage, when a gap in collective interpretive resources puts someone at an unfair disadvantage when it comes to making sense of their social experiences. An example of the first might be that the police do not believe you because you are black; an example of the second might be that you suffer sexual harassment in a culture that still lacks that critical concept
>
> (2007, p. 1)

Let us explore the significance of these two in relation to Social Work specifically.

Testimonial Injustice

Fricker notes that Testimonial Injustice occurs when a speaker 'receives an unfair deficit of credibility from a hearer owing to prejudice on the hearer's part' (2007, p. 21). This represents a situation when an unfavourable perception is imposed onto a speaker resulting in them being 'less believed'. In such a situation the explanation of the person listening to them is imposed onto the speaker in a way, diminishing or disregarding the speaker's credibility. This can involve a straightforward experience of a person's views not being listened to, but the question of not being heard can also be connected to wider questions of identity power.

Consider the following case study:

> Robert is a social worker who is called upon to assess the situation of Sian and Idris, an older couple in their 70s. Sian and Idris are a retired couple without children who have an active social life, involving a wide network of friends and connections in their community. Both play tennis and are involved in the running of their local tennis club and Sian also volunteers with the local foodbank. Idris had a career in Local Government and still has many former work colleagues with whom he maintains regular social contact. Sian was a teacher for most of her life, and also has many former colleagues who she sees regularly, as well as a wider network of friends. Idris is being assessed for support following a severe stroke. He now requires significant support in managing everyday tasks including his personal and practical care needs, having lost all movement in one side. While his Physiotherapist has said he is likely to regain some movement, both Sian and Idris are both dealing with the huge changes to their lives which this is going to involve. Sian is present throughout the assessment and shares with Robert her concerns that she will be unable to cope with her husband's needs which she feels she must have additional support to manage. She is now the only driver and on her own is not strong enough to lift the wheelchair which has been provided for Idris into the car, and she is concerned that both she and her husband will be increasingly isolated in their house and unable to maintain the social networks which are such an important part of their lives. During the assessment Robert asked Sian if they had any family support which they could access, and Sian feels she is judged negatively in saying they do not have any – both of their parents died long ago and neither maintains any contact with siblings. The social worker concludes the assessment and explains that

they will send this once it is completed. On receiving the completed assessment, Sian sees that they have been allocated one hour of care for the morning to assist Idris in getting out of bed, washed and dressed, and a brief call in the evening to assist him getting to bed. However she is upset to see that the social worker has simply assumed Sian will be carrying out all other personal care for Idris, and as well as having to manage all of the housework, shopping and cooking on her own, particularly in the context where it is clear that both her and her husband are now going to be significantly isolated from the wider connections which have played such an important part in their lives.

Reflection Break

- Why do you think Sian has experienced her concerns being disregarded by the assessment she has received?
- Consider some possible scenarios as to why might Robert have assessed the couple's needs in this way. How might this have been done differently?

Hermeneutical Injustice

The second dimension of Epistemic Injustice which Fricker outlines is Hermeneutical injustice. She characterises this as a more of injustice which take place in advance of Testimonial Injustice. Hermeneutics are the branch of knowledge concerned with interpretation and hence this concept is defined as "the injustice of having some significant area of one's social experience obscured from collective understanding" (2007, p. 154). Like Testimonial Injustice, Hermeneutic Injustice also reflects the connection between questions of power and 'knowing' but while Testimonial Injustice is concerned with the credibility of testimony, Hermeneutical Injustice is concerned with the way we understand and interpret social experience. This manifests social injustice in the sense that less powerful groups in society are less likely to have their social experiences recognised and understood in wider society, and as a consequence of this, people who are members of these groups are less likely to have been offered the resources to make sense of those experiences.

Now, consider this other case study:

Kwame, a black male social worker arrives at the home of the Griffiths family, a white British family, to undertake an assessment. This is being undertaken following reports from the children's school that the two children aged 6 and 8 are showing signs of neglect. On arrival at the house Kwame meets Arnold Griffiths, the children's father, however on looking at Kwame refuses him access to the house, saying he only prepared to talk about his children with 'an English social worker'. Kwame explains to Mr Griffiths that while he was not born in England, he has lived almost the entirety of his life there, and that he is a very experienced social worker who has worked with many families over many years. Despite these efforts, Mr Griffiths continues to refuse him access. Kwame returns to the office and explains to his team leader and line manager Phillipa what has taken place. Phillipa expresses immediate frustration with the situation saying she is currently under "massive pressure from Senior Management to get all the assessments of the children on her list assessed as soon as possible". Given this, the work is going to have to be re-allocated as a priority and she asks Lisa, a white female social worker, to undertake the assessment that afternoon. Phillipa says nothing further to Kwame about the situation, leaving him feeling that he was at fault for not having been allowed to undertake the assessment.

Reflection Break

Fricker describes Hermeneutical Injustice as a situation which 'puts someone at an unfair disadvantage when it comes to making sense of their social experiences'. Is this a useful way of understanding this situation?

- One of the other Social Workers who observed this encounter later comes up to Kwame and seeks to offer him support. She describes Phillipa as 'a complete stresshead who just gets ridiculously bossy when things get to her'. While Kwame doesn't disagree with that, does an explanation of this situation at that level explain how he might be left feeling?
- Imagine you were the manager faced with the situation Phillipa was in. How would you address this situation?

Within both of these scenarios, we see the presence of active and passive power as Social Workers and their managers perform their duties within the constraints of current policy and resources. It is important in thinking about these examples to situate them within a context. For example, Robert, Sian and Idris' Social Worker, may have been recently challenged by his manager over the high cost of the applications for funding he makes compared to all the Social Workers in his team. Regarding the second example, it could have been the case that the Social Work agency which Phillipa and Kwame work for has been recently criticised by the Social Work Inspection authorities for the number of cases of child neglect in their area, and for the need to be addressed as a matter of urgency. To say this is not to justify those actions – rather the point of Epistemic Injustice as a concept is not simply to lay the responsibility at the door of particular individuals. What this concept points to is the way questions of justice and injustice are about the way individuals make decisions within a social and institutional context, including the current pressures on Social Work practice. At the same time, it is crucial to understand the impact of this can have for those more directly on the receiving end of those situations, as well as in terms of the overall ethical position of Social Work as a profession.

As we have noted in previous chapters, under conditions of neoliberalism, state-based Social Work is governed by workload management systems which place frontline workers under considerable pressure not just to ensure the safety and wellbeing of the children and/or vulnerable adults, but also to complete all of their case recording, assessments, court statements and legal reports in specific time frames. Many Social Workers find themselves working under conditions where it is simply not possible, no matter how well organised they are, to complete the work allocated to them to the standard they want. In situations where the pressures on practice escalate, we can see the following things taking place:

- **Demoralisation** – As Social Workers people feel unable to meet the assessed needs of the people, they are working towards caring and protecting in their communities, and simply give up on caring so much about these people.
- **Blame** – A culture of blame can develop when the pressure on a group of staff intensifies and management have made it clear that they do not want to hear about the problems associate with the pressure on staff.

- **Isolation** – Both of these processes above can lead to people adopting a 'survivalist' mentality where staff are only able to focus on what is immediately in front of them, leading them to reduce or even cease communication with colleagues, feeling that there is no point or benefit to this.

All of the above create conditions where instances of Epistemic Injustice are more likely to take place. If Social Workers are placed under pressure about reducing the costs of care they are delivering as the primary objective of their work, their capacity to engage with and validate the perspective of vulnerable service users will be impaired. This makes 'Testimonial Injustice' more likely. Thinking about 'Hermeneutical Injustice', it is clear that good Social Work practice requires a collaborative approach in practice where 'professional curiosity' is nurtured, and that Social Workers are supported to think through and reflect on the situations in which we as Social Workers find ourselves. Rather than something which is an add-on in Social Work practice, evidence shows that this is directly connected to the fundamental focus of contemporary practice.

Read the following excerpt from a news article published in *Community Care*, a UK professional magazine:

Leaders Must Foster Professional Curiosity and Challenge to Improve Child Protection, Finds Review.

The Child Safeguarding Practice Review Panel said senior managers needed to give practitioners the 'time, resources, and training' necessary for effective safeguarding, as well as promote 'safe professional challenge' within and between agencies. In an echo of previous studies, the panel's 2022–2023 annual report found that a lack of professional curiosity and challenge were among key deficits flagged up in rapid reviews of serious cases carried out by local safeguarding partnerships over the past year. The panel, which examined 393 cases, found an over-optimism concerning parents' capacity to give safe care and an over-reliance on parental self-report, with missed 'opportunities' to triangulate this information with that from other sources.

Not Seeing Underlying Issues Behind Behaviour

The panel also criticised a failure to see behind a child's behaviour to identify underlying causes, an issue that was evident in cases of extra-familial harm. "In these cases, behaviour was viewed as the issue to deal with and manage as opposed to exploring and understanding the underlying cause, which was often associated with vulnerabilities such as mental health", the report said. "There were examples where practitioners referred to children as 'troublesome' or 'problematic' and where victim-blaming language was used in reports or case records". This also applied to some practice with families from black and minority ethnic communities, with 'missed opportunities' to consider the wider social harms and inequalities they faced. This included the practice of 'adultifying' some black children, by treating them as responsible for their actions and not recognising their needs, and emphasising criminal behaviour over their welfare.

https://www.communitycare.co.uk/2024/01/30/leaders-must-foster-professional-curiosity-and-challenge-to-improve-child-protection-finds-review/

The final paragraph in the above article points to the ways in which pressures on practitioners can so easily create situations of Hermeneutical Injustice, in that they are not bringing a holistic understanding of the situations of service users into their assessments, leading them to fall back on blaming and pathologising 'difficult' service users. Fricker points to the way that when processes like this take place, those most likely to be worst affected by this are groups which are themselves the most marginalised:

> it is generally socially powerless groups that suffer hermeneutical marginalization, and so we can say that, from the moral point of view, what is bad about this sort of hermeneutical marginalization is that the structural prejudice it causes in the collective hermeneutical resource is essentially discriminatory: the prejudice affects people in virtue of their membership of a socially powerless group, and thus in virtue of an aspect of their social identity.
>
> (2007, p. 155)

We noted above that in situations where organisations are under severe pressure to meet their objectives and that that organisation does not allow the space for staff to articulate the pressures they are under and for them to be meaningfully addressed, that cultures of demoralisation, blame and isolation can easily become established. This creates the conditions for 'Testimonial Injustice' amongst Social Work staff themselves, where those who continue to raise 'difficult' issues for the organisation become classified as 'difficult' members of staff who are dismissed accordingly. This also can lead to situations where those service users who are already most marginalised in their identities are also the most 'hermeneutically marginalised', that is the specific knowledge which practitioners most need to address in order to genuinely support these individuals and communities is disregarded, with the result that those people are problematised and labelled rather than understood in the context it needs to be.

Let's now look at a final couple of case study and see how epistemic injustice can materialised.

Case Study 1

Asad is a young boy of 11 years old with severe learning disabilities who attends a Special Needs School, Willow Green, which is based in the same suburb of a large city where he lives with his mother, Fatima. Fatima is a single parent who has looked after Asad on her own after her husband left the family home when Asad was three years old, and who now has no further contact with his wife or son. Fatima has a large Pakistani Muslim extended family network in the city in which she and her son live, but she earned considerable disapproval from her parents after her husband left their marriage. Fatima felt she was blamed for the fact that he left the marriage, in spite of trying to explain to them that it was her ex-husband's failure to recognise the realities of raising a child with severe learning disabilities. Asad is non-verbal and autistic and spends large amounts of time on his own playing on his iPad. He can occupy himself for long periods of time in this way and be very contented; however, if he feels that there is something he wants that he is being prevented from having, he becomes anxious and upset and if this escalates, he can lash out. He has hit his mother and staff at the school several times in situations like this. Asad is in general happy in the school once he has formed relationships with staff and they have got to know him and become used to the way he conveys his needs using a communication system which is on his iPad, which he can use effectively.

Unfortunately, the academic year at Willow Green School has not begun well. Asad's class has been unable to recruit a permanent teacher since the term began several months ago. While some of the Teaching Assistants have been doing their best to maintain the teaching in the class, the school has also had difficulties recruiting Teaching Assistants, and the class has experienced a large number of agency staff who arrive and sensing the difficulties in the class have not remained in the school. The frequent changing of staff is a source of significant anxiety to Asad, and this contributes to difficult behaviour at home. Fatima has been on the receiving end of this and has phoned the school in tears many times pleading with them to establish regular staff in her son's class. Recently, she arrived at the school without an appointment shouting at the reception staff and demanding that school head "do what he is paid to do". On one occasion when she was not informed as to why Asad came home with a large scratch on his arm, she came to the school and made her way past the School Reception and straight her son's class, shouting at staff calling them 'uncaring'. The most recent difficulty involved a situation in class where Asad became very agitated and hit one of the newly arrived teaching assistants on her forehead, leading the School Head to seek to permanently exclude Asad from the school. As a Duty Social Worker, you have been called on to assess this situation.

You begin your assessment interviewing staff in the class. They describe Asad as 'hard work' and his mother Fatima as a 'complete nightmare' as she 'can never say no' to Asad which 'makes it impossible to manage him in class'. These views are echoed by the School Head, though in more polite language.

When you visit Fatima at home, you do observe the way will give into to all of Asad's demands; however, you are also conscious of how isolated she is, with no adult contact other than a few of the other parents at the school. You also note that her whole life is organised around the care of Asad. She cries quietly through much of this meeting and pleads with you to keep him in the school.

- Using Fricker's concept of Hermeneutic Marginalisation, how would you make sense of the range of presenting issues in the situation at School?
- How might you work with the school in helping them appreciate the wider circumstances of Fatima's life, as well as the way they have contributed to the presenting situation with Asad?
- Think about what the interpretative resources which a Social Worker needs to allow them to understand this situation holistically. What are these?

Case Study 2

Noor was discovered by security guards at a port on the south coast of England late at night appearing lost and alone. She was cold, thin, dishevelled, as well as being confused and frightened when she was discovered. Though she spoke very limited English, the security guards were able to ascertain that she had been travelling for about two months before arriving in the UK from Afghanistan. She was not with any other family members at the time she was found. The security guards were instructed by their manager to contact 'Border Force', a UK government department which monitors all goods and people who cross national borders. 'Border Force' officers took Noor to a holding facility where she was detained and questioned by them as to how she came to arrive in the UK, why she had travelled alone, and whether she posed a risk to UK security. Despite being exhausted and distressed, Noor engaged with Border Force staff as well as she could via a telephone translator. Whilst Noor was reluctant to share information, Border Force staff ascertained that Noor was presently separated from her family and that she had no means to contact them, or they her, due to the war-torn state of her home country of Afghanistan. Border Force staff contacted Social Workers whose role was to conduct an Age Assessment to determine whether Noor would be eligible for support from Social Services. During this assessment, Noor had again to speak to people she had never met before and share the distressing details of her journey. The outcome of the assessment was that Noor was considered to be an 'unaccompanied minor', meaning that she is considered a child in the eye of the law. As a consequence, she was placed in an emergency foster placement in the local area. On arrival at the foster placement, Noor felt safe enough to eat for the first time in several days without fear of retribution. She remained at the foster placement for three days and was then assigned a Social Worker, and moved to a more permanent placement.

- Using Fricker's concept of Hermeneutic Marginalisation, how would you make sense of Noor's situation arriving in the UK?
- From the perspective of the Social Worker assigned to her, what are the interpretative resources which they will need to allow them to appreciate the circumstances which led her to leave Afghanistan and undertake such a dangerous and traumatic journey to the UK?
- You are at a family dinner party and you end up telling people about some of the work you are doing with Unaccompanied Asylum-Seeking young people. After describing their difficulties and issues, your cousin states 'I think these people just come here because they think Britain is a land of milk and honey!' What key points might you want to get across to this person in problematising such a view?

Fricker has noted that "hermeneutical injustice most typically manifests itself in the speaker struggling to make herself intelligible in a testimonial exchange raises a grim possibility: that hermeneutical injustice might often be compounded by testimonial injustice" (2007, p. 159). As Social Workers who want to use our power to ethical ends and challenge Epistemic Injustice where do we go next? Fricker argues in answer to such a question that:

> The form the virtue of hermeneutical justice must take, then, is an alertness or sensitivity to the possibility that the difficulty one's interlocutor is having as she tries to render something communicatively intelligible is due not to its being a nonsense or one being a fool, but rather to some sort of gap in collective hermeneutical resources. The point is to realize that the speaker is struggling with an objective difficulty and not a subjective failing. Such a sensitivity involves, once again, a certain reflexive awareness on the part of the hearer, for a speaker whose communicative efforts are hampered by hermeneutical injustice may seem to be making no sense at all to one hearer.
>
> (2007, p. 169)

If we think about these two case studies, the situation of Noor and that of Fatima, we can see how pertinent this description is of their situations. The school where Fatima's son is attending is experiencing wider organisational problems which have become problems for her. In trying to articulate the problems she is facing, she faces dismissal and pathologisation. This builds on the rejection experienced within her own family which manifests both Testimonial Injustice – in the way her explanation of account of the decline of the marriage was seen as a problem with her – and Hermeneutical Injustice – in the way her family has failed to acknowledge the specific experience involved in caring for a profoundly learning-disabled child.

Similarly, in the second case study we can see the way global problems of war, invasion and the rise of authoritarian political movements, like the Taliban in Afghanistan come to be refracted on the treacherous journeys that individuals like Noor undertake. In seeking to escape these profound difficulties through which they lose their connections with their families, communities and a country, they arrive and subjected to complex assessments and often detention as they seek asylum according to internationally recognised treaties. In spite of the traumatic nature of their departure and the danger and violence that are frequently experienced on journeys like this, they are treated as objects of suspicion and danger upon their arrival.

Conclusion

Epistemic Injustice in essence is a concept that allows us to be better attuned to the to the situations we find ourselves in as practitioners, and able to facilitate the respectful conversations which allow the many voices which need to be heard in Social Work practice to be heard and validated. As Social Workers, we are importantly positioned to make a difference in situations like this. The concept of Epistemic Injustice is also so significant for Social Work because the profession is itself is a profoundly epistemic endeavour; in other words the bodies of practice wisdom, theory and research which has been developed over time represent crucial hermeneutic resources which Social Workers can bring to bear on the situation of a service user. The role of Social Work education is so important as Universities are such important gatekeepers of this body of knowledge. However, the development of Social Work agencies, Social Work research and Social Work education are key aspects of a functioning democratic society which is based in a context of legal recognition of equality. But what would happen to Social Work if this context were removed at the macro level of politics? It is these sorts of questions which we look at in the next chapter on radicalisation and the rise of the Extreme Right in politics.

5 Radicalisation, Social Work and Society

Introduction

In the introduction of this book, we began by noting the extent to which the world has changed since the publication of the first edition. The emergence of the phenomenon of 'radicalisation' – the rise of the violent Islamism and the Extreme Right, which will be the focus of this chapter, is one of the most profound and depressing markers of this change. At the beginning of this book, we also noted that many of the issues we are dealing with in Social Work practice today are global issues with local manifestations. This is true of the problems of homelessness and mental health, as we have discussed in previous chapters; and it is also true regarding the rise of these authoritarian political movements, whether these take the form of violent Islamist groups, or that of white supremacist political groupings of the Extreme Right. These are global movements, often organised through online spaces, but which have had profound impact in particular places. In the face of these developments, various governments have sought to set up prevention work, which in some places has been situated as a safeguarding responsibility for Social Workers. In this chapter, we discuss the ethical basis of our involvement in these activities. These safeguarding activities were set up to deal with preventing ongoing involvement of often vulnerable individuals, many of whom are isolated or who have significant mental health issues, in acts of terrorism and hate crimes. However with regard the Extreme Right more specifically, we are seeing some situations when political parties and movements which promote these sorts of supremacist ideas and policies have taken up power within the state. Where does this leave ethically based forms of Social Work practice in these situations? We conclude by thinking about the nature of the current threat to democracy and legal forms of equality, which we are now facing.

The Historical Context: 9/11 and the End of the 'End of History'

We begin this chapter by seeking to historically contextualise the unstable times in which we are now living. We can trace this back to the events which took place at the end of the 1980s with the end of Communism and the Cold War. In 1989, the Berlin Wall which separated Communist East Germany from the capitalist West came down, and two years later, the Soviet Union was dissolved and ceased to exist as a state. The countries of Eastern Europe which had been contained within the Soviet orbit for decades were now on an entirely different path. While China was still governed by its Communist Party, it became integrated into global capitalist production in an entirely new manner, a phenomenon would have seemed inconceivable even ten years earlier. Communism, as it had

DOI: 10.4324/9781003458715-8

been known throughout much of the twentieth century, and the Cold War, which had controlled governments across the world throughout the twentieth century, was from thence forward, nothing like the kind of force it had been, and this was hugely significant in thinking about the form of global politics in the post–Cold War period. In 1989, the American political scientist Francis Fukuyama sought to capture the significance of this new period in an article, later a book, which argued that humanity had now reached 'the End of History'. With the collapse of the Soviet Union, the Cold War over and capitalist markets now spreading throughout the world, we were, according to Fukuyama, living in a world defined by the ongoing global ascendancy of capitalism and Western liberal democracy. He argued,

> What we may be witnessing is not just the end of the Cold War, or the passing of a particular period of postwar history, but the end of history as such: that is, the end point of mankind's ideological evolution and the universalization of Western liberal democracy as the final form of human government.
>
> (Fukuyama, 1989, p. 4)

What Fukuyama offered here was a vision of a world where capitalism and liberal democracy would from now on benevolently and peacefully work their way across the world, a world which he saw as having transcended political, class, social and ethnic divisions, and where there were to be no further political developments in history. It was this vision which was abruptly terminated on the morning of 9/11 with the terrorist attack launched by Al-Qaeda on New York and Washington. Early on that Tuesday morning, 19 members of Al-Qaeda hijacked four commercial flights in the United States and deliberately crashed them; two of those planes struck the World Trade Centre in New York City, leading to the collapse of both towers and the deaths of 3,000 people; a third plane crashed into the Pentagon building in Washington later than morning. While the death and destruction caused by this event were devastating, it was the fact that an event of this nature and magnitude had *even taken place*, and the way the consequences of this reverberated across the world, that were the most significant. The period in which the 'End of History' could be imagined as a possible global future was buried under the rubble of the World Trade Centre in New York. This was replaced by a new and much darker Zeitgeist theory – the 'Clash of Civilisations' – which was the title of a new work by another US political scientist, Samuel Huntington. Huntington argued that what the 9/11 attacks and the rise of violent Islamist political movements across the world illustrated was that while the world of the Cold War was divided between Capitalism and Communism,

> the great divisions among humankind and the dominating source of conflict will [henceforth] be cultural. Nation states will remain the most powerful actors in world affairs, but the principal conflicts of global politics will occur between nations and groups of different civilizations. The clash of civilizations will dominate global politics. The fault lines between civilizations will be the battle lines of the future.
>
> (Huntington, 1993, p. 22)

According to this theory, it was now 'culture' rather than different social and economic divisions of the world which would determine the shape of global politics. In US and Western policy what followed 9/11 was what US President George Bush Junior called 'the War on Terror'. The first act of this saw the US military and its European allies in

NATO invade Afghanistan, at that stage led by the Islamic fundamentalist government of the Taliban which was sheltering the leader of Al Qaeda, Osama bin Laden, who they refused to hand over to the US. It was ironic that despite Afghanistan's role in supporting Al Qaeda, the majority of the terrorists involved in 9/11 came not from countries which were hostile to the US, but from Saudi Arabia, a country which was then and which continued to be closely allied with the US and Britain (Keay, 2021). This was only one of the many contradictions and distortions of the 'War on Terror' period within world politics. In 2003, the US military led a combined force of troops from the United States, the United Kingdom, Australia, Spain and Poland in the invasion of the Republic of Iraq. Iraq was at that stage run by the brutal dictator Saddam Hussein and despite the horribly authoritarian nature of the regime, it was a secular regime which was in no way related to the violent religious fundamentalism of Al-Qaeda. Nonetheless, these events were folded into the aggressively interventionist model of the 'War on Terror'.

The wars in Afghanistan and Iraq witnessed devastating levels of civilian deaths, but alongside this, one of the most appalling consequences of the War on Terror were the abuses of Human Rights which took place; both through the actions of states as well as actions of terrorist organisations. In seeking to capture violent religious fundamentalist fighters in 1990s, the US introduced a programme of illegal 'extraordinary rendition', whereby individuals considered to be involved in terrorism were abducted and transferred across national borders and detained without any legal due process. The interrogation techniques used in these places would be illegal in the US and most of Europe and represented severe abuses of human rights. The U.S. government set up the Guantanamo Bay detention camp at a US Military Base in the Caribbean in 2002 and in setting this up President Bush declared that the Geneva Convention, which protects prisoners of war, would not apply to Taliban and al-Qaeda detainees captured in Afghanistan. These inmates were detained indefinitely without trial and several detainees have allegedly been subjected to cruelty and torture. Most prisoners of Guantanamo were eventually freed without ever being charged with any crime, and were transferred to other countries; however, there are other prisoners who to this day have never been criminally charged, but who continued to be detained indefinitely; a situation which has been widely condemned by Human Rights bodies (Amnesty International, 2024).

At the same time, as US and its allies undermined Human Rights and the rule of law through actions such as this, jihadist groups grew across the world, undertaking further violent attacks on public space and civilian life across the world. Attacks by Al-Qaeda and its affiliates across the world were evidenced through events such as the Bali Bombings of 2002, an attack primarily directed against Australian civilians (but which also killed numerous Indonesian civilians as well as people from many other countries), the Madrid train bombings of 2004 and the 2005 7/7 bombings of the London Transport system. In their global campaigns, jihadist groups drew in countries with no direct involvement in the 'War on Terror', such as the terrorist attacks carried out in Algeria, Libya, Nigeria, Morocco and Cameroon. The combination of the events described had deeply destructive, chaotic and traumatising impact on individuals, communities and societies across the world. Under the impact of wars, health systems break down, systems of education and social support are unable to function, supplies of food and water are placed under threat, the legal system is undermined, and political accountability for abuses by both state and non-state actors can disappear. The rights accorded to children, women, minority groups and refugees may have been fragile enough in times of peace; these are even more so in times of war. The loss of accountability for crimes and violence carried out in these time by both state and non-state actors has the impact of undermining the most basic experience of personal security. Under the impact of terrorism ordinary people going about their daily lives suddenly become 'collateral damage' in acts of random violence.

What Is 'Extremism'?

Alongside these political developments, a new terminology has developed to the situation we were now in. One of the most widely used terms used to characterise jihadist groups is the term 'Extremism'. This isn't a new term at all – rather it was a term that gained a new lease of life in the post 9/11 period. J.M. Berger, an academic who researches this area, has noted that while we now live "in a world where violent extremism is widely noted to be a defining feature of our age" (2018, p. 2), it is remarkably difficult to define exactly what this means in our present context. Berger notes that one of the issues in characterising what is 'extreme' implies a yardstick of 'normality' against which the 'extreme' can measured, but what is that 'normality'? In other words, the definition of 'extremism' can never be a value-free exercise. The present system of liberal democracy has many critics; does the aspiration to radically change this or even overturn this make a person an 'extremist'? Is extremism defined by the ideas people have or the methods they use to enact these? Berger notes that there is a huge tendency to imply in the use of this term that extremists are always 'the other guys' rather than 'people like us'. Yet if we look back through history, this "provides ample evidence that extremism is part of the human condition and not the exclusive province of any single race, religion or nation. Not all violence is extremism, nor are all of humanity's countless wars, conflicts and atrocities" (2019, p. 4).

The UK Government's 2024 definition of Extremism defines this as

> the promotion or advancement of an ideology based on violence, hatred or intolerance, which aims to:
>
> 1 negate or destroy the fundamental rights and freedoms of others; or
> 2 undermine, overturn or replace the UK's system of liberal parliamentary democracy and democratic rights; or
> 3 intentionally create a permissive environment for others to achieve the results in (1) or (2).

Here extremism is defined as an attack on the status quo of the UK's system of parliamentary democracy and the rule of law. The US government by contrast defines a 'domestic violent extremist' as:

> actors who conduct or threaten activities that are dangerous to human life in violation of the criminal laws of the United States or any state; appearing to be intended to intimidate or coerce a civilian population; and influence the policy of a government by intimidation or coercion, or affect the conduct of a government by mass destruction, assassination, or kidnapping.
>
> (US Dept of Homeland Security, 2021)

So while the U.K. definition is primarily concerned with ideologies which seek to undermine liberal democratic practices and values, the US definition focusses on violent behaviour and actions. Berger's definition offers an alternative to both of these which seeks to grasp what is distinctive in the thinking or ideologies of contemporary violent authoritarian movements. He sees these as essentially concerned with the framing grievance through the exploitation of identities, defining extremism as a "belief that an in-group's success or survival can never be separated from the need for hostile action against the out-group". Here the in-group represents people who share an identity (such as religion or ethnicity) while the out-group represents those whose different religious belief, nationality or ethnicity defines them as 'other' (2019, p. 4). The strength of this definition is the way it focusses on the inherent supremacism and chauvinism involved in contemporary forms of extremism – the most significant of which are Salafi-jihadism of groups such as Al-Qaeda and Neo-Nazi groups, which have now become prominent after decades on the fringes of politics. In these sorts of authoritarian movements, people don't just view their understanding of the world as superior to others, they seek to have their identity group defined as supreme over other groups, which they view as degenerate or evil. Berger's definition also distinguishes these sorts of ideologies from others which are commonly described as 'extremist'. Communists and Anarchists, for example, would both argue that liberal democracy should be overturned and replaced, but what they seek is – in theory – a political system which offers a far more profound and universal form of equality than capitalist liberal democracy. They could be thought of 'extreme democrats', but this represents a very different kind of politics from the supremacism of neo-Nazis and jihadists.

Many politicians and commentators have described the Irish Republican Army (IRA) as 'extremist', but here it is important to distinguish between terrorism and extremism. As Berger notes "terrorism is a tactic whereas extremism is a belief system" (2019, p. 30), so while they often travel together, they are not the same thing. In other words, there can be political movements which are ideologically extremist, but which insist on non-violent methods. There are also nationalist movements, such as the IRA, which adopted terrorism as a tactic in their battle against the British Army in the 1970s, but whose ideological advocacy of a 'United Ireland' would be shared by many Irish people – the vast majority of whom would at the same time deplore the terrorism of the IRA. When thinking about the term 'terrorist', it is also important to remember the adage that 'one person's terrorist is another person's freedom fighter'. Take the example of Nelson Mandela, leader of the African National Congress (ANC) in the fight against Apartheid in South Africa. The British and US government considered Nelson Mandela to be a terrorist throughout the 1980s, while he was a hero to most black South Africans. However, once Apartheid ended in the early 1990s, Mandela was democratically elected president of South Africa and went on to be awarded the Nobel Peace Prize, with politicians of many different views rushing to be photographed alongside him. Similarly, after the cessation of violence brought about the Peace Process in Northern Ireland in the mid-1990s, former members of the IRA such as Martin McGuiness went on to become government ministers and worked effectively alongside those who they had once considered their sworn enemies. These examples illustrate a transition from terrorism to peaceful democratic participation in government. One of the factors which contributed to this change was that both the IRA and ANC had defined political objectives concerned with specific historic injustices, and over which they were able to negotiate with those they once fought when the political space for this arose. The political objectives of the ANC and IRA are very different from those of the Extreme Right and from Salafi-jihadist groups like Al Qaeda, since rather than a concern with historic injustices, these groups have a deeply conspiratorial view of the world, discussed further below.

Reflection Break

British Prime Minister Margaret Thatcher stated in 1981 regarding the IRA: "There is no such thing as political bombing or political violence... Crime is crime is crime". In this view, groups which use terrorism, as the IRA did, are simply criminals.

Do you agree? How are groups like the IRA both different and similar the violence of common criminals?

Do you think the perspective of the victims of terrorist attacks is important in this discussion?

Radicalisation

Radicalisation has become another key term in describing contemporary 'extremist' movements. The UK government definition of this is "the process of a person legitimising support for, or use of, terrorist violence" (Gov.uk: 6/3/2024). McCauley and Moskalenko offer a more useful definition of this as a "change in beliefs, feelings, and behaviours in directions that increasingly justify intergroup violence and demand sacrifice in defence of the in-group" (2008, p. 416). This definition is valuable for the way it points to the fact that radicalisation is not simply concerned with undertaking terrorist acts; rather it is about trying to get people to adopt particular kinds of conspiratorial and supremacist political views in the first place. Once the person has been acculturated into this way of thinking, they come to accept that violent actions are 'necessary'. Consider the following quote from the ISIS recruit, Aqsa Mahmood:

> The family you get in exchange for leaving the ones behind are like the pearl in comparison to the Shell you threw away into the foam of the sea. [But] the first phone call you make once you cross the borders is one of the most difficult things you will ever have to do. Your parents are already worried enough over where you are...However when you hear them sob and beg like crazy on the phone for you to come back it's so hard.... But as long as you are firm and you know that this is all for the sake of Allah then nothing can shake you Insha'Allah (God willing).
>
> (Frantz and Schubert, 2015)

This points to the way Aqsa Mahmood's radicalisation involved a complete break from her old life from her family in Glasgow and the privileged life she led there to travel to Aleppo in Syria to join the Islamic State in November 2013. Once there she became infamous for her role in recruiting many other young British women to join ISIS. Central to this were her prolific postings on Twitter and Tumblr, which included images of brutal ISIS executions in Syria, praise for 'revenge' terrorist attacks in France and Tunisia; she even celebrated the brutal rapes which ISIS carried out on the Yazidi women (McDonald, 2018, p. 65). Yet a year before she arrived in Aleppo, she was completing her final year at school and planning to go to university to study medicine. As Tehmina Kazi notes, "Privately educated Aqsa had every benefit a young British girl could ask for, yet still trod a path of subservience, dehumanisation, and collusion with barbarism" (Kazi, 2019, p. 133). It is probably something of mystery even to those who knew Aqsa Mahmood very well why it was that she went from such apparent normality to the advocacy of such brutal violence in such a short time.

In December 2020, police arrested Matthew Cronjager, a 17-year-old white British young man who was successfully completing his A-Levels at a school in Essex. On raiding his house, Police seized a large collection of neo-Nazi literature, with bomb instructions and combat manuals found on his computer. For the previous year had been active in far-right online chatrooms, where he had posted about his hatred for gay people, Muslims and 'powerful Jewish figures in banks and stuff', calling for a 'revolution' based on his fascist beliefs. Cronjager did not know that one of the extremist groups he was part of – the encrypted Telegram messaging app 'The British Hand' – had been infiltrated by an undercover police officer. He sent the officer money and planned obtaining 3D-printed guns, as well as a shipment of firearms from Europe. Cronjager also discussed his plans to 'execute' one of his best friends, an Asian young man, after finding out he had slept with white girls. He informed the undercover officer:

> I've found someone I want to execute…I know it's an overall target and he's a sand n***er that f***ed a white girl…In fact I think 3 of them…I figure we could just 'find' a double barrel shotgun and saw it down for things like this.

He admitted they had been friends 'for ages' but 'I can just kill him like that' (R. v. Matthew Cronjager – Sentencing Remarks).

In court, Cronjager's solicitor referred to the fact that the young man was on the autistic spectrum, and denied he ever meant to do anything and has now 'renounced his extremist views', saying they were borne out of loneliness and misery (BBC News 3/9/2021). However the Judge in his case was unmoved by this and he was sentenced to 11 years in prison. His Asian former friend attended the court case where Cronjager was sentenced and commented in court that:

> Matt and I shared a strange humour, but I never for one moment thought that he held racist views, especially against me…This has significantly changed me as a person [and] affected how I trust people or more importantly how I don't.
> (R. v. Matthew Cronjager – Sentencing Remarks)

Why Do People Become Involved?

One of the key things that research about radicalisation demonstrates is that there is no single path into radicalisation within the movements we have been discussing so far. While most people recruited are male, recruits come from all social classes and religions. Some are from apparently happy and functional families while others come from families where they have been neglected and mistreated. While ideologies adopted in the two cases above are very different, the thinking they demonstrate is very similar. In both cases, we can see that radicalisation involves inculcating people within a universe of meaning in which acts of violence against 'the other' are not just seen as acceptable but are morally right. While political violence is as old as human society itself, there are some distinct patterns that can be seen in today's radicalised individuals. With earlier forms of political violence throughout the twentieth century, violent tactics tended to develop following the repression of political demands initially expressed non-violently. The IRA, discussed earlier, is an example of this. Catholics in Northern Ireland were discriminated against in housing, employment, and throughout Northern Irish society, and in the late 1960s, civil rights protests took place to raise these issues. However, after peaceful protests were violently suppressed by the British government, the paramilitary IRA emerged, supplanting the role previously undertaken by peaceful protest. Today's radicalised individuals follow a different trajectory to this in that most of them have "no background in solidarity organisations or political activism of any kind" (McDonald, 2018, p. 5). While contemporary neo-Nazism and Salafi-jihadism are most definitely political projects, their recruits are often people like Aqsa Mahmood and Matthew Cronjager with no previous interest in politics at all. Recruitment can take place through social networks, such as university societies, places of worship or football supporters' groups, but equally many are socially isolated individuals whose only contact with political ideologies is through the internet. The role of the internet is crucial for understanding radicalisation as this has become not just the primary means of recruitment, but also the way the central platform these groups use to inspire and gather a global audience of supporters. Caolan Robertson, a former far-right activist who was drawn into this world on social media, believes algorithms on social media were crucial in bringing neo-Nazi material into his social media feed. He also noted that in far-right video material that

> the production values have increased and that entices a lot of young people who are on the internet who might not know the difference between legitimate media and extreme media anymore because it's all starting to kind of look the same.
>
> (Johnson, 2021)

A UK government report from 2021 on '*Safeguarding and Radicalisation* also notes that "the significance of online influences through discussion forums, social media platforms and games has potentially been exacerbated by the increased isolation and amount of time young people spent online during the pandemic" (Gov.uk, 2021, p. 27).

Many converts to Salafi-jihadism have backgrounds in criminality or previously lived hedonistic lifestyles with partying, casual sex and drug taking prior to their conversion to a religion they had previously paid little or no attention to. Similarly, many neo-Nazis are isolated people with histories of mental health problems or autistic spectrum condition which are exploited in their recruitment. As noted earlier, while the ideologies adopted by Matthew Cronjager and Aqsa Mahmood express sworn enmity towards each other, the structure of the thinking they adopted is remarkably similar. The journalist Khadija Khan has described this as 'supremacist' thinking, where people come to believe that

> their ideology is superior to all others, that their efforts to impose that ideology are essential, and that this can be achieved through a rampage of horrific crimes against humanity… Be they white or Islamist, supremacists are on the march.
>
> (Khan, 2019)

The writer Arun Kundnani argues similarly that

> What draws recruits to ISIS is not so much religious ideology as an image of war between the west and Islam. This is a narrative of two fixed identities engaged in a global battle: truth and justice on one side; lies, depravity and corruption on the other.
>
> (Kundnani, 2015)

The fact that you can substitute the image of war between 'the White and Black Races' for 'the West and Islam' shows how similar the structure of thinking associated with Salafi-jihadism and neo-Nazism are.

There is much media commentary which presents the violent authoritarianism of Salafi-jihadism as a product of the religion of Islam. Critical examination of these claims shows how false this claim is. While Salafi-jihadists (as well as people on the Extreme Right) make this claim, their version of Islam is not just distinct from, but is deliberately destructive of the mainstream and heterodox historic forms of Muslim religious practice and belief practised throughout the Muslim world. The Iranian Koranic scholar Navid Kermani has described Salafi-jihadism as a travesty of the 'multi-ethnic, multi-religious and multi-cultural Orient' and a form of 'religious fascism' which is destroying Islam (2015, pp. 80–81). The extent of opposition to Salafi-jihadism throughout the Muslim world is captured extensively by the Algerian writer Karima Bennoune in her book *Your Fatwa Does Not Apply Here* (Bennoune, 2013). She has noted that: "Many people of Muslim heritage are staunch opponents of fundamentalism and terrorism, for good reason... they are much more likely to be the targets. Only 15% of Al Qaeda's victims in 2004–2008 were westerners" (Bennoune, 2014). ISIS ideologist Anwar al-Awlaki stated that "if a Muslim kills each and every civilian disbeliever on the face of the earth he is still a Muslim and we cannot side with the disbelievers against him" (Bennoune, 2010). It is in the name of such a project that these groups seek to 'purify' Islam, which they achieve through disciplining, repudiating, expelling, and murdering those who believe in a more tolerant, pluralist, and hybrid conception of Islam. Salafi-jihadism is, like Neo-Nazism, a fundamentally authoritarian political movement, and their claims of wanting to 'purify' Islam are identical to the way neo-Nazis want to 'purify' the 'white race', through violently attacking hated 'others'. In this sense, one of the best ways we can characterise the politics of these movements is through the term 'violent authoritarianism'.

The sociologist Farhad Khosrokhavar has noted that radicalisation cannot simply be seen through the lens of national security, but that it 'must become a problem entailing our understanding of society'. (Khosrokhavar, 2015, p. 7). It is common to hear radicalisation described as though it is simply about 'bad people' – a view epitomised in British former PM David Cameron's description of ISIS as a 'bunch of psychopaths' (Black, 2016). What this discussion omits is an understanding of the societal factors which have led to the emergence of violent authoritarian political movements. Khosrokhavar, whose research concerns young people in the segregated and impoverished suburbs of metropolitan France, argues that while the 'humiliation, frustration, social and economic exclusion and racism' experienced by French Muslim youth is real, that those who become jihadists "do so by ideologizing their internal experience; they expand their hatred of 'non-Muslims' by adopting a jihadist vision". He goes on to argue that for these people "Islam proposes an alternative that far-left ideologies are no longer able to provide" (2015, p. 17), adding that

> the decline of the Communist Party has occurred within a historical conjuncture when social advancement can no longer occur for a large portion of the lower classes, who are reduced to economic exclusion. When exclusion is accompanied by stigmatisation, an explosive mix can result. Groups that are both mistreated and stripped of the means for expressing their social situation have a tendency to retreat into passivity or silence, or express their revolt through violence.
>
> (2015, p. 11)

This connects to our introductory discussion in this chapter about the significance of the decline of Communism and socialism as ideologies which previously provided the political vehicle for people who were dissatisfied with poverty and exclusion.

We can understand the growth of anti-immigrant far-right political parties across the world in a similar light. These groups gain power by blaming Muslims and immigrants for the decline in living standards and for the deteriorating state of public services. These parties appeal to people who have a definite sense of the way there are winners and losers in the world and that politically the world is heavily stacked in favour of those winners. While these people often have justified grievances about the state of the world, they are drawn into a politics of blame as they lack an understanding the social and political forces which have generated this situation; these were forms of explanation which were historically associated with trade unionism and the politics of the left. In a context where the political parties of the left have moved to the centre and no longer provide a voice for the working classes in politics, this creates disillusionment which the Extreme Right are adept at exploiting. It is in such a situation that people are open to adopting conspiratorial forms of explanation. Conspiracy theories take root in a context where

> the world is experienced as a frightening and confusing place, where the anchoring reference points of meaning seem to have been wrenched from their moorings, [thus allowing] these conspiracy narratives form a powerful rallying call for their supporters and offer new anchors. The far right has created a community of shared meaning and acceptance around this. In this sense, conspiracy theories, despite their irrational substantive contents, are not irrational at all and their growth poses a dilemma for feminists and the left in finding ways to present alternatives to these
>
> (Cowden and Yuval-Davis, 2022, pp. 109–110)

In conspiracy theories, real problems are over-simplified into blaming an 'other' onto which the distress and frustration a person feels about the present can be projected. This sits alongside a nostalgic memory of the happy days in the past when people felt their lives were better. Blame is the praxis that results from this toxic combination and the forces of the extreme right are mobilising this into a dangerous force, driven as it is by real frustration and a lack of understanding of political and economic forces which are generating the problems which people experience. In a state of blame, people also refuse having to think about their own involvement and responsibility for the way the world is now, and what they could do to make things better.

We can summarise this discussion by pointing to three central features of the violent authoritarian movements we see today:

1 **A Manichean Worldview**: In Manichean thinking, the world is seen through a deeply polarised and simplistic lens of good and evil, corrupt and innocent, pure and impure. The horrific violence undertaken is seen as necessary to 'cleanse' society from its 'impure' elements.
2 **Social Media Anti-heroes**: Radicalised individuals have often experienced a sense of 'humiliation and victimisation', but rather than campaign to change this collectively, they seek to regain a sense of status through acts of violence which allow them to become "heroes for all who share their credo, notorious public enemies for everyone else" (Khosrokhavar, 2017, pp. 17–18). This violence is often carefully choreographed to be shared on social media. Think of the theatrical cruelty of ISIS member Mohammed

Emwazi's ('Jihadi John') decapitation of British Aid Worker Alan Henning. Similarly, the horrific mosque murders in Christchurch New Zealand in 2019 were 'livestreamed' by the neo-Nazi Brenton Harrison Tarrant as he moved around the mosque murdering worshippers (Evans, 2019). This dissemination on social media points to the centrality of the internet in the world of radicalisation today. Researchers investigating this have also noted the way radicalised people often gain huge satisfaction from the notoriety they gain (McDonald, 2018, pp. 149–172), becoming 'internet celebrities' in a macabre mirror to the way this happens in mainstream society. Faisal Devji has noted that acts of martyrdom on jihadist social media are presented less as 'religious events than part of a global culture of reality television' (Devji, 2005). So rather than being separate from the global media culture in which now all live, the violence of radicalisation is very much part of this.

3 **Hatred of democracy – hatred of women**: People who seek to radicalise others home in on the things that are missing in people's lives and people recruited have often suffered from mental illnesses, learning disabilities and other vulnerabilities. While this understanding is crucial to Social Work's safeguarding role, we also need to recognise that as well as seeing radicalisation as something which is *done to someone* that it also involves something *a person does* (Macdonald, 2018, p. 189), that is, through the conscious adoption of a set of political attitudes. For both neo-Nazis and Salafi-jihadists, nothing epitomises that which they see as debased and depraved about contemporary society more than the idea that women and LGBT people should be able to occupy an equal place in society. Many have argued that the Manchester Arena bomber, Salman Abedi, deliberately targeted the concert of a young female singer with a largely female fan base. Those he killed on 22 May 2017 were primarily women and girls, seen by Abedi as deserving of punishment for their 'immoral' lifestyles (Dhaliwal, 2019; Afzal, 2018). The bombing of the London gay pub *The Admiral Duncan* in 1999 by the Neo-Nazi David Copeland represents an identical phenomenon. The violent authoritarianism of these movements is rooted in what Kevin McDonald has called 'antidemocracy' (Macdonald, 2018, p. 47).

The Safeguarding Role in Radicalisation

Given the prevalence of these violent authoritarian movements and their success in recruiting people to carry out atrocities, many countries across the world have developed state-based prevention programmes to address this. The UK has developed such a programme, known as 'Prevent' (gov.uk, 6/3/2024) following the London bombings in 2003. In 2015, the Prevent policy became a legal duty for public sector institutions, thus drawing Social Work directly into its orbit. The UK's Prevent programmes has been contentious with some writers considering this to be a continuation of the human rights abuses undertaken as part of the 'War on Terror', discussed earlier. These programmes have also been criticised for the way they focus on Muslim communities, communities already marginalised by racism and poverty, and the writer Arun Kundnani has characterised the UK's Prevent programme as a form of state surveillance towards Muslim communities (Kundnani, 2014). Similarly, within Social Work, others have asked whether involvement with Prevent is 'securitising' Social Work interventions (McKendrick and Finch, 2017) and therefore undermining trust-based relationships with children and families. The Department for Education report *Safeguarding and* Radicalisation (2021) represented the first attempt to gather evidence on experiences of staff involved in this work, and while Social Workers reported that while they did encounter suspicion about Prevent amongst Muslim families, they felt they were largely able to be overcome this through explanations which addressed people's fears about the intention of the programme. It has also been found that while Muslim parents can be suspicious of Social Work involvement in this area, they were at the same time acutely aware of the dangers regarding their own children. One Social Worker noted that:

> A lot of the families cry out for help as well, you know, you could be sitting in there dealing with one matter and you will have built up a relationship with Mum and they might say, "Well actually, I'm worried about my child or young person". And it starts the dialogue.
>
> (Cowden, 2021, p. 6)

Patel has similarly noted that "many of the referrals to Prevent are made not by the authorities but by ordinary families, and who are concerned about the impact of radicalisation on their children" (Patel, 2019, p. 61). Other research in this area suggests Social Workers saw the work undertaken under the Prevent Duty as largely similar to other safeguarding work they undertook with Child Criminal Exploitation or Child Sexual Exploitation (Cowden, 2021). It is also that case now, the greatest number of referrals into the UK's Prevent programme concern people involved with the Extreme Right rather than violent Islamists. The case studies below illustrate examples of the way in which young people, often with particular vulnerabilities, are being recruited into violent authoritarian groups. In a safeguarding context, it is important that Social Workers understand both ideologies that people are being drawn into adopting, but also the life circumstances which can be leading them to adopt these ideas.

Case Study 1: Phillip

Phillip is a 15-year-old white British teenager who lives with his mother; he is the only child whose father has had little or no involvement with him. Phillip was diagnosed with autism as a child and though he is high functioning on the Autistic Spectrum, he has always been within the Special Needs education system as he has been unable to manage within mainstream education. He and his mother were recently forced to move after they were evicted from their previous house when she was made redundant from her job. They had lived in a vibrant multi-cultural area adjacent to a street market where a number of the stall holders got to know Phillip and often let him help on the stalls after school, a role that Phillip really loved. After being evicted they moved some distance away to where his mother was able to get further work, and ended up living on a quite isolated new housing estate on the edge of town where they do not know anyone. Phillip has felt angry and depressed since the move, and really misses the people he used to see and talk to at the market. As part of his Autistic Spectrum Condition, Phillip tends to hyper-focus, and has started to become obsessive about the idea that they were forced out of their previous home because 'Muslims' were taking over the area they previously lived in.

Geraldine, one of the teaching assistants in Phillip's class at his new school, has been trying to get know Phillip and has been concerned by how withdrawn and disengaged he has seemed in class. She was taken aback when after spending quite a lot of time with him in class, that he commented that he didn't have a problem with other races in general, just Muslims because they were not like 'us' and that they wanted to run Britain 'doing their Sharia law'. When she asked him what he meant by this, he explained they were taking over British cities, making white people leave, and that this was had happened to him and his mum. Geraldine, aware that the family had recently moved, tried to reassure Phillip saying he would soon find other friends and nice people in the new area and that this probably wasn't why they had had to move.

A few weeks later, Geraldine was again spending one-to-one time with Philip and again he told that white people had to prepare themselves for the time when Muslims would get them thrown out not just of the city where they had lived but also from the 'whole of England'. Embarrassed, Geraldine changed the subject and asked him how he was settling in. He told her he was now part of a group called the 'Young Patriots' on Facebook. Geraldine assumed the Young Patriots were a social group like the British Legion and was reassured. However, a week later, Geraldine saw Phillip in the school canteen at lunchtime and noticed that he was looking at pictures of hunting knives on his phone, though he put his phone away once he saw she was looking at him. Later that day, she looked up the Facebook page of the 'Young Patriots' and was shocked to realise they were a white supremacist group which used many of the same phrases Phillip was using about white people being 'forced out' of British cities by Muslims on their social media site.

Questions for Discussion

1 What are the factors in Philip's life that has made him vulnerable to recruitment by the Extreme Right?
2 It is significant that large numbers of people recruited to both far right groups through the internet are people with Autistic Spectrum Condition. What do you think the Extreme Right offers these people?
3 Geraldine has contacted the local Social Services department with concerns about Phillip. If you were to begin working with Phillip as a Social Worker, what would you be focussing on?

Case Study 2: Jade

Jade is a young woman who grew up on a council estate and had a troubled relationship with her parents. In her early teenage years, she was deemed 'beyond parental control' and entered the Local Authority care system following a pattern of behaviour where she repeatedly went missing from home for days on end, not attending school, as well as having multiple incidents of involvement with the police concerning possession and distribution of drugs. She became involved with a group of young people with similarly troubled family backgrounds, while being moved to a series of different foster placements, none of which had any success in engaging with her. A youth worker who worked her commented that the group of young people she spent all her time with became like 'her real family'. The focus for the group's activities was a gym where they all met. After about a year of her involvement with this group, one of the group's leading figures, a young man called Tariq with no previous interest in religion of any sort converted, or as he told them 'reverted', to Islam. This surprised everyone as it was strange to see a young man who had barely attended school lessons now practicing Qur'anic verses in Arabic. Jade was very drawn to the transgressive image associated with Tariq's new identity, and from previously wearing only jeans and crop tops, began wearing a hijab around town. Tariq subsequently invited her to 'learn more about Islam' and the two of them spent time together watching the YouTube videos of the ISIS ideologue Anwar-Al-Awlaki, who explained that any true and virtuous Muslim needed now to be prepared to actively join the jihad to 'defend Islamic lands'. The group's Islamic identity grew as others adopted Islamic dress, stopped taking and dealing drugs and began to discuss whether they would heed the call of Anwar Al-Awlaki to help their Muslim brothers and sisters in Syria. Jade was very much in favour of this though when it was pointed out that women could not join the mujahideen, she said that this didn't matter – she would go to Syria as a bride, where she could "settle down as a bride, living as a true Muslim".

Questions

1 What are the factors in Jade's life that has made her vulnerable to recruitment by jihadist groups?
2 Many people who are recruited to these groups are heavily influenced by what is happening in their friendship networks. Why do you think these can be important?
3 After hearing from another young person that Jade is planning to go to Syria to become a 'jihadi bride', her Youth Workers contacts Social Services to set out his concerns. If you were to begin working with her, what issues would you be focussing on?

Conclusion

This chapter has sought to offer a discussion of the issues thrown up in the period we are currently living through; a time in which social life is increasingly impacted by violent attacks on public space, demonstrations of hatred directed towards women, sexual minorities and migrants and refugees, as well as the growth of the right wing political parties which were once consigned to the political fringe but which are now in many places influential in government and forming state policy. These developments are fuelled by a widespread dissatisfaction with the status quo; what Wendy Brown has aptly called "the ruins of neoliberalism" (Brown, 2019). Disillusionment and distrust in politics and in public institutions is growing, largely as a consequence of the way rampant individualism and the logic of the marketplace have frayed the fabric of civil society and democratic life. These feelings are being targeted and mobilised ideologically to produce radicalisation. Research has demonstrated that Social Workers have the skills and understandings to steer vulnerable individuals away from the violence and hatred promoted by the authoritarian movements that we have discussed in this chapter (Cowden, 2021). Many governments across the world have initiated national prevention and deradicalisation programmes, and without wanting to deny the problems with these programmes, they have had a significant degree of success in tackling at situations where the agents of ideological violence are isolated 'lone wolves'. What we need to see much more of is governments developing policies concerned with reducing poverty and inequality and thus fostering a sense of commonality and the common good in society. While there are instances of this, we are also seeing the growth of right-wing anti-immigrant politics which is not simply located in the darker corners of the internet but is "interconnected with communities, non-violent agents and legal entities" (Ishchenko and Varga, 2021). In other words, we are now in a situation where many in government are prepared to encourage the blaming of minorities for declining living standards and underfunded public services rather than develop policies that address social-economic disparities and the grievance and alienation which fuels radicalisation. As Social Workers, we have a crucial contribution to make to these problems; this is not just in our safeguarding role which prevents people from being drawn into nihilistic violence and hatred, we also have a direct interest in rebuilding and safeguarding the principles of political democracy itself, principles on the which the profession of Social Work is itself based.

6 Empowerment

What Is Empowerment?

We have already noted the IFSW definition of Social Work as a profession which "promotes social change and development, social cohesion, and the empowerment and liberation of people" (IFSW, 2014). If, over the past few decades, many Social Work authors have written about empowerment, this was not the case before 1990 (Adams, 2008). Why then has this term taken centre stage not just in Social Work theory and practice, but in contemporary Social Policy and political rhetoric? What does our present preoccupation with the 'empowerment' tells us not just about the way Social Work is being framed and understood, but also about what is happening in society that gives this term such significance and cache?

When it comes to defining 'empowerment', there are a number of difficulties we immediately encounter. One is that the term carries such an aura of self-evident 'goodness' and positivity about it, it is often hard to question its use. But once we look beyond the assumption that empowerment is by definition a 'good thing', what we find is the fact that the term is used to mean very different things in different contexts. Ward and Mullender were amongst the first to note this when they argued in 1991 that

> empowerment has become the current bandwagon term in social work and is being used to justify what are, in fact, varying ideological and political positions...Broadly, empowerment is associated at one end of a continuum with the New Right's welfare consumerism, and at the other with the user movement which demands a voice in controlling standards and services themselves. One is the 'essential expression of individualism', the other rests on a collective voicing of universal need.
>
> (1991a, p. 21)

Ward and Mullender's argument is that the term is confusing, because it is being used to mean different things within different political rhetorics: it is about an idea of individual 'consumer choice' within a neoliberal social welfare discourse, but in the context of grass roots service user movements, it is about disempowered groups having a voice. Alison Zippay (1995), writing in a US context, has made the same observation. She notes that while historically "efforts to empower poor people have traditionally been associated with liberal reformers (...) in an ironic turn of events, conservative Republicans have been amongst the most vocal and enthusiastic proponents" of the concept of 'empowerment'. She notes that this apparent paradox makes sense once conservatives have re-positioned themselves as "advocates of minimal

DOI: 10.4324/9781003458715-9

government intervention in social problem solving", as they have from the 1980s onwards, since this allows them to "hail the encouragement of self-initiative and individual choice and applaud the concept of local autonomy" (Zippay, 1995, p. 263). In other words, ideas about self-help and community activism, while being historically associated with progressive and radical politics, have now been harnessed within the language of neoliberalism as part of an overall attempt to reduce the role of the state in areas of social provision.

Zippay notes that in this context, the concept of 'empowerment' appeals to contemporary policy makers and politicians as to them it represents people 'taking responsibility for their own lives', instead of 'looking to the state' to resolve those issues. However, as Zippay has noted, this represents a major shift from the terms historic roots where it referred to the idea of greater community participation to "enhance the democratic process", and ideas about "the empowerment of disenfranchised community residents as a radical force for the redistribution of resources" (1995, p. 264). These latter views are distinct from the individualised view of empowerment expressed within the language of neoliberalism in that for progressives, there is always a social dimension to problems of disempowerment (such as poverty, unemployment or domestic violence), rather than simply 'bad choices' or fecklessness. The radical view of empowerment is therefore also about making demands on the state, including demands for more democratic access to resources. Both of these arguments from Zippay and from Mullender and Ward imply that the success of the term 'empowerment' is that it is able to appeal to a wide range of positions across the political spectrum – almost everyone is in favour of it – but in reality, it is being used to mean entirely different things in practice; hence when it comes to looking at concrete strategies to implement 'empowerment', the consensus around what empowerment means breaks down.

A key example which was used in the UK and the USA was the sale of state or local government owned housing stock to the residents living of those estates. This was presented by conservatives in both countries as means towards making people more 'empowered'. What this meant was that instead of being so-called 'passive recipients' of state-owned and state-controlled services – in this cases, welfare houses – the residents would be given the opportunity to own them, and therefore, have a supposedly more direct interest in improving the quality of life in those areas, instead of 'looking to the government' to do this for them. However, this proposal for the sale of state-owned housing was opposed by those on the left for the reason that, while it may be beneficial for people who were able to purchase the properties, the long term impact of this policy would be to remove a significant quantity of housing which had previously been available for people on low incomes from the wider housing stock, making the poorest people more vulnerable in the housing market and leading to a major increase in homelessness. This reveals the different ways in which the term 'empowerment' was being used: in neoliberal discourse, the market is presented as empowering, while for the left, the market is seen as causing disempowerment, since state authorities which once accepted responsibility for reducing homelessness no longer have the resources available to do this. There is indeed considerable evidence that the sale of formerly state-owned housing as it occurred in the UK in the 1980s had exactly this impact on the housing market, and that the sale of this property, as well as creating a new class of owners-occupiers, also created another group who were excluded from the housing market altogether, creating a long-term increase in homelessness. The Australian researcher Alan Kohler has noted the extent to which these problems of housing shortage, homelessness and people who are unable to obtain access to the housing which they and their families need are profoundly connected to the insistence on market-based models of housing provision (Kohler, 2024).

If we stay with this concrete example for a moment, we could ask what this means in terms of how we might define 'empowerment'. Robert Adams defines empowerment as "the means by which individuals, groups and/or communities become able to take control of their circumstances and achieve their own goals, thereby being able to work towards helping themselves and others to maximise the quality of their lives" (2003, p. 8). While this sounds on the face of it a progressive and democratic definition, the problem is that it could be argued that the policy of selling off council houses is entirely consistent with this definition; in other words those people who were fortunate enough to be able to have benefited from this initiative have been 'empowered'. However, what falls out of view, if we look at the situation simply in terms of this definition, is the wider more general picture of housing and homelessness. This illustrates a point made by Mary Langan regarding the use of term 'empowerment', which is that it implies "an individualistic conception of power, which, by reducing social relationships to the interpersonal, obscures the real power relations in society" (1998, p. 114). Adams defines 'empowerment' as individuals, groups and communities taking action taking action to improve the 'quality of their lives'. But to address Langan's point, one of the problems with this definition is that is directs our focus to the group which is the beneficiary of a particular area of state policy, and in doing so obscures the reason why this policy has been adopted by the state, not to mention the implications that this has for other groups. If we look at the picture of homelessness across the world, we can see the way, as Kohler (2024) has argued, there are significant sections of the population who are locked out of the private housing market. This raises an important question about the meaning of empowerment, since if it is defined in terms of the benefit to a particular group or community, what does it mean if their empowerment is secured in a way that is to the detriment of another group or community?

- **What Is Empowerment?**
- **Think about the following situation and the ways in which it manifests 'empowerment'. In doing this exercise, read only Part 1 first and consider the questions posed. Once you have done this, then look at Part 2 and consider those questions.**

Part 1: JANE'S STORY: Jane lives with her family in a small village in a rural area south of Birmingham. She is informed by her local Residents Association that there is a likelihood of attempts to erect buildings for which the planning permission has not been granted on an area of Green Belt land near her house. She feels concerned about this and is determined to stop it, and hence gives her details to the Association to inform her of any activities they are organising in opposition to this. One morning, Jane is telephoned by activists from the Residents Association telling her that builders have arrived on the site and would she be willing to join people from the village who are organising a blockade of the site. Jane drops what she is doing and joins the resident's protest. When the Builders show the demonstrators documentation that proves the organisation behind attempt to build on this land does actually own it, the leaders of the Residents Association respond by asserting that the owners do not have planning permission. Some of the builders turn back, but others try to continue working until residents block the Access roads around the site, until the demonstrators are removed by police. The Residents Association vows that the fight against the builders and the group behind them will go on even if it means facing arrest by the police.

1 Does an incident like this demonstrate an empowered group of residents? How is this empowerment being manifest? What kind of motivation do you imagine these residents had in acting in the way they did?

Part 2: ANNA'S STORY: Anna is part of large family of Gypsy Roma Travellers. She was born in Yorkshire but for some time she and her extended family have been travelling in an area south of Birmingham. Anna has five children all of school age. For some time she has been trying to get them into various schools, but this has been hampered by the lack of a permanent residence, and bullying at a number of schools at which her children have attended. One of her sons also has asthma which is at times severe, and Anna would like him to be able to see the same doctor over a period of time instead of always visiting different Accident and Emergency departments when he has a severe attack. A group of the men in her family have been trying to acquire some land as a solution to the problem of always getting moved on by the police and hostile residents. However, the problem is that whenever they buy land and seek planning permission for building they find this is always denied once it is clear that the owners of the land are Gypsy Travellers. In frustration, the group of travellers has simply decided that if planning permission is denied, they will go ahead and build without it. Hence a piece of land is purchased outside a small village, and planning permission is sought. Not surprisingly this is rejected; however, the group goes ahead and engages a building company to begin work as planned. On the morning the builders are due to begin work the group's caravans are parked next to the site, but the builders are prevented from beginning work they are stopped by local residents blockading the site, carrying banners saying 'Keep off our Green Belt' and 'Stop the Invasion'.

- **Has your understanding of the situation changed at all having read Anna's story? What attitude might you take to the situation now?**
- **What might such a situation tell us about the meaning of the term empowerment?**

The Empowered Citizen/Consumer

Both Ward and Mullender and Zippay have pointed to the significance of the 1980s as a period where the term 'empowerment' was mobilised with very different meanings within different political discourses. This can be linked to the insights of Gail Lewis, who has argued that the 1980s was a turbulent period in which the welfare state was being criticised both from 'below' – from user groups, grass roots campaigns and social movements like feminism and anti-racism, as well as from 'above' – from governments with a 'New Right' agenda for reducing the role of the state in social provision (Lewis, 1998). Both of these political groupings were talking about 'empowerment', but with very different meanings and implications. These issues were resolved through the dominance of the consolidation of a neoliberal agenda concerning the reduction of the role of the state.

In the context of neoliberal social policy, the concept of 'empowerment' has not only become central but has been linked to ideas about 'citizenship'; defining the roles and responsibilities of citizens. The emphasis on the market, consumer choice and reduced role for the state in social care provision are now experienced as permanent features of the welfare landscape. John Clarke argues that this ideological reconstruction of welfare has in effect 'de-collectivised' service users from being seen as citizens with entitlements, as they were understood under the Welfare state, to individuals seeking choice in service provision. In this context, 'empowerment' has become part of the rhetoric of 'choice', and he notes the way that:

> The imagery of choice both condenses and articulates a variety of desires for public service change and improvement – not all of which are about individualised consumerism. But choice links them as though they could be met through the singular means of empowering citizen- consumers to make choices.
>
> (2005, p. 450)

Clarke is making the point here that people's desire for good public services which genuinely respond to their needs has become reconstructed as simply about the need for 'choice' in public services, and in this framework, to be 'empowered' comes to be defined as the capacity to act effectively within a market of consumer choices. The ideal of the citizen has thus become one who seeks to be an "independent agent, rather than a dependant subject" (2005, p. 450), who wants to 'decide for themselves' rather than expecting the government to provide for them. While this rhetoric of 'community empowerment' sounds on the face of it progressive and democratic, the notion of the 'good citizenship' on which it is based implies a norm in which experiences of dependence come to be viewed in highly negative terms. This ideal of the 'empowered citizen', as Cowden and Singh have noted, often bears little relationship to the actual circumstances in which people come into contact with social welfare services; who is it who will:

> (...) represent the interests of those significant proportions of the population that are denied the status of citizen, such as asylum seekers or individuals with severe mental health difficulties? [With the State] having conceptualised its role as the facilitator and empowerer of essentially privatised communities, what happens when people in those communities fail to demonstrate "appropriate" understandings of their role?.
>
> (2007, p. 13)

The point here is that this new conception of the 'empowered citizen' makes particular assumptions about individual capacities, wants and needs which often acts to obscure the reality of new forms of exclusion and social division which are taking root as a consequence of neoliberalism. Clarke develops this point when he argues that within our current economic and political situation there are broadly three different categories of citizens, whom he characterises as:

2 The law abiding and hardworking majority, who are named, incentivised and rewarded. They are offered forms of choice and 'voice', provided this choice is exercised 'responsibly'.

3 Those who would like to be in the above category but are struggling to manage this. For these people what the state offers is 'a hand-up, not a hand-out' – that is there are government sponsored interventions which seek to address their attitudes, character and motivation in areas in which they are seen as lacking.
4 Finally there are those who are perceived as actively refusing to enter the world of the hard working and law-abiding. These people become "objects of intensified surveillance, criminalisation and incarceration in the drive to extend civility, reduce anti-socialness and enhance community safety" (Clarke, 2005, pp. 457–458).

Clarke's work suggests that our contemporary world of Social Work and social care in a post-welfare state situation is one where the Victorian distinction between the deserving and undeserving poor has returned with a vengeance. His argument about the way different groups of citizens are classified and addressed differentially by the state is one that has also been discussed by the social policy analyst Bill Jordan. Jordan's work is distinctive for the way he has sought to understand the power and significance of ideas about deserving and undeserving within the history of Social Work and social welfare. He argues that under these conditions where the gains of the post-war welfare state have been so substantially eroded, a new version of what it means to be a 'good citizen' has emerged accordingly:

> In relation to mainstream citizens, the government is trying to nurture and develop certain psychological characteristics – motivation, self-esteem, confidence, entrepreneurship and self- development...to promote a self-improving form of citizenship [which] works on each individual to get them to have the right attitudes toward themselves, and to make the most of every opportunity that comes their way (...) Self-improvement, through work and in our private lives, becomes a requirement of citizenship.
>
> (Jordan, 2004, p. 9)

Jordan notes that these expectations are manifest through things such as education, where we are expected to get the most for our children, through health services, where we are expected to do all we can to maximise our own and our families' physical and mental health, and as workers, where we are expected to make ourselves as employable and flexible as possible. Following Michel Foucault, whose work was discussed in the previous chapter, Jordan calls this new approach to citizenship a 'project of the self'. This means that a sense of duty to fulfil these obligations is instilled 'internally', thus creating a situation where people aspire to live their lives according to these principles. Barbara Cruikshank argues that this process has become a key aspect of our present mode of being governed, which now concerns:

> (...) securing the voluntary compliance of citizens...Technologies of citizenship do not cancel out the autonomy and independence of citizens, but are modes of governance that work upon and through the capacities of citizens to act on their own. Technologies of citizenship are voluntary and coercive at the same time; the actions of citizens are regulated, but only after the capacity to act as a certain kind of citizen with certain aims is instilled.
>
> (1999, p. 4)

The people in Clarke's first category above are people who are seen to be the 'right kind' of citizens, and hence are encouraged in this. This means that for the people in the latter two categories come to be understood not as people suffering particular sorts of structural in equalities, but as problematic individuals who require who need to be "motivated and instructed in how to get their projects of the self started" (2004, p. 9). This latter point has major significance for Social Work since it works almost entirely with those sections of the community seen as least capable of acting in accordance with these norms of citizenship. In this respect, Jordan notes that there is an irony about Social Work's current rhetoric about empowerment and inclusion, since:

> (…) in local authorities and other statutory agencies it is charged with motivating and cajoling these service users toward projects of the autonomy and self-development, while controlling those deviant and self-destructive aspects of resistance strategies (crime, drugs, benefit fraud, self harm, mental illness).
>
> (2004, p. 10)

Is Empowerment 'Good for You'?

This interrogation of the term empowerment leads us to further question – is it meant to be something that you do for yourself, out of your own choice, or it is something that is done to you of for because someone else has decided that it is in your best interests? In other words, has come to be seen as such a good thing, that if you don't have it, it needs not just to be offered to you, but could be imposed on you? This situation may seem paradoxical, but it emerges out of the way in which 'being empowered' has come to be positioned as an imperative of good citizenship in the landscape of contemporary health and social welfare interventions. Karen Baistow has argued that in the current period:

> Taking control of one's life, or particular aspects of it, is not only seen as being intimately connected with the formation or reformation of the self as empowered, it is increasingly becoming an ethical obligation of the new citizenry. Not being in control of your everyday living arrangements, your time, your diet, your body, your health, your children, suggests there is something seriously wrong with you ethical constitution. Empowerment is not only good for you, it seems to be becoming essential to leading a better life.
>
> (1994, p. 37)

Baistow notes that this sense of empowerment as an 'ethical obligation' changes the way it is seen from an idea of empowerment as something which is good when people choose it for themselves, to the idea that if you do not choose it, this is because there is something wrong with you – we all 'need to be' empowered, and indeed if you don't want to be, then there must be some kind of flaw in your attitude or personality. It follows from this that if you are unwilling act in a more empowered manner by yourself, then you may need to be 'empowered' by someone else:

> My current reading of empowerment discourses indicates that (…) empowerment is something that is done to you by others, or that you do to others who thus become empowered by your actions not their own. Those who do the empowering are increasingly likely to be health and welfare professionals: social workers, health visitors, nurses, community clinical psychologists, psychotherapists etc. and

> managers in a variety of organisational settings. Those to whom empowerment is done are most likely to be users/clients/patients or employees. These are candidates for empowerment because in professional estimations they need it doing to them.
>
> (1994, p. 37)

In other words, those who experience poverty, depression, poor housing or dysfunctional relationships are now seen to have a primary responsibility as individuals to empower themselves and solve what are now seen as problems related to the choices they have made, rather than structural features of the economy. This illustrates the shift in the definition of empowerment within the neoliberal policy universe: empowerment has come to be about creating an ideal of citizenship where the citizen is an "independent agent, rather than a dependant subject" (Clarke, 2005, p. 450). Yet there is at the same time something deeply paradoxical about the way that it is professional assessments which designate who firstly who needs to be empowered as well as the means by which this is be realised:

> (…) far from being left roleless, or less powerful, by the process of user empowerment, professionals are increasingly being seen as central to it in a number of ways… [which] confirm the mutual dependence of the of the professional and empowerment; firstly [through] the detection of suitable candidates in need of empowerment and secondly, the empowerment of them.
>
> (1994, p. 39)

Baistow concludes her analysis by noting the "confusing and confused irony" of the fact that "deciding who is to be empowered" is itself one of the most significant "signs of power" (1994, p. 41).

The new discourse of 'empowerment' can therefore be thought of as one which adopts the mantle of being progressive and democratic, but which essentially makes sense in the context of the state seeking to divest itself of historic responsibilities for redressing social problems. As previously noted, this way of thinking about empowerment implies a particular version of citizenship – that of the hard working and law abiding – which is seen as that which needs to be adopted, or at the very least aspired to, by people living in situations of material deprivation. But what this ignores is the different realities people experience; not just at the level of income, but also experiences of education, the kinds of ways in which people encounter the power the state and how they experience that. Hence, professionally defined empowerment strategies, which Jordan entirely realistically characterises as "motivating and cajoling" service users against their deviant and self-destructive behaviour (2004, p. 10), are often unsuccessful. This is because this individualised conception of empowerment fails to grasp the way those problems, while manifested at the individual level, are socially produced. In the lives of people for whom 'begging, borrowing and stealing' are strategies for survival, it is the grinding reality of poverty which defines assumptions about what is possible. And what is particularly insidious is the way when those strategies are seen to fail, it comes to be seen that it is those people themselves who are the failures, rather than our understanding of the issues.

The Khan Family

In the context of work in your Children and Families Team, you are referred to the case of Mrs Khan. Mrs Khan is 38 years old and originally from Pakistan. She lives with her husband, aged 54, who was born in the UK. The couple are married and have five children, aged 1, 4, 5, 8 and 11. Up until two years ago the family was getting along reasonably; however, a number of simultaneous difficulties have caused considerable problems for them. Mr Khan has worked for the last 15 years as a forklift driver in a factory not too far from where they lived. Two years ago he sustained an injury to his hand and arm which means he is no longer able to drive a vehicle or carry out manual work involving the use of both hands, such as lifting. Though the injury was caused through an accident at work he has been unsuccessful in obtaining compensation and has had to go onto Jobseekers Allowance (JSA). Though there have been some jobs he could have done, the money he could have obtained for this work was less than the benefits he currently has, and therefore he has not seen any point in accepting them. One of Mr Khan's brothers has a shop and has offered some work to him. This does not bring in much money, but because he does not declare these earnings, he is able to use this to supplement his JSA. Mr Khan is extremely frustrated by his difficulty in finding work and as a result of his boredom and discontent he has begun spending many of his evenings at a local club where cheap alcohol is on sale and where many of his friends go.

Mrs Khan speaks little English and since she came to the UK she has spent most of her life looking after her children. Her caring responsibilities have increased in the last year since her mother was diagnosed with Alzheimer's disease; something which has caused considerable distress to her and her family. Whenever her father needed help he would telephone Mrs Khan in a state of considerable alarm, and she would feel it was expected of her to drop what she was doing and immediately offer support to her mother. The Khan family came to attention of Social Services as neighbours noted that the oldest child, the 11-year-old Harbinder, was regularly looking after the younger four children while Mrs Khan was round at her parent's house, dealing with her mother, and Mr Khan was either working at his brother's shop or out at the club with his friends.

Questions:

1 **You have been given the case of the Khan family to work with regarding concerns around neglect. When this piece of work is allocated to you as a Social Worker, your team leader informs you that a Duty Social Worker who made an initial visit to the family describes Mrs Khan as 'very disempowered'. In terms of thinking about how you understand the issues here, how useful is 'empowerment' as a way of understanding and working with the difficulties she faces?**

2 **Looking at the issues she faces and the resources available to her, would you say that the strategies she has adopted for dealing with the demands on her are a realistic response the situation she finds herself in, or an expression of her 'disempowerment'? Why?**

Empowerment and Power Relations

While strategies based on this understanding of empowerment can sound attractive, we need to be aware of the dangers in seeing this simplistically as the panacea for social problems. Firstly, it can easily slide into the blaming of those seen not to want to be 'empowered'; that their rejection, either actively or passively of professional interventions, leads to the conclusion that there is nothing more than they are capable of. In this way, the individualised means of conceptualising the term can end up reconstructing the distinction between deserving and undeserving service users – this is empowerment as a discourse of 'regulation'. Secondly, by focussing exclusively on individual behaviour, we fail to grasp the significance of the way individual difficulties are socially produced. Under conditions of neoliberalism, as we have discussed in this chapter, the economy has changed such that a significant section the population is either excluded altogether from the labour market, or has only a tenuous relationship with the world of work – low wages, hugely reduced levels of job security. At the same time, these people's experience of seeking state benefits is that they are both inadequate and punitive – and it is through processes like this that classes of disempowered people are 'systemically' created. In order to understand the problematic aspects in the behaviour of these people which bring them to the attention of professionals, we need to be able to ask the more fundamental question about what it is that leads people to act in ways that are violent, destructive or anti-social. The social theorist Slavoj Zizek addresses these issues in an interesting way in his book *Violence* (2009). In his investigation of this as a social phenomenon, Zizek argues that while we focus primarily on what he calls immediate 'subjective' violence – the violence that has a clear and obvious perpetrator – what we fail to see is the 'objective' violence – the violence which is "inherent to the 'normal' state of things" – which forms the backdrop to the former, but is rendered invisible by its very 'normality' (2009, pp. 1–2). The challenge is to be able to understand the relationship between the two, and this brings us back to this question about the 'two souls of Social Work' discussed in Chapter 1. Do we understand people's problems as caused by the way they have 'failed to adapt' to the world in which we live, or are we able to locate the immediate problems in the wider context of the impersonal 'systemic' exclusion which defines so many lives? What do these different understandings mean in practice?

A key issue in all of this is putting a critical understanding of power back into the equation. In the previous chapter, we discussed the problem with seeing power only as a 'generalised capacity to act' is that this takes our attention away from the underlying assumptions about who feels they are or are not entitled to act; as it is these which define the everyday and 'normal' operations of power. The individualised empowerment discourse which we have been questioning in this chapter not only obscures these wider questions but also makes the mistake of understanding power as a possession, which can be passed from one person to another. We consider the idea that you can make someone empowered is confused. In this sense, it is crucial that we adopt a critical approach to the use of terms of like 'empowerment', which cannot be properly understood without first thinking about power and the nature of disempowerment as they are experienced in people's lives.

The Case of David Fairbairn

David is a young man of 15 years old who has been referred to you for a Court Report for his criminal behaviour. He is also likely to be excluded from school for repeated incident of violent behaviour. David is part of a gang of boys his age which has been involved in a number of robberies of Kebab shops in the area of

Birmingham where he lives. It has also been alleged that David has used a knife to threaten other boys at school to obtain mobile phones and leather jackets. David is white, but all the other boys in the gang are from black African-Caribbean backgrounds, and this is something which is commented on in the case notes you read before meeting him.

When you meet David you are struck by how friendly and charming he is. With little encouragement from you, he recounts his activities with the gang with great pride, and you are intrigued by the way David he tells you how he has rejected the idea that he as a white boy should not be associating with black gang members – he is proud to be allowed into that world. David boasts to you that there are many criminal activities he is involved with that he has not been convicted for – particular theft of car stereos. He tells you that he only steals these from particular kinds of 'posh cars' and says that the people who lose them will 'get the money on insurance anyway'. He claims that he can get into a car and get the stereo out in less than 30 seconds, faster than anyone else in his gang and has the nickname 'Lightning' in his gang for precisely that reason.

In attempting to write your court report you feel a strange mixture of feelings towards David. On the one hand you are appalled by the violence involved in his gang's attacks on the kebab shops and other pupils; on the other you cannot help but feel admiration for him. Further conversations reveal his family situation. He has no contact with his father and his mother has raised him on her own. His mother is currently studying Accountancy to try to improve her circumstances and spends much of the time studying, often leaving David and his sister to manage on their own with little food or money in their flat. You cannot help but note that she has more or less left him to care for his younger sister, aged ten, and you are impressed by how caring and protective he is towards her.

Questions:

1. **Discuss your overall response to this young man and his situation.**
2. **As Social Workers encountering people like David we often feel trapped between an idea of 'individual responsibility' and an idea of seeing someone's behaviour relative to the world or circumstances they are in. What are the arguments in favour of the 'individual responsibility' argument versus the 'relative circumstances' approaches? Which of these approaches do you feel is the most sound 'ethically'?**
3. **Might there be another way of working with a young person like David? What might an empowering intervention with him look like?**

In this chapter, we have argued that while the concept of empowerment has continues to be important in Social Work today, the predominance of neoliberal policy assumptions has shifted the meaning of the term. If that use of the term did represent an appropriation of an earlier usage, this raises the question of whether the term can be reclaimed more in line with its original usage for Social Work today. We want to conclude this chapter by thinking about this issue specifically in relation to case study above. One point noted earlier is the confusion involved in thinking of power as an object which can be passed from one person to another. We have argued that power is a relationship – and Patricia Hill Collins expresses this in an interesting way when she talks of power as "an intangible entity that circulates within a particular matrix of power relations and to which individuals stand in varying relationships" (2000, p. 274). The operation and experience of power in service user's lives is often quite complex and it is important for Social Workers to be able to recognise this. In his book *Challenging Oppression: A Critical Social Work Approach* (2002), Bob Mullaly argues that "although there may be distinct categories of oppression, there is no oppression that creates a distinct group of oppressed people who are unaffected, one way or another, by other forms of oppression" (2002, p. 151). Power and oppression are only rarely about groups of oppressors and groups of victims confronting each other – it is more useful to think about the way power circulates not just between individuals and groups but also within a particular person, so an individual can be simultaneously an oppressor and a victim.

The second key point we would make is that though power circulates it is also located. What this means is that it is exercised as well as resisted in specific contexts – in families, in workplaces, in schools, in social settings. Empowerment therefore needs to be about the way individuals and groups situate and re-situate themselves in relation to specific located power relations. As Collins notes: "As people push against, step away from, and shift the terms of their involvement in power relations, the shape of those relations changes for everyone" (Collins, 2000, p. 275). What is crucial about this conception of empowerment is that people's capacity for self-realisation does not exist in a vacuum, but needs to be understood within the particular social relations and networks of relationships in which individuals find themselves. Empowerment in this sense can involve questioning and challenging the assumptions made by other people, and the assumptions of social institutions in the way they interact with people.

The Brazilian educationalist Paulo Freire has offered some insightful ways of thinking about these issues in Social Work (See Cowden et al., 2020 for a recent discussion of these in relation to Social Work). The Brazilian educationalist Paulo Freire has offered some insightful ways of thinking about these issues in Social Work. Freire is one of the most influential educational thinkers of the late twentieth century and he advocated a conception of education based on dialogue between student and teacher. He argued that this changed the dynamic of education offering the potentiality for the oppressed to regain their humanity and overcome their condition of inferiority. His most famous work, *Pedagogy of the Oppressed* (1972), argues for a system of education that emphasises learning as a practice of freedom. Freire began this book by characterising the disempowerment many people experience as based in what he called a 'double consciousness', and this is expressed by the way people are

> at the same time themselves and the oppressor whose image they have internalized. Accordingly, until they concretely 'discover' themselves and in turn to their own consciousness, they nearly always express fatalistic attitudes toward their situation.
>
> (Freire, 1972, p. 61)

Freire saw this of 'fatalism' as a consequence of people having internalised the dominant logic, and because the dominant logic dominates people's thinking and their perception of what is possible, it is very difficult for change to occur unless people have some space where they can critically reflect on how things could be different. Without this space, it is very difficult to even accept that there are other ways of doing and being. At the micro level, people become locked into the perceptions and expectations or other people, while at the macro level, it is endlessly repeated that there is 'no alternative' to the rule of the market over all aspects of social and economic life. In such a context, it is really so surprising that people's responses reflect this fatalism towards their wider situation?

Freire went on to define empowerment as the "the deepening and widening of the horizon of democratic practice" (Freire, 1990). We want to conclude this chapter by thinking about the implications of this understanding in relation to the case study above. A key implication of this 'deepening and widening' is the idea of Social Workers being able to see the humanity within a service user, even if this humanity is not reflected in all of their actions. David Fairbairn embodies the contradictions of an individual who on the one hand demonstrates considerable insight, understanding and empathy, but who on the other appears to be able to switch this off and engage in acts of random cruelty and violence. His current situation is that he is on the path towards a career in the Criminal Justice System, which will reinforce, at both a subjective and objective level, that he has nothing useful to contribute to society. He comes to us not out of choice, but out of a lack of alternatives. We would suggest that a starting point for work is recognition of the real relations of power which shape the relationship between ourselves as professionals and him as the service user. A key concept in Freire's definition above is the idea of 'democratic practice', implying not just recognition of his humanity but also that he is a citizen with political rights and the capacity for meaningful participation. However, this latter point would be meaningless to him in the absence of a space in which he can develop a wider understanding of his situation. In this sense, he needs to be politicised – based on an awareness of both the way the cards are stacked against people like him but also of the destructive and abusive nature of his own criminal behaviour – as part of a process of developing moral agency. The role of the Social Worker could be to initiate a dialogue which is based on uncovering or 'naming' the operations of power in his life, including the Social Work role itself, and in doing so creating a space where he can think about the significance of the way he uses and abuses power himself.

One possible objection to this course of action might be that it is 'patronising' to work with David in this way; he knows his world and how to survive in it, what do you know about that? In an attempt to develop Freire's insights on empowerment, McClaren and De Silva make the point that:

> A major consideration for the development of contextual critical knowledge is affirming the experiences of [service users] to the extent that their voices are acknowledged as an important part of the dialogue; but affirming [these] voices does not necessarily mean that [Social Workers] should take the meaning that [service users] give to their experiences at face value, as if experience speaks romantically or even tragically for itself. The task of the critical educator is to provide the conditions for the individual to reflect upon and shape their own experiences and in certain instances transform those experiences in the interest of a larger project of social responsibility.
>
> (McLaren and Da Silva, 1993, p. 49)

This quote is important for the way it emphasises the importance of a critical understanding of power and disempowerment as the basis for thinking about empowerment. Social Workers hold power over Service Users, yet that power can be used in positive ways. As practitioners, we may not understand everything about the worlds someone like David lives in, but one of the things we may be able to offer is a way of thinking about the wider social political and economic relationships which frame the choices he has. The social theorist Cornell West argued the purpose of this critical perspective is that it creates a space which "allows suffering to speak. That is, it creates a vision of the world that puts into the limelight the social misery that is usually hidden or concealed by the dominant viewpoint of society" (West, 2000, p. 551). A dialogue between the Social Worker and David could begin to address the unhappiness in his situation, as well as an understanding of what being in his gang offers him in terms of a positive form of self-identity. At the same time, David's activities within the gang are based on treating his victims in a cruel and dehumanised way. It is this ethical contradiction that offers the Social Worker a way of talking about what is wrong with his gang activities which does not simply involve seeking to 'motivate and cajole' David towards a more respectable existence, an existence he has rejected just as it this has rejected him. This form of dialogic Social Work both respects and interpolates his capacity to make ethical choices, at the same time as developing his wider awareness of his own situation, and in that process, creating the possibility of other ways of being. The course of action proposed above may not have a guaranteed outcome – what interventions in Social Work do? In this sense, it involves a risk, but not just the risk that it may be unsuccessful. It also opens up the risk that the Social Worker's position becomes open to interrogation from the outside, from the service user. To take this risk requires us to have confidence not just in our skills and abilities, but in the authenticity of our own critical understanding, and it is perhaps this which is the most important element in any discussion of empowerment.

Part Three

Ethical Perspectives for Social Work

7 Decolonial Ethics

In many parts of the word, we are witnessing a growing interest in understanding Indigenous realities, and an increased awareness of the many adversities faced by Indigenous people and communities. However, engaging with Indigenous communities requires not only a good understanding of the historical context and present-day realities of these communities but also a change in approach in order to avoid repeating the oppressions that came with colonialism. In this chapter, we examine how non-Indigenous Social Workers can meaningfully and ethically practice with Indigenous people and communities by challenging some of the unequal power relationships that contribute to maintaining oppression.

Situating the Context

Today, we can still observe the very negative and long-lasting consequences of colonisation. These include lateral and interpersonal experiences of violence that plague many communities, lack of access to clean drinking water in many places and the over-representation of Indigenous children in child protection services, to name only a few. Many of the adversities faced by Indigenous communities can be directly traced back to the implementation of colonial policies. As we will see in this chapter, these policies have resulted in many difficulties are still faced today by Indigenous people, such as family separation, forced adoption and sterilisation, intergenerational trauma and violence. Social workers who work with Indigenous people and communities therefore have to be cognisant of this history of colonialism and acknowledge the impact it had, and continues to have, on Indigenous people, as well as being aware of their colonial standpoint and how it can impact the work they undertake.

The chapter begins by briefly presenting Indigenous worldviews. We will also examine some of Canada's colonial history, its impact on Indigenous populations and the more recent ideas of reconciliation and decolonisation. As such, because Indigenous cultures and histories are diverse, Social Worker should take time to understanding the specifics of the community or Nations they will work with.

Next, the chapter will examine how a value such as justice can mean something different for Indigenous and non-Indigenous people, and how non-Indigenous perspectives currently dominate contemporary society, debates and policies, leading to experiences of epistemic injustice by Indigenous people. Drawing from a case study of a Social Worker working in education, the chapter examines how a policy to reduce Indigenous student attrition in a higher education institution can be developed in a more ethical manner. The chapter will conclude by a discussion on ethical practice based on a decolonial standpoint as one that centres the importance of Indigenous people's full participation and on redistribution of power.

DOI: 10.4324/9781003458715-11

Indigenous Worldviews

While there are many ways to present Indigenous worldviews, and while they can differ from one community to the next, they are often characterised by the idea of the circle and the interconnection between all the elements that surround us, as well as the respect, reciprocity, responsibility and relationships between them all (Kirkness and Barnhardt, 1991). In Indigenous worldviews, no element – water, animals, humans, insects, plants or the cosmos – has power over another. Instead, all elements making up the world are said to thrive because they are interconnected and because they engage with and take care of one another. Teachings like those are passed on from generation to generation through oral traditions in the forms of stories, myths and legends. For many Indigenous communities, these constitute the basic knowledge from which they understand the world around them and the relationship that they cultivate with it. Drawing from the Anishinaabe tradition, Borrows (2019) explains how oral traditions and stories are used to transmitted values. Citing Basil Johnston's book *The Gift of the Stars*,[1] he writes,

The importance of oral tradition and informal knowledge transmission

Many Indigenous communities around the world have kept their knowledge and traditional cultures alive through what we call the oral tradition.

Values are often passed down through myths and legends, and knowledge and skills are conveyed through living practices and day-to-day activities. All these important teachings are also kept alive through Indigenous languages and cultural practices, which still today are very important to many Indigenous communities.

> [Through stories] Our ancestors intended to prepare the minds of their children to look for and see relationships between plants, weathers [*sic*], seasons, insects, birds, animals, and fish and to make stories out of what they had perceived; to animate their spirits to reach out to the spirits of the dead and those of the upper world; to inspire their hearts to espouse compassion, selfishness, courage, love, respect, honesty, tenacity, and all their kindred attributes; and their inner senses to perceive things beyond the reach of their physical senses.
>
> (Johnston, 2013 cited in Borrow, 2019, p. 5)

This is also true for other nations, such as the Huron-Wendat Nation. In the preface of *La Femme Venue du Ciel, Mythe Wendat de la* Création, Sioui-Picard (2016) explains, "The Wendat creation myth is at the heart of the Wendat philosophy. The story of Aataentsik and her descent is certainly one of our most important myths. This story helps us understand our place in Creation" (p. 5).[2] Myths such as that of Aataentsik are essential to many Indigenous communities to transmit important oral history and values and to explain their worldviews.

Some Indigenous nations in North America, such as the Algonquin and Cree Nations, sometimes use symbols such as the medicine wheel to explain their worldviews. While the meaning and understanding of the medicine wheel may vary between nations, they can provide insight into some principles of Indigenous worldviews, including the notion of circular thinking (Mashford-Pringle and Shawanda, 2023). The medicine wheel is often illustrated in the form of a circle with four quadrants, in which each of the quadrants represents different dimensions that form a whole. These quadrants can cover many dimensions and their interconnections, such as health (mental, physical, spiritual and emotional health), the stages of life (infant, child, adult, elder) and the elements of nature (fire, air, water and earth), among other things.

For many Indigenous people and Nations, worldviews present values that continue to be important today. They shape the way Indigenous people understand and organise their society, and this is also true for Indigenous communities for whom parts of their culture and language have been decimated by colonisation. As Mohawk author Taiaiake Alfred explains:

> Knowing the history of European colonialism in North America demands recognition of the damage that has been done to the vitality of our traditional cultures. But we must also honour the fact that indigenous peoples have survived: the frameworks of their value systems remain intact and vital. Indigenous governance systems embody distinctive political values, radically different from those of the mainstream. Western notions of dominion (human and natural) are noticeably absent; in their place we find harmony, autonomy, and respect. We have a responsibility to recover, understand, and preserve these values, not only because they represent a unique contribution to the history of ideas, but because renewal of respect for traditional values is the only lasting solution to the political, economic, and social problems that beset our people. To bring those roots to new fruition, we must reinvigorate the principles embedded in the ancient teachings, and use them to address our contemporary problems.
>
> (Alfred, 2009, p. 29)

It is therefore of upmost importance for Indigenous communities to revive and preserve their ways of knowing, their culture and, closely link to this, their language. If so many Indigenous communities today struggle to revive or preserve their culture, it is because of the deep history of colonialism.

Colonialism and Its Impacts on Indigenous Communities

From the 1400s to early 1990, many European nations set sail from the continent to discover the New World. While this chapter draws specifically on Canadian history, colonisation happened much more broadly. For example, England sent many settlers to North America, Asia, Oceania and Africa; the Netherlands sent colonists to Southern Africa, Indonesia and beyond; France sent settlers to North America, the Caribbean, Africa and Indonesia; and Spain and Portugal sent settlers to South and North America.

Motivated by the Doctrine of Discovery and Terra Nullius, many European people settled into newly 'discovered' lands, despite the already strong presence of Indigenous communities living on the land. While each part of the world has its own specific context and history, this period in time marked the beginning of colonisation for many Indigenous populations at the time.

Colonisation is characterised by domination of a group over another. It is defined as

> a project of territorial expansion by powerful states that typically involves resettlement into the newly claimed lands of the colonizing state's people and the displacement, if not eradication, of the people who had previously lived there. It is not the only basis of justice claims made by and to states, but colonial displacement and eradication remain a very real source of lingering sentiments of injustice.
>
> (Nicholls, 2011, p. 161)

In addition to settling on a land, a colonisation process will generally involve the colonisers imposing ways of life by passing new laws and regulations, such as the Indian Act *(1876)* in Canada. The Indian Act, which has been amended several times but is still in place at the time of writing this chapter, defines the rights of Indigenous people, and also defines who is considered to be an Indigenous person according to lawmakers.[3] But laws such as the *Indian Act (1876)* had other purposes, including to annihilate Indigenous culture and ways of life.

The Doctrine of Discovery and Terra Nullius

In Latin, Terra Nullius means 'vacant land'. The Doctrine of Discovery is a Christian concept indicating that upon discovery, the land is deemed vacant and can be claimed as such and occupied by the person who discovered it. This doctrine was instrumental in the history of colonisation because it made it legal for the colonisers to strip non-Christian people, such as Indigenous people, of their sovereignty.

While many Indigenous communities have long demanded the repudiation of the Doctrine of Discovery, it took over 500 years before this was finally done. Pope Francis finally rejected the Doctrine after a visit to Indigenous communities in North America, and after making a series of apologies to First Peoples in Canada. An official statement now asserts that the Doctrine "did not adequately reflect the equal dignity and rights of Indigenous peoples" (Vatican, March 30, 2023).

As Bob Joseph, a member of the Gwawaenuk Nation, eloquently explained in his book *21 Things You May Not Know About the Indian Act* (2018), settlers drew on multiple strategies to achieve their goal of eradicating Indigenous Nations. Notably, they created a reserve system and imposed a colonial system of government within communities, they forced entire Nations to change their names for European ones, and they forbade Indigenous people from holding ceremonies – in other words, from practicing their culture and traditions. Those who did not respect the law were subjected to punishment. For example, between 1884 and 1951, Ceremonies were banned and people performing them had their material confiscated and were arrested (Wilson, 2018).

Assimilation was one of the clear aims of the Indian Act, as Deputy Minister of Indian Affairs Duncan Campbell Scott put it: "Our objective is to continue until there is not a single Indian has not been absorbed by the body politic, and that there is no Indian question, no Indian department. This is the whole object of this Bill" (Campbell Scott, as cited in Standing Committee on Aboriginal Affairs, Northern Development and Natural Resources 2002).

The *Indian Act* and its impacts on women

The *Indian Act* included many sections which were particularly discriminatory against women. For example, until 1985, Indigenous women who married non-Indigenous men were stripped from their Indian status and all the rights associated with it such as the right to live on reserve (with her community). In 1985, a successful Charter of Human Rights challenge attempted to repair this discrimination by allowing women to regain their status as registered Indians and by allowing their children the right to obtain their Indian status. While this amendment allowed many people to rejoin the Indian Register, it also clearly illustrates the control that the government continues to exercise over Indigenous peoples today.

Among the many drastic measures contained in the *Indian Act* to strip Indigenous people of their culture and their language, the legacy of the residential school and day school systems continue to cause deep pain and trauma among Indigenous people in Canada. Neuroscientist Kimberley Matteson and her colleague (2022), who looked at Indigenous communities in Canada and in the US, explain how the impacts of residential school systems are felt not only by people of the generations who experienced them directly, but also by their children. They explain that the impacts not only include the loss of land, language, culture and traditional ways but also bring about a range of health issues directly related to the trauma, such as high blood pressure, increased inflammation, and cognitive and emotional challenges, including anxiety, fear and problems with concentration. Residential school survivors and their descendants are the living proof of Indigenous people's strength and resilience.

What Is a Residential School?

To evangelise and assimilate Indigenous children, the Canadian federal government set up a system of residential schools. By resocialising the children, this system would impose European values on them, with the aim of "killing the Indian in the child" (Truth and Reconciliation Commission of Canada, 2015a).

Two Distinct Ways to Understand the World

In the introduction of this book, we have presented the idea of values and the fact that they can be interpreted and hierarchised differently from one person to the next, and these interpretations will affect the way the person understands their world and what is important to prioritise within it.

Reflection Break

Think about the word 'justice' and write down how you understand it.

This is a good illustration of *your worldview* with regard to how you see the concept of 'justice' overall.

Now, reflect back on the Indigenous worldview we covered earlier in this chapter. How could justice be understood, or achieved, according to an Indigenous worldview? Write down your answer and compare the two interpretations of the same concept according to these worldviews.

We will now reflect on how ideas such as justice and social justice can be understood differently depending on the worldview that is set forth. These concepts are interesting to examine since many Social Workers claim to hold them as a professional or even personal value yet they may hold different meanings for different Social Workers (Hawkins et al., 2001).

First, let's examine how such concepts may be understood from an Indigenous standpoint. Earlier, we discussed how an Indigenous worldview stresses the importance of reciprocity between humans, animal, sprits and the earth. If you weren't raised with an Indigenous worldview, the idea of justice could have a very different meaning that what you wrote down as your own. Different Indigenous Nations and communities also have different visions of justice. As one example, Mohawk author Taiaiake Alfred understands the concept of justice as "a perpetual process of maintaining that crucial balance and demonstrating true respect for power and dignity of each part of the circle of interdependency" (Alfred, 2009, p. 66). According to this Indigenous worldview, justice aims to restore harmony following an injustice, considering that injustice as a form of dysfunction, "an erosion at some point that disturbs the crucial balance" (Alfred, 2009, p. 66). How does this compare to your understanding of justice?

Differences in perception or worldviews are not themselves an issue. Indigenous and non-Indigenous people have the right to think freely and understand the world in their own way. Issues may arise when one worldview is imposed, or seen as more valid, in comparison to others. Unfortunately, settler societies often invalidate Indigenous worldviews. Dominant groups often consider Indigenous knowledge and values to be less credible than the dominant group's knowledge and values. Because policies and laws are often passed by non-Indigenous people and based on colonial values and ways of knowing, Indigenous people are often placed in a position of *epistemic injustice*. For example, research on child protection practices with Indigenous families have shown that Indigenous parents' knowledge and opinions are less valued and that Social Workers and lawyers often speak on their behalf in court (Leckey et al., 2022). We covered the idea of epistemic injustice proposed by Miranda Fricker in Chapter 4 so you may want to return to this chapter and reflect on how Indigenous people are experiencing various forms of epistemic injustice.

Reflection Break

Think about how much you know about of the history and current situation of Indigenous people and communities that are in proximity of where you live. How can you be better informed about the histories of Indigenous people?

If no Indigenous people live in your countries (e.g. England) and that you are one of the colonising countries, how do you feel this content applies to you?

How can you, as a person and professionally, engage in principles of respect of Indigenous people?

Think about two or three actions that you could take.

A Call for Action and for Reconciliation

Following a class action lawsuit from Indigenous people who were still affected by their experiences in residential schools, the Truth and Reconciliation Commission was set up in 2008 to document the history and lasting impacts of residential schools and to give survivors opportunities to tell their stories. The final reports, published in 2015, included 94 far-reaching calls to action to further reconciliation between Canadian and Indigenous people, such as providing better training for professional civil servants to recognise the legacy of residential schools, for professionals to be better trained in cultural competency, as well as a call to respect Indigenous people's right to self-determine as guaranteed by Article 12:1 of the United Nations Declaration on the Rights of Indigenous Peoples.

The calls for action in the Truth and Reconciliation Report as well as the government's recognition of the hurts caused to Indigenous people by colonialism have led many organisations, including Canadian universities, to recognise and attempt to repair some of the damage that was inflicted on generations of Indigenous people.

We have seen so far that there exist many Indigenous cultures and Nations in Canada, and across the world, as well as different worldviews. We have also mentioned that Indigenous cultures and realities may be different from one community to the next: some people have always been able to preserve a large part of their culture through the language that is still spoken in their community, others have reconnected with their communities after being separated from their families as a result of residential schools, and some have reconnected with their culture after their families were almost completely separated from their communities because of the ravages of colonisation. Each story is both singular and collective. One common feature in this history of colonisation is the oppression experienced by Indigenous communities. Intervening ethically as a Social Worker will therefore require a special consideration of power imbalance, and much care to avoid repeating the imposition of colonial worldviews while doing so. Interventions should also focus on respect and self-determination of Indigenous people and communities as enshrined in the United Nations Declaration on the Rights of Indigenous People (2007), which set out the rights of all Indigenous people, wherever they are located in the word. But how can we act in accordance with the notion of self-determination for Indigenous people and with respect for their worldviews, considering the way in which society is currently organised? To do this, adopting a decolonial perspective can be helpful.

Did You Know?

While the United Nations Declaration on the Rights of Indigenous People (2007) has no legal value for UN members, it nevertheless put forth the principles and ideals that should be followed to uphold the rights of Indigenous people. As such, it functions more like a code of ethics.

It was adopted by on September 13, 2007, by a majority of member states (144). At the time of the vote, four countries opposed to its adoption (Canada, New Zealand, Australia and the United States) and 11 abstained.

The Declaration contains 46 articles, including the right to self-determine, to preserve their cultural identity, and to be protected against discrimination.

Adopting a Decolonisation Perspective to Engage in Ethical Practice

There are various ways to understand the concept of decolonisation, but some will articulate it as an ongoing process requiring critical reflection about the ways the social and structural aspects of a given society are set in place to benefit non-Indigenous people at the expense of Indigenous people. Earlier, we discussed some of the goals and features of the *Indian Act*, which is a good example of a colonial law. To engage in a process of decolonisation therefore requires that we think critically about how the law benefits non-Indigenous people over Indigenous people. For example, Hauskeller et al. (2022, p. 735) discuss how to engage in decolonisation, or what they call decoloniality scholarship: "Decoloniality scholarship makes central the question of how knowledge is produced, arguing that knowledge production is an epistemological, political, and methodological matter infused with power".

Thinking critically about the *Indian Act* therefore means reflecting on what principles underpin it, why and how it was put in place and how it has negatively impacted Indigenous people. It also requires that we reflect on the power relationships in which non-Indigenous people hold power over Indigenous communities, which have been crystallised in the law, (e.g. the Indian Act that decides who is considered Indigenous and who is not, or having one or two non-Indigenous official language spoken government), and on how this system has been maintained in place over time.

Decolonisation also requires time, as well as a long-term commitment, from people and institutions trying to engage with it (Stein et al., 2021). Decolonisation is not theoretical. It requires to people to set in motion a process of change in the way we think, so that Indigenous worldviews, values, cultures and ways of doing become more visible and valued, to the point that those changes are reflected in the structure of the institution going through a decolonisation process (Stein et al., 2021).

Finally, decolonisation requires that people and institutions authentically engage Indigenous people and, more broadly, Indigenous communities in the process (Howitt, 1998). In other words, decolonisation cannot happen without Indigenous participation. Even if you engage in critical thinking about power relationships between Indigenous and non-Indigenous people in the context of your institution, without their participation, you will only repeat the process of colonisation by imposing your way of thinking – even if it is radically different than what was thought before. It is not possible to engage in decolonisation without the participation of Indigenous people in the process.

Some authors have proposed the idea of a *decolonial ethics*, which is a commitment to critically challenge colonial ways of thinking while fostering the development of relationships grounded in a different understanding of the world. Decolonial ethics can also be applied to other populations that have been oppressed as a result of colonialism, such as in the context of anti-Islamophobic Social Work (Moosa-Mitha, 2022).

Decolonial ethics offers a framework for critically reflecting on and challenging the current colonial way of thinking and organising social life, and in the process of doing so, engaging simultaneously with Indigenous people so that their worldviews and values can be fully considered as part of a different way of thinking and organising society (Hauskeller et al., 2022).Social workers need to engage in critical reflection, including efforts to understand their own history and lived experiences, and the way these contribute to maintaining colonial structures. As part of this critical reflection, Social Workers also need to carefully explore the context around them, and how, for example, current structures and systems are built on worldviews that neglect or even ignore Indigenous

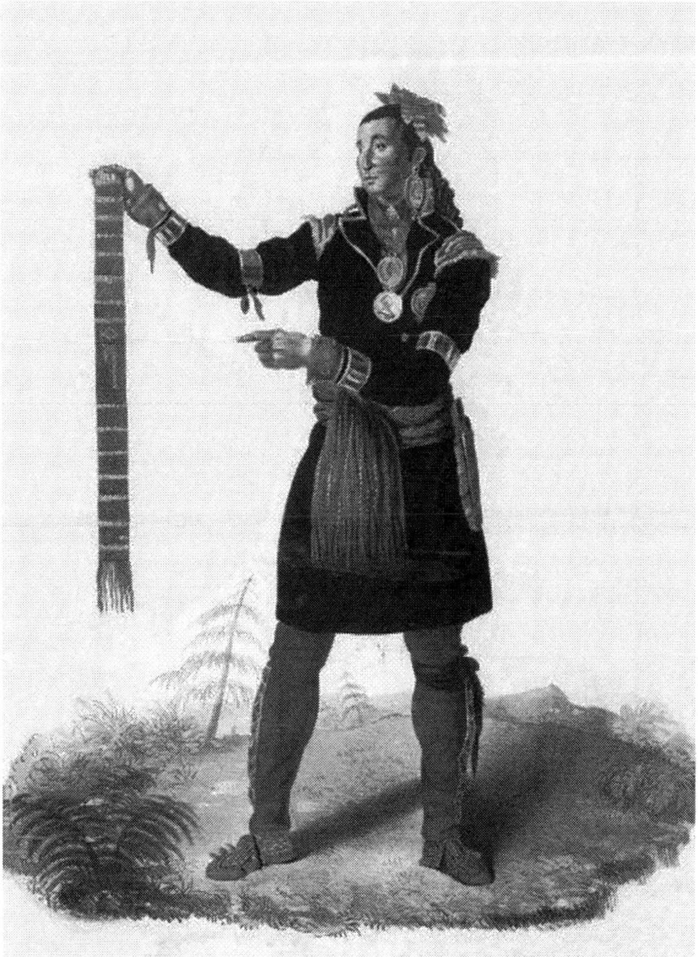

Figure 7.1 Nicholas Vincent Tsawanhonhi, principal Christian chief and captain of the Huron Indians established at La Jeune Lorette near Quebec[4]

Source: Library and Archives Canada, number 2837382

ways of knowing. An analysis of the social landscape or the structure with regard to power dynamics will be essential as part of the process of decolonisation (Figure 7.1).

A decolonial ethics standpoint also stresses the importance of engaging the population or the group Social Workers work with, such as an Indigenous community, in the process of decolonisation. This engagement should be done not only as a way to give a voice to the excluded others, but instead, from ground up, so that "those voices, reorient our thought in relation to them, and thereby see how this changes our vision of the world" (p. 84). In adopting a decolonial ethics standpoint, it will be important to pay attention to the type of engagement that Social Workers draw from in the decolonisation process. Engagement should be meaningful rather than instrumental. Arnstein's participation ladder (see Figure 7.2) can be pertinent to think about Indigenous engagement, and has already been adapted to working in this context by Indigenous scholars such as

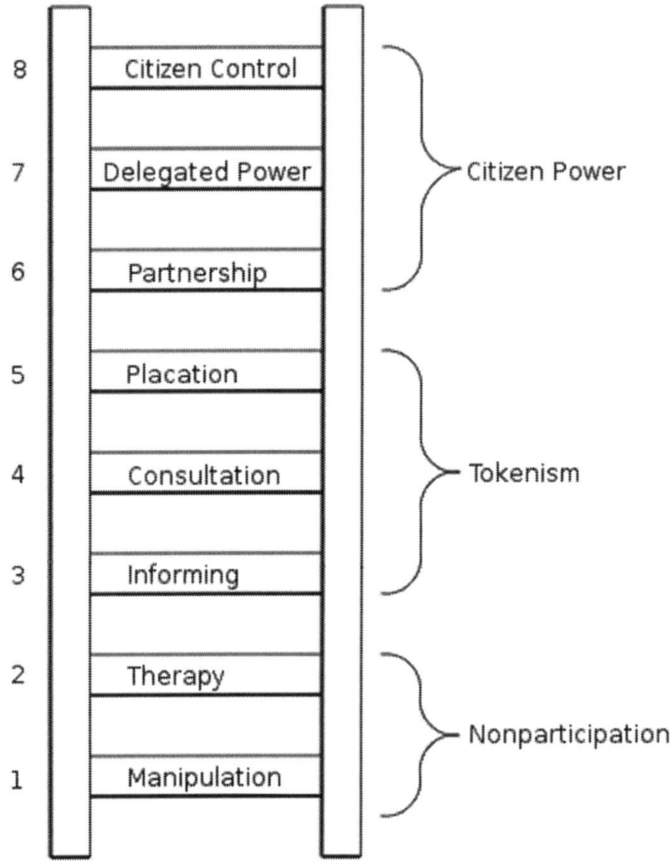

Figure 7.2 Arnstein's original ladder of participation (1969, p. 217)

Huron-Wendat professors Millaire and Pullen Sansfaçon (2023) who have adapted this framework by drawing on the Wampum necklace, whereby each rung of the ladder is a Wampum row. Wampum necklace was made of seashells and were used by different Nations to remind them of the terms of an agreement as well as mutual commitment, stressing the notion of agreement and mutual respect (Gardacz, 2020).

Based on this understanding, decolonial ethics would require Social Workers to involve Indigenous people and communities to participate at the highest level possible and ensure that the conditions are set in place to facilitate this participation throughout the process.

Let's now turn to a case study to examine how decolonial ethics could be deployed.

Case Study

Jacques is a non-Indigenous man of Irish descent working in a university in Eastern Canada as a student welfare officer. He completed his training in Social Work in 1995 in Toronto but decided to move to the coast five years ago to be closer to his husband's family who live there. He is managing a team of two other student welfare officers who are also trained as a Social Worker locally. As a manager, one of Jacques' roles is to accompany faculties and departments in developing strategies that improve students' wellbeing as well as a prompter access to student services when needed.

Since 2015, one important dimension of the university's strategic plan is to support each unit to increase their enrolment of Indigenous students in their programme. Targets have been set by various regulators and funding organisations. The university sees this as a way to respond to some of the recommendations of the Truth and Reconciliation Report.

So far, the various recruitment strategies put in place seems to be successful, as student numbers have steadily increased at enrolment points. However, new issues have emerged in the process.

Over the last two years, some programmes are now reporting a high level of attrition. More Indigenous students enrol, but many of them leave within the first year or two without a diploma. The university decides to mandate Jacques and his team to work with the units that are faced with the problem. Jacques has to propose a strategy to reduce the attrition and ultimately to improve the support offered to Indigenous students until they graduate.

Questions

- What conditions needs to be put in place for Jacques to be in a position to work from a decolonial ethics standpoint while completing his mandate?
- What steps should Jacques take to deliver the strategy to the senior administration of the university?
- What would such a strategy look like?

Write Down Your Ideas

In the context of applying a decolonial ethics standpoint, Jacques would need to engage critically with the question of colonialism, its manifestations in the institution, and the power dynamics that contribute to maintaining it. Jacques will also have to ensure that Indigenous voices are centred from the outset.

Engagement in Critical Reflection

Before doing anything, Jacques needs to think about his own social and institutional position, and how this could impact power relationships. As a non-Indigenous person, it is very possible that his own conception of the world (his beliefs and values) are drastically different from those of the students who will be affected by the strategy he has been asked to develop. He therefore needs to learn as much as possible about Indigenous culture and worldviews before engaging in this work so that he can be better prepare to engage with Indigenous students.

It's important to educate yourself about Indigenous cultures and realities as a starting point for critically engaging in decolonial ethics. This will help you to prevent unconsciously subjecting Indigenous people to microagressions.

A microaggression can take many forms, including actions and words that, intentionally or not, come from prejudices that are grounded in racial oppression and domination (Canel-Çınarbaş and Yohani, 2019). Microaggressions have serious consequences on Indigenous people. They may make them feel invalidated as Indigenous people, prevent them from publicly identifying as Indigenous, or make them feel that the environment they are in is hostile to Indigenous people (Houshmand et al., 2019). In their research, Canel-Çınarbaş and Yohani (2019) found that microaggressions were very common in universities and that students experienced high level of discrimination in these settings. They propose that people who work in these institutions should be self-aware about their own attitudes. They also say that it's important for institutions to recognise institutional racism in order to prevent discrimination and microaggressions. In Jacques' situation, an essential first step is for him to engage in an in-depth reflection on his own social position as a white man of Irish descent and the way that can lead to power imbalances. He should attempt to become aware of his prejudices and how the institution may contribute to perpetuating them.

Example of a Conversation That Could Be Experienced as a Microaggression

During the first meeting with students, Jacques welcomes them and explains what they will work on together. During the break, Jacques is speaking with Alice, an Indigenous student, and in a friendly manner, tells her that he would have never guessed she was Indigenous: "Wow, you don't look Indigenous! Are both of your parents Indigenous?"

This sort of comment may look like it comes from healthy curiosity, but may have the effect of invalidating Alice with regard to her Indigenous identity and ancestry. But this can be prevented by Jacques ensuring that he reads and learns about some of the prejudices that are held against Indigenous people.

Various resources help to challenge some of the prejudices against Indigenous people, such as the leaflet "You don't look Indigenous! And other prejudices" (Amnesty International, 2021)

Indigenous Students' Engagement

Next, Jacques will need to think about how he can fully engage Indigenous people in the development of the strategy. The first thing he will need to think about is who he needs to engage: Indigenous students? Indigenous staff? Indigenous community? He will also need to think about what constitutes an appropriate form of engagement. Proper engagement from the outset of a project is key to a decolonial ethics standpoint. Proper Indigenous engagement will make it possible to centre Indigenous realities and worldviews throughout the strategy and will contribute to the process of institutional decolonisation. This is particularly important in the context of reconciliation work, as described earlier in this chapter.

For the question of who should be engaged. As a baseline, it would be important that Jacques engages as many Indigenous people as possible, and from the widest possible range of backgrounds and cultures. Ensuring meaningful and sufficient participation and engagement of communities and people, whatever the project Social Workers engage with, is no simple task. But as we have seen previously, meaningful participation is key to truly engaging in a process of reconciliation, integrating Indigenous worldviews into whatever work is being done, and more broadly, to begin to decolonise Social Work practice with Indigenous communities. Because decolonisation is also about a change in power relationships, it is important to facilitate a process of participation that allows this to happen, and to promote respect for all forms of knowledge and values equally, regardless of the identity of the participants.

Jacques will therefore want to facilitate the participation of Indigenous people in the policy development, but he will also have to be careful not to fall into the trap of inadequate participation, reflecting the bottom rung of the ladder of participation (Arnstein, 1969) or the Wampum necklace (Millaire and Pullen Sansfaçon, 2023).

In this sense, to achieve meaningful participation, Jacques will need to go beyond simply inviting Indigenous people to attend a one-off meeting and nothing more. This type of participation could be akin to a form of instrumentalisation. Instrumentalisation and tokenism should be avoided at all costs when working with Indigenous people as it greatly harms the institution's reconciliation efforts and the development of a trusting relationship with Indigenous communities.

With this in mind, Jacques would also need to avoid only involving student in a way that is illusory. In our case study, this could happen if Jacques decided to write the strategy with his team and then simply invite one Indigenous person to have a look at it, without fully explaining to the person how the institution works or what is expected of them. If he took this illusory approach, then even if the person made some comments and suggestions about the strategy, Jacques would not really take them into consideration but would brag about the fact that the consultation was done and perhaps would put the person's name on the document as having participated in the project. Notwithstanding Jacques's policy-writing skill, or how knowledgeable he is about Indigenous students' realities, or the amount of praise he may get from people about the document, including from some Indigenous people or from the administration, the level of involvement of Indigenous people as illustrated in this example would be unethical from a decolonial ethics standpoint because the participation and engagement are inadequate. This approach does not contribute to increasing the respect for Indigenous knowledge and worldviews, nor to redistribute power.

A different vision of participation is therefore essential to engage ethically with Indigenous people and communities. The level of *citizen control*, on the other hand, is one where people who are concerned by the issue are fully participating in decision-making and management of the project (Arnstein, 1969).

Looking again at Jacques' situation, this would mean that in order to develop the policy, he would form a committee of Indigenous students and Indigenous staff, and involve, as much as possible, community partners that are concerned with student academic perseverance. He should also try to involve an Elder in the process. Indigenous Elders are people who are "recognized for their wisdom and their ability to advise their community on issues and problems, in accordance with rites and customs" (Millaire and Pullen Sansfaçon, 2023, p. 8) and can be invited to attend, with appropriate compensation for their knowledge and time, in the context of reconciliation. People invited to engage with the work that will lead to the strategy development should be given the time and space to discuss and reflect on student attrition, come up with a different understanding of the problem and propose solutions so that students' needs are better met at the university. If Jacques is involved in writing the strategy, he will adjust the content to so it is pertinent to the institution, but will not control the content. He will openly discuss how he is presenting the work of the committee and will be doing so in a way that he remains fully conscious of the power that he may wield in making suggestions about how to present it. He will facilitate the process rather than lead it. When the strategy is ready, Jacques will facilitate a meeting for the committee to present it to the administration, with him, and will facilitate the adoption of the policy within the institution. He will be keeping the lines of communication open with the committee to ensure that they understand that they remain in control, but that his skills and knowledge of the institution can help to convince the administration to adopt the policy. In doing so, he will make sure that the voices of Indigenous people continue to be heard, understood and valued as an equally important worldview and source of knowledge.

In a project aimed at understanding the realities of trans and Two-Spirit youth, Pullen Sansfaçon et al., (2024) have proposed a combination of Indigenous methodology (Strega and Brown, 2015) and Social Action methods (Fleming and Ward, 2004) to facilitate the meaningful engagement and empowerment of Two-Spirit youth in the process. To do so,

What Does It Mean to Be Two-Spirit?

'Two-Spirit' is an umbrella term specifically used by some Indigenous people and communities to self-identify as having sexual orientations that are not heterosexual, or a gender identity that is not cisgender. Two-Spirit identity is deeply rooted in Indigenous culture (FNQLHSSC, n.d.) and can include a political standpoint that recognises the role of colonisation in the contemporary experience of transphobia and homophobia present in many Indigenous communities (Cook-Meyer and Labelle, 2004) (Figure 7.3).

they drew on the notion of Talking Circles, in which participants talk, using a talking stick, ensuring a culturally relevant approach to discussing their realities. One after the others, youth were invited to share about their experiences, looking at *what, why* and *how* questions, as suggested by the Social Action method; apart from that initial meeting, participants were invited to take part in all the decisions related to the project (meeting modalities, how to disseminate data and so on) and an Elder was also invited open and close the Talking Circle meetings and facilitate discussion. They were involved until the end of the project and, in addition to more traditional forms of dissemination, they were invited to choose their own dissemination strategy, which resulted in the production of a podcast – *Mamu: A Two-Spirit Podcast* (*mamu* means "together or in a group" in Innu-aimun). To disseminate their podcast, one of the youths created an art piece and stickers were created with a QR code linking directly to the podcast, which was posted on Spotify.

(https://open.spotify.com/show/5MEulHpoxYCs7VDJCaIgRG)

In this example, we can see that youth are supported in making decisions about the form of consultation they want, whether they decided to participate, the content of what

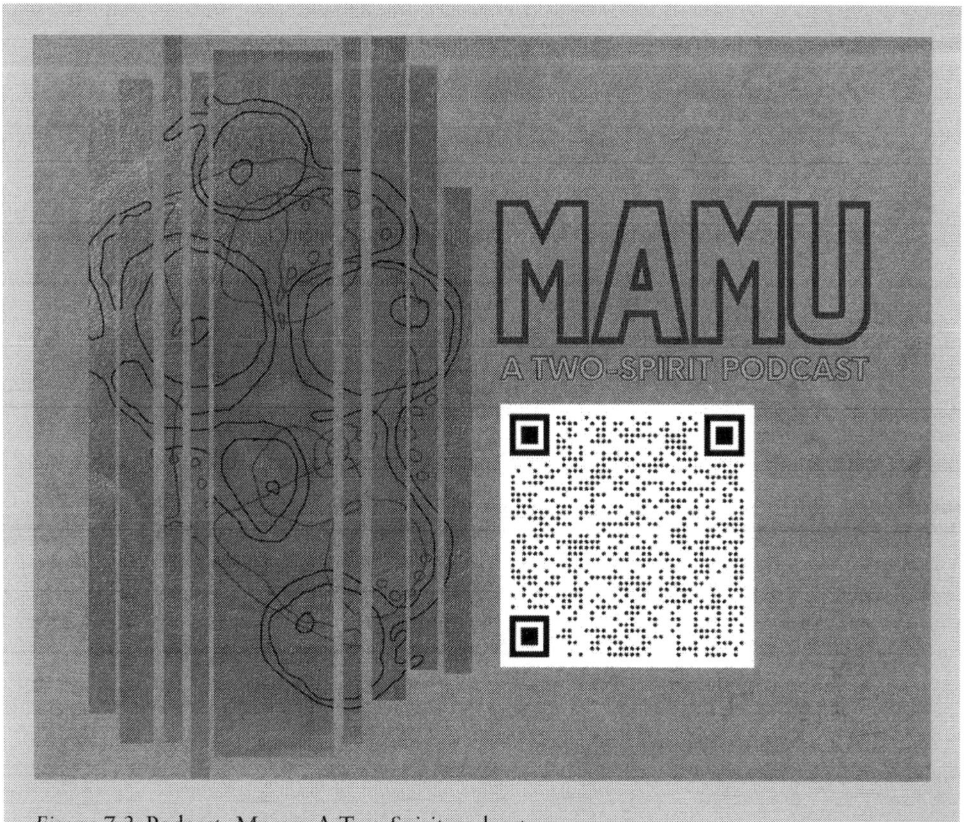

Figure 7.3 Podcast: Mamu: A Two-Spirit podcast

they see as the most important to share, and the modality for doing so. In engaging with Indigenous students, Jacques could adapt his methodologies to facilitate the process in a way that is not only participative and democratic but also culturally safe so that all participants can fully engage in the process of defining strategies to increase student perseverance at the university.

Conclusion

In this chapter, we have briefly examined different Indigenous worldviews, and how colonialism has contributed to the devaluation of Indigenous people and their knowledge. We have also examined, through a discussion of a value of such as justice, how Indigenous and non-Indigenous worldviews differ. We have also presented how a decolonial ethics standpoint that emphasises critical thinking and meaningful engagement of Indigenous people can help move forward in a process of decolonisation and reconciliation.

Notes

1 Basil Johnston, *The Gift of the Stars*, Cape Croker First Nation, ON: Kegedonce, 2013.
2 Translated from the French by the authors.

3 For an example of amendment of the *Indian Act* and its impact on Indigenous people, see Assembly of First Nations (2019).
4 The title of this image in Figure 7,1 contains terms that are now considered outdated and inappropriate. The word "Indian" reflects historical usage and does not align with current respectful terminology. Today, we recognize and refer to the Wendat Nation rather than using the term "Huron", which is no longer appropriate. This wording remains for historical reference only.

8 Kantian Ethics, Respect for the Person and Self-Determination

Respect for the person and self-determination have come to be seen as core values of Social Work practice, both nationally and internationally. Directly or indirectly, these concepts are central to many professional organisations' codes of ethics such as the Canadian Association of Social Workers (CASW), the National Association of Social Workers (NASW) and the British Association of Social Work Code of Ethics.

This chapter begins with the exploration of Social Work's underlying roots in the moral philosophy of the Enlightenment. As discussed in Chapter 1, the Enlightenment was eventful in terms of the development of philosophy and science, and was a period in which people were attempting to think about the human condition in new ways. The thoughts and ideas that developed in philosophy, politics and other sciences continue to have a major influence on contemporary society.

Anchored in the work of Immanuel Kant, an important Enlightenment philosopher, this chapter examines the concepts of self-determination and human dignity and discuss how his work continues to be perceivable today in modern codes of ethics. The chapter begins by outlining key concepts of Kant's work and examines how these concepts have played such an important role in framing ideas about ethics in modern Social Work. The concepts are then applied to a Social Work case study to illustrate how it can helps managing a complex ethical dilemma that highlights issues around self-determination and respect of the person.

Who Was Immanuel Kant?

Immanuel Kant was born in Prussia in 1724. He was not from a powerful or aristocratic family; rather, his father was a labourer, and the family's financial means were very limited. He nevertheless studied mathematics, physics, philosophy and religion at the University of Königsberg at the age of 16. It was, however, only after publishing a number of unsuccessful books that Kant published his first major work on moral philosophy, entitled *Groundwork of the Metaphysics of Morals* (1785). This publication went on to have a major influence on contemporary philosophy and established Kant as one of the most influential philosophers of all time.

Practical Reasoning and Moral Autonomy

For Kant, the search for and the finding of *truth* can only occur through a critical examination of reality which he calls 'practical reasoning'. What does practical reasoning means?

DOI: 10.4324/9781003458715-12

What Is Practical Reason?

Practical reason is the general human capacity for resolving through reflection the question of what one is to do (Wallace, 2003).

As we have seen so far throughout this book, Social Workers work with people, groups and communities that are experiencing complex situations. Our values sometimes intuitively lead us to feels 'right' or 'wrong' about sometimes. However, Kantian ethics requires to engage in practical reasoning when faced with a complex situation, or an ethical dilemma. This means that you must reflect about the situation thoroughly before making your mind up. This concept of practical reasoning probably seems fairly simple to you, but you must remember, from reading the previous chapters, that many factors influence your decision. In addition to your personal values, aspects such as the organisational values and the culture of your workplace, or the power relationships between you and your manager can all affect the way you think about a situation. All of those can stifle your practical reasoning ability, so you must remain aware of it.

For example, think about a situation in which you would be accompanying a young woman who currently live on the street and who frequently uses heroin. This young people just found out that she is pregnant. Despite expressing that she does not want to keep the child, she has decided that she will be going through with pregnancy instead of having an abortion. She is contemplating having the child adopted at birth. Take time to think about this situation and write down how you intuitively feel about it. How do your values affect how you think about the situation? As a professional, you may favour one specific course of action. But even if you feel that you have well considered all the elements in the situation, it is possible that your personal values or those promoted by the organisation unduly influence your evaluation of the situation. Practical reasoning requires you to examine the situation carefully and think about all the possible elements that could affect your decision.

Some of your personal experience may, according to Kant, affect your understanding of the situation as well as how you may think about it. For example, if you were adopted as a child, this experience may affect your perspective on adoption and on abortion. Not being adopted or coming from a loving family, or having experienced a situation of abuse as a child may also affect how you perceive the situation presented above. The same is true if you yourself had an abortion in the past, or know someone who did. All those experiences can affect the way you understand this situation and think about it. You can see that depending on your worldviews, and of your experience, a situation can be understood very differently from another person.

In Kantian terms, knowledge does not exist in a vacuum, as reality is constructed through each of our various experiences in the world. Therefore, as a starting point, Kantian ethics requires to realise that 'knowledge' of something does not always equate with *truth*, even when you think, you have found a proof which seems difficult to argue against. Let's have a look at a case study.

Case Study

Sylvia is a clinical Social Worker working in private practice. Over her career, she has worked with many gender-diverse young people. When deemed competent to make decisions for themselves, she has always supported their autonomy and accompanied them in their journey to find the best way to meet their needs. Sometimes, this means that she accompanied them to access specialised medical care to undertake a gender transition. As a member of the World Professional Association of Transgender Health (WPATH), she stresses the importance of informed consent and follows the international guidelines – the Standards of Care Version 8, published in 2022.

Recently, she has noticed a lot of news reports about youth who 'detransition' or who have 'sex change regret' (Slothouber, 2020). While Sylvia has only encountered one youth who have since regretted her transition and detransitioned, she hears more and more about those youth and is starting to be worried about her own. She is also aware of increasing resistance against access to medical transitions for minors, and she has learned that some countries like in England, Finland and Sweden, they have started to restrict access to gender affirming medical. Recently, she has come across a report that was commissioned by a government to understand the reasons for the growth in referrals, and changes to population accessing gender identity clinics in the UK. As she reads the conclusion of the report, she is wondering if she should continue to support youth people journey towards a gender transition. Indeed, the report mentions that there is no reliable evidence base upon which to make clinical decisions, or for children and their families to make informed choices as no evidence to support long-term outcomes of interventions to manage gender-related distress.

Reflexion Break

If you were Sylvia, how would you feel about working with gender diverse and trans youth at the moment?
When faced with conflicting evidence, how can you decide on what to base your intervention?
Why is this?

Until 2010, the issue of gender diversity among young people were largely relegated to the realm of psychology, psychiatry and paediatrics: a 'health' issue diagnosed as 'Gender Identity Disorder'. Nowadays, gender diversity is no longer pathologised and trans and non-binary youth who experience 'gender incongruence' or 'gender dysphoria', a form of distress that occurs when a person feels an incongruence between their gender and their sex assigned at birth, can access medical care to meet their needs. The medical care that are provided are usually based on the Standards of Care published about every ten years by the WPATH since 1979. Many well-established professional organisations around the world support access to gender affirming care for transgender youth such as the Canadian Paediatric Society (Vandermorris and Metzger 2023) and the American Association of Clinical Endocrinology (2022) despite the fact that some countries have, since 2023, started to restrict those. However, a few highly mediatised reports, such as the Cass Review in the UK, are increasingly cited and used to ban access to gender affirming care in some jurisdictions. But those critiques have not been making the headlines in most part, even if British Medical Association has undertaken their own review of the report and the European Federation of Sexology and the World Association of Sexual Health have reiterated the importance to follow evidence as presented in the Standards of Care V8 published by WPATH (Coleman et al. 2022). How can Sylvia move forward with intervening with trans and non-binary young people from the Social Work discipline? How would practical reasoning help Sylvia see more clearly in what seems to be a complicated scientific landscape dominated by contrasting evidence?

First, in this situation, or any other situation where it is possible to competing evidence, it is important examine the different types of evidence, as well as the weight each of them are given in a situation. For example, in many areas of medical research – think of vaccine, or cancer treatment research – systematic reviews are often used as the 'Gold Standard of evidence'. Because Sylvia is working with youth who are considering a gender transition and that some of them may at some point ask for medical interventions such as hormone therapy, relying on such type of evidence may feel reasonable at first sight.

However, practical reasoning would require Sylvia to further engage in critical reflection and ask herself some further questions: Is there other type of evidence that need to be taken into consideration? Is it always possible to conduct double blind randomised control trial in an ethical manner? Why cumulative evidence published in care guidelines published periodically by an international association since the late 1970s would now be considered inadequate? What do research that employs different methodologies report on this subject? Is quantitative research should be considered more trustworthy and rigorous than qualitative research? Why is systematic review considered a gold standard and the best evidence possible?

By reflecting on questions such as those, by engaging in practical reasoning, and avoid only considering what caught her attention recently, Sylvia will continue to critically review all the available evidence and consider the evidence more holistically. She will continue to guide her intervention based on international guidelines, while at the same time, remain aware and open to emerging evidence that may be published over the following month and years. She will also remain critical of the discourse that could circulate as the media seem to play an important role in polarising and politicising debates around transgender youth (Pang et al. 2022). She will remain aware that what is presented in the media about gender transition, like any other social issue, is often only partial (Billard, 2023). As such, practical reasoning will help her pay attention to all those various aspects and how they can affect her reasoning behind it.

You can see from this discussion that trough practical reasoning, we can begin shedding lights on ethical questions. Exercising practical reasoning will allow you to question different facts and/or taken for granted in a process of reflexion and critical thinking. It is through practical reason that a person can develop what Kant calls the 'moral autonomy', which is the ability to decide for one's self.

Moral Autonomy, Human Dignity and Self-Determination

Kant`s notion of practical reasoning is central to his theory because he believed that everyone was capable of practical reason. Because everyone is able of practical reasoning, that is, to think for themselves, everyone should also be considered auto-determining, and able to make decisions for themselves. Indeed, according to Kant, people should be treated with dignity because they are rational agents, that is, free agents capable of making their own decisions, setting their own goals, and guiding their conduct through reason (Rachels and Rachel, 2023). A Kantian approach, therefore, supposes that all individuals, because they can think, should be seen as having the ability to make decisions for them, in other words, to be self-determining.

You must be wondering if practical reason, as understood by Kant, is really something that everyone could undertake. Indeed, because Social Workers intervene with different service user groups, some of which have, for example, power of attorney (that means that they cannot decide for themselves in certain or all areas of their lives), it may be legitimate to ask whether this principle can really apply to everyone.

What Is 'Moral Autonomy'?

Moral autonomy is a Kantian term that means the capacity to make morally right decisions. Moral autonomy is only possible because all people have the ability for practical reasoning. In Social Work, this means that even when someone prescribes a rule to follow, a 'morally autonomous' person will be able to think critically and reason before deciding to apply the rule or not.

To answer this question, it is useful to examine the social and historical context in which Kant lived while developing his theory. In Europe, in the eighteenth century, many groups of people, such as the disabled, those with limited cognitive abilities, immigrants, and even women, did not have citizenship rights like men. Therefore, it is not likely that these groups were taken into consideration in Kant's original theory. In other words, when he wrote his book, Kant probably had in mind only middle-class males of German descent. However, this does not mean that groups that were not part of Kant's original understanding should be excluded from this principle. Indeed, while some groups of service users may not be legally able to make decisions for themselves in some areas of their lives, it does not mean they are unable to be self-determining in other areas. While Kant's emphasis on self-determination may not mean the same for all user groups, all individuals have the ability to be self-determining in at least certain areas of their lives.

Reflection Break

If, according to Kant, everyone has at least some level of moral autonomy and is able to carry out practical reasoning, it would be legitimate to ask the following:

Is practical reason sufficient for defining a right action from a wrong one? (you may want to return to Sylvia's story to think this question through)

Can you think about any challenges, opportunities or even danger in just using 'practical reasoning' when making a decision?

Kant explains that the process of practical reasoning must always be undertaken in relation to three key principles:

- The intentions behind the action must be good.
- The action must be done out of a sense of duty.
- The action must be based on the 'good moral law'.

These three elements, when combined with the process of practical reasoning, will help define the morally right course of action according to Kant. We shall now examine these three principles briefly.

1 The principle of good intention

The first principle concerns the intention of the person in undertaking an action. We recall from the above discussion that when we are faced with a situation in Social Work and are required to make a decision, we must use our practical reason and question all the different aspects of the situation to help us make that decision. However, moral autonomy and practical reason are not sufficient, according to Kant, for performing good actions. We also need to examine what is the intention behind the action, that is, 'why we want to do such and such' and ensure that the action derives from what Kant calls the 'good will', that is that the intentions are good.

What Is the Concept of 'Good Will'?

A central feature of Kant's work is the idea that for an action to be good, it must have been undertaken on the basis of good will and good intentions. If this is the case, then the action can be considered good, regardless of the consequences that result from it.

To illustrate this point, let us take the example of a Social Worker who usually displays good judgement in her practice. One day, after careful consideration, she decides to slightly bend a rule to help a person who needs a particular service but does not fully meet the criteria. She was later reprimanded for her decision, and a note was added to her file at Human Resources.

In Kantian ethics, bending the rule is not intrinsically good or bad. To assess, one needs to look at the intention behind the action. Bending a rule could be right if the intention that led the person to make this decision is a good one (i.e. to help someone who really needs it) but could also be considered wrong in other situations, such as in the case of a person who bend a rule to conceal an information, for example.

Let's look at another example. On the other hand, a person may be very generous and always give money to charity. If the person does this with no other intention than to help the charity, then, for Kant, the action could be considered morally good. However, if the person gives money to charity only for tax purposes, then the action would not be considered good in a Kantian sense because it is not performed out of good will, even if the charity still benefits from the donations of this particular person.

In other words, what constitutes goodness should not simply be evaluated on the basis of the result of an action. Instead, a Kantian approach examines the basis of the intention or motivation behind the action to decide if an action is morally right or wrong. Therefore, according to Kant, it does not matter how many qualities a person has: If the intention behind the action is wrong, then the action cannot be morally right.

The Milgram experiment is a good example of this principle. In this experiment, conducted in the 1960s, Stanley Milgram, then researcher at Yale University, wanted to examine how people responded to authority. He asked a number of participants to administer an electric shock (simulated) to another person they could not see, every time that person responded incorrectly to a question. Most participants, though feeling quite uncomfortable, administered the electric shock because they were asked to by a man in a white coat. Since this was only an experiment, the electric shocks were not real, and nobody in the experiment was actually hurt. Now, even though this was the case, does this make the participants' actions right? We must remind ourselves that the participants were only acting out of respect for authority. Though it seems obvious in this example, it is very likely that Kant would say that the actions were morally wrong. The actions would not be considered good because the intention behind the actions was not good. While we all agree that it would be hardly possible to find a good intention behind administering an electric shock to someone, what is important to note here is that it is really the intention behind the action that counts and not the consequence of the action itself. Indeed, Kant believes in the assertion that nothing is unconditionally good except good will. It is therefore the intention behind the action that matters, not the action itself. Thus, for Kant, it is the intention, rather than the consequences, that are crucial, even though, and unfortunately so, the good intention may not result in good consequences. To remind ourselves of this point in a single phrase, in Kantian ethics, "the end never justifies the means". In other words, the consequences of an action, though positive in the end, can never be justified by an action that is not well intentioned.

2 The Principle of Duty

We have seen, thus far, that the morally right action, or in the case of Social Work, an ethical intervention or decision reflecting Kantian principles, is an action that involves thought and questioning through practical reasoning; it is undertaken out of good intentions or, as Kant calls it, out of 'good will'. The ethical Social Worker will therefore be called upon to challenge the many assumptions that are likely to be observed in practice, will refuse to take anything for granted, and will do so for the right reasons.

What Is a Duty?

A duty is something that someone ought to do and implies a moral obligation. For example, duties in Social Work are usually articulated within codes of ethics and codes of practice, but also within certain laws.

This brings us to a discussion regarding another important concept in Kantian ethics, that of 'duty'. Kant tells us that every action must also be undertaken out of a sense of duty. "Duty to what?" we might ask. Let have a look at the concept of duties, in the context of Social Work.

For Social Work, action out of duty means following what is in your code of ethics, as long as you do not take the latter's contents for granted and always commit yourself to thinking it through by carefully examining its application to different situations through practical reasoning. The concept of duty is therefore important and relates, in this regard, to the principles of ethical practice set out in codes of ethics that applies in your jurisdiction. For example, the code of ethics from the Canadian Association of Social Workers (2024) lists that the first duty of Social Workers is to Respect the Dignity and Worth of All People. Six other principles that emphasise the value base of Social Work are then outlined. We shall return to some of these principles later in this chapter, but for the moment, we can observe that the Canadian Association of Social Worker's code of ethics is formulated around different duties that are relevant to the profession. In this sense, we can talk about a 'duty-based' ethics.

However, we discussed earlier that, in a Kantian sense, behaving a certain way out of pure social conformity or in response to authority, for example, does not necessary add up to a good action. In other words, doing something because we have been conditioned to do so is not right, even though we may have been told that it is. Furthermore, Kant reasoned that setting out to do the right thing because one feels 'happy' to do so is not as worthy doing the right thing because one feels a moral obligation to do so and rationally thought about the action beforehand (the notion of intention).

So how do we know that what is in the code of ethics is really 'the duty' we should undertake as a Social Worker? We may see here a paradox in interpreting Kant's moral theory. On the one hand, Kant tells us not to take anything for granted and always use practical reason in examining evidence. On the other hand, he also tells us that we ought to act out of a sense of duty to moral law. Can we just apply codes of ethics in Social Work to any situation? Where does this leave us? What if a 'duty' conflict with another one? For example, what if a Social Worker is faced with a situation whereby, on the one hand, she has the duty to protect someone from harm, and on the other hand, she has to the same person to make their own decisions? In order to shed some light on this aspect of duty, we shall have to look at what, according to Kant, is good moral law.

3 Defining and using 'Good Moral Law', or commands

For Kant, to live according to a sense of duty, as described above, is to live an ethical life. Ethical life does not depend on our feeling of rightness or wrongness, but instead on our pursuit of practical reason. To do so, we must think about our sense of duty as being formulated around 'moral laws' that Kant believed were essential to ethical life. However, we may wonder if a certain incompatibility exists between, on the one hand, Kant's arguments in favour of practical reason, and on the other hand, his insistence on adhering to moral laws. The answer to this lies in the way Kant understands the concept of moral law. Moral laws, according to Kant, are not rules that directly influence actions; rather, they put in place the principles that allow people to act out of good will, out of a sense of duty, while at the same time using their ability for practical reasoning. These principles, in Kant's theory, refer to that of 'imperative' or, *rules to adhere too* as we shall refer to it in this book.

What Is a 'Moral Law'?

A moral law is a principle that is define by the person who is making a decision, through practical reasoning. The articulation of the moral law should always respect two basic conditions or principles:

It must underpin a *fundamental respect for the person*, and you must be able to make it *universal to all*.

Kant considered two basic types of rules: the *hypothetical rule* and the *categorical rule*. Hypothetical rules *advise* you on a course of action, but that generally implies a condition, meaning that it is usually formulated using an 'if' and 'then' structure. For example, a hypothetical rule might be something along the lines of "if you want to be a good citizen, then exercise your right to vote". This example stresses the conditional aspect of good citizenship through voting. It also stresses that if you do not want to be a good citizen, you do not need to vote. It is therefore conditional in nature.

A categorical rule, on the other hand, is a rule that instructs people what to do regardless of the reason or without reference to any other end (Kant, 1785). For example, a categorical rule might be "always participate fully in society". This is a categorical rule because it proposes a direction that must be followed regardless of the possible outcome. In this case, it would include voting, but do not exclude other forms of citizenship participation like volunteering for example. For Kant, categorical rules are central to the articulation of good moral laws because, unlike the hypothetical one, it is not a means to something else; as you will remember, good actions in Kantian morality must be undertaken because they are right in themselves, rather than a means an end. For Kant, it is the categorical rule that people must follow to lead an ethical life, since it is the only command that does not involve a means to an end.

To illustrate the difference between a hypothetical and categorical command, consider the following example from Social Work practice.

Imagine you are about to leave the office at 5 p.m. when a service user, who appears extremely distressed, arrives. Your manager asks you if you would be good enough to stay a little longer to deal with the situation. Let us imagine that you decide to stay on and help her. What is your reason for doing so? You may decide to stay on and help the service user because you want to impress your manager with your dedication, which would be looked upon positively in the event of a promotion or salary increase. You may also decide to see the service user because you would feel guilty if you did not, that something might happen to her and you would feel responsible. Alternatively, you may accept to see the service user simply because she is distressed and in need of help, even though you were about to leave the office. In other words, you may see her out of respect for her as a person. The first two reasons for agreeing to see the service user are based on Kant's *hypothetical rules* because the service user is merely seen as a means to an end, whether for your own self-interest in gaining a promotion or for avoiding your own feelings of guilt (if you want a promotion, you must work harder.... If you want to have good appraisal, you must see the service user...). On the other hand, seeing the service user simply because she is distressed and needs help, even though it may be inconvenient for you, represents a *categorical rule*; your motive for seeing the service user is not based on any other end than to respond to her need, and in this sense, you are acting solely out of a sense of moral duty.

However, how can a person be sure that a rule, even if it is 'categorical', will lead to ethical life? Kant defines two principles in which the rule must fit:

- It must always be based on the respect for the person
- It must always be universal, that is, applicable in all situations.

Respect for the Person

'Respect for persons' is a principle that presupposes that the rule should never use another person as a means to an end. This is consistent with the concepts of 'good will' and 'paying little attention to consequences' discussed above. This principle tells us that a person should never be treated as a means to an end but must always treated as an end in itself. To understand this, consider again the example of the manager who asks you to stay at work later than usual to see a service user who is distressed and needs immediate attention. A categorical rule for this example would be "always help people who are in need". If you applied this command to the situation, then you would either see the service user right away or you would arrange for an alternative solution so that she could eventually get the help she needed. Helping someone only because one wants to impress others would not be acting in accordance with respect for that person and constitutes treating him or her as a means to an end.

Universality

Universality, for Kant, is principle that determines a right action on the basis that if it is right for one, it is right for all, and may thus be adopted as a 'universal law'. This means that whatever you intend to do, you must make sure that your action would be ethical regardless of the context in which it takes place and could thus be universalised. This categorical rule therefore emphasises that a good action will be good to whomever, wherever, and whenever. Again, the command given in the example of the Social Worker that is questioning herself about staying or not to help the distressed service user, would clearly meet the universality criteria, as whatever situation, a person would be happy to be in the receiving end and get help with their situation. In line with the Social Work 'duties' discussed above, you can also see that combined, they form an interesting way of 'universalising' good Social Work practice.

As you can see, the command that are emerging as part of the practical reasoning process are not ready-made rules that we pick and choose whenever we need to make a decision. Instead, they give an orientation to the development of the rule that can be applied to a given situation. Combined with the notion of good intention and developed through the process of practical reasoning, these two principles (respect for the person and universality) ensure that the rule you define in a given situation will lead to the right action. We shall now examine each of these categorical commands before drawing conclusions about Kantian ethics and considering how such an approach may help in the analysis of ethical dilemmas in practice.

Reflection Break

Thinking back to the principles of Kantian ethics:

1 Summarise what you consider the main point of Kant's ethical theory.
2 How might these principles be used in Social Work practice?

For Kant, an ethical life is possible because people have the ability for practical reasoning and are therefore morally autonomous. Because of this quality, people who are acting out of good will and out of a sense of duty to the moral law are able to perform morally right actions. It is through the ability to reflect and think critically that a person can assess whether an action is ethical. To do so, the person will formulate rules that will guide them in making their decision. These rules, which are called categorical imperatives, must be taking into consideration two principles, that is 'respect for the person' and 'universality'. It is by combining these elements that Kant believe that all people can live the ethical life.

Let's now examine how we can apply Kant's theory to a practical situation in Social Work.

Case Study: Mark's Story

Gabriella is a 27-year-old woman from Spain. She came to the Quebec, Canada, a little more than four years ago to work. One night, when she was returning home from work, she was attacked and raped by a group of men. Despite an extensive investigation, the police were never able to find the perpetrators of this crime. Shortly after the incident, Gabriella started to suffer from depression; at the same time, she discovered she was pregnant as a result of the rape. Because of her religious beliefs, Gabriella felt she had no choice but to continue with the pregnancy, and she gave birth to Juanita. Gabriella asserts that without her religious beliefs, she would 'never have made it up to now'.

Following the birth of her daughter, Gabriella had been in touch with Mental Health Services because her problems with depression worsened. It was noted that she had not responded significantly to either medication or the work undertaken by the community psychiatric nurse and psychologist. Things rapidly deteriorated for Gabriella when Juanita born: Gabriella was diagnosed with post-partum psychosis a few days after the birth and was taken by force to a psychiatric hospital so that she could receive care. As Gabriella was unable to look after Juanita during this time, Juanita was temporarily placed in the care of a foster family. Gabriella remains in hospital for one full month. As she returned home, she felt increasingly isolated. She has very few friends and no family in Canada. She feels unable to return to Spain. Since the first episode, Gabriella has been in and out of psychiatric hospitals and has found it increasingly difficult to care for Juanita. Realising she could no longer cope, Gabriella have decided to consent for Juanita, who just turned one year old, to be adopted.

Justina and Lucie have been in a relationship for seven years and have lived together for five. Justina is originally from Spain but has been living in Quebec, Canada, since she left university ten years ago. Lucie is French Canadian. Lucie was raised as a Catholic but is not particularly religious. Justina is also Catholic and is fully involved in her local Catholic church. Lucie sometimes accompanies Justina as their Church is LGBT friendly. For some time now, Justina and Lucie have felt the desire to have a child. After carefully exploring the different options, they decided that adopting a child, as opposed to sperm donation, would be the best choice for them. They felt that this would be a more equal solution because neither of them has the desire to carry and give birth. Justina and Lucie have been on an adoption waiting list for nearly two years, and no child has been matched with them so far.

However, this is just about to change. Justina receives a phone call from their Social Worker at the local agency they are registered with. The Social Worker, Mark, explains that a one-year-old baby Juanita will be placed for adoption. Since Juanita is of Spanish origins, Justina and Lucie are keen on the idea of adopting the baby. When the Social Worker explains to Gabriella that she has found potential parents, she is very happy, that is, until she understands that the adopting couple are lesbians. She then becomes adamant about her daughter being adopted by a Roman Catholic heterosexual couple as according to her faith, only married heterosexual couples should have children. She insists that for her, it is important that Juanita "will be raised in the values she dearly believes in". As she signed the consent 20 days ago, she threatens to withdraw her consent for the adoption if Social Services proceeds with Justina and Lucie as the adoptive parents. She is well aware that she has 30 days to act.

Reflection Break

Looking back through the case study:

1 Identify the ethical dilemma facing Mark.
2 Identify the various courses of action Mark could take.
3 Write down what you feel are the most important elements to take into consideration in each course of action you identified above. Why do you feel they are important?
4 How would you express the issues facing Mark in terms of Kantian ethics?

Analysing the Ethical Dilemmas from a Kantian's Perspective

The dilemma facing Mark in the above case study raises many difficult issues regarding individual rights, welfare, self-determination, and autonomy, as well as discrimination against all or some of the individuals involved.

A Kantian approach may be helpful in casting light on these issues. We now propose to look at the case study and to apply Kantian principles to its various aspects of the situation discussed above. As mentioned before, Kantian ethics focuses on a person's ability to engage in practical reasoning, the motivation and sense of duty behind an action, and whether the action is compatible with 'good moral law' in terms of it adhering to the two principles of respect for the person and universality.

How do these elements relate to the situation facing Mark in this case study? The focus of the analysis will be on the Social Worker, Mark, and his actions, rather than on the issues facing Gabriella, Justina, and Lucie, since it ultimately falls upon Mark to decide what course of action to take. After the analysis of Mark's situation through Kantian principles, we will pose some further questions and then examine the possible courses of action. We shall conclude this chapter by looking at various codes of ethics and practice in relation to Kantian ethics and then discuss the possible challenges that emerge in practice.

In order to examine the situation facing Mark and to analyse it in light of Kantian principle, we must, as with any ethical dilemma, first identify precisely what the dilemma is. There are many perspectives in which this dilemma could be analysed, but we will now focus the analysis on the dilemma as being articulated as a conflict of values between the right of self-determination of Gabriella as Juanita's birth mother relinquishing her child and the possible discrimination towards Justina and Lucie as a same sex couple wishing to adopt. Mark could take the following courses of action:

a Let Justina and Lucie know that the placement is not viable and that he will be in touch with them soon when another suitable child becomes available. In this way,

Gabriella does not revoke her parental consent for Juanita to be adopted. However, Mary and Justina are discriminated against on the basis of their sexual orientation.

b Continue with the adoption process and undertake all necessary procedures with Justina and Mary, but at the same time run the risk of Gabriella revoking her parental consent for Juanita's adoption. If this were to occur, Juanita would likely be placed in temporary foster care until an adoption order was obtained from the court and new suitable adoptive parents were found.

This situation illustrates the nature of Mark's ethical dilemma in that he now has to make a decision one way or the other. While you may hold your own views about the best decision, it is clear that there are significant problems regarding either course of action.

Mark's Moral Autonomy

In what sense can a Kantian ethical framework help us resolve this dilemma? In this light, the first point is that Mark is capable of moral autonomy. Indeed, according to Kant, all individuals should be perceived as having moral autonomy, i.e. that they are capable of deciding for themselves, or self-determining. They are able to make their own decisions because they are able to think. Mark received a degree in Social Work and is therefore capable, one assumes, of critical and independent thought. Mark is also registered as a Social Worker in his province and as such, he adheres to his provincial code of ethics and Canadian Association of Social Workers (CASW) code of Ethics. For example, in the CASW Code, it is clear that qualified Social Workers are expected to think for themselves and draw from evidence and reflective practice:

> Social workers engage in lifelong learning, professional development, and self-reflection to provide evidence-informed inclusive services to diverse service users and to enhance their professional knowledge, skill, and expertise.
>
> (CASW, 2024, p. 24)

We therefore assume that Mark has an ability for practical reasoning with regard to this situation, as well as a good level of moral autonomy.

Mark's Motivation and Good Will in Making a Decision

If we continue with the application of the Kantian perspective to resolve this ethical dilemma, the other element to examine is Mark's motivation in acting in this particular situation. Again, one can only make assumptions with regard to Mark's motivation. When the time comes for you to face an ethical dilemma in practice, it will be very important for you to have some real insight into your inclination to act in a certain way or another and to carefully examine your motivations for acting. As we explained above, only good motives can justify a good action in a Kantian sense.

Therefore, only the person making the decision can truly have this insight. With regard to the case study, only Mark or the Social Worker facing such a dilemma is able to examine their deepest motivations in acting one way or another. This is the very basis of being able to engage in critical reflection with regard to an ethical dilemma. You should therefore ask yourself the following questions: Why am I inclined to act in such a way? What are my motives behind my chosen course of action? Am I *free* to act in this particular way? If not, do I have sufficient moral autonomy to challenge my own decision? Am I about to undertake this action out of a sense of duty? You must ask yourself such questions when faced with an ethical dilemma and using a Kantian framework for ethical reasoning. In order to answer the questions in Mark's situation, we must also decide who is the central focus: Justina and Lucie, Gabriella and Juanita, or both parties.

In order to analyse Mark's motivation in this case, we will again make some assertions and base our reasoning on Mark's commitment to the profession and his CASW's Code of Ethics.

We can assume that as a Social Worker, Mark is committed to a set of values common to Social Work practice. As discussed in the introduction to this section, three Social Work values tend to appear in the literature on Social Work ethics, namely, respect for persons and the self-determination of service users, commitment to the promotion of social justice, and the concept of "professional integrity" (Banks, 2020). Therefore, we can assume that Mark's inner motivation for practising Social Work is compatible with these core values and the various codes of conduct and ethics.

In examining the CASW (2024) Code of Ethics, a relatively large number of articles may be pertinent to Mark's situation. However, our purpose here is not to name them all, but instead, to focus on those that we feel are particularly relevant to motivation in this case. First, Mark has the duty to respect the inherent dignity and worth of all people (CASW,) and to promote the self-determination and autonomy of all people (CASW, 2024). This could be illustrated by his wish to work with both Lucie/Justina and Gabrielle/Juanita. Mark advocate for the rights of all individuals, families, groups and communities to be free from oppression, exclusion, racism and discrimination (Article 2.3 CASW, 2024) and upholds the principles of social justice related to the rights of individuals, families, groups, organisations and communities to receive fair and equitable access to services, resources, and opportunities and to be free of oppression, racism, and discrimination (Article 2.1 CASW, 2024). Therefore, in assuming that Mark is a qualified Social Worker who builds his practice around these core values and respects the above codes of practice and ethics, we may assert that Mark's motivation in this situation is to undertake Social Work practice within the boundaries of his profession and to leave aside any personal values he may hold. We could also posit that his motives are good because he would like to help Justina and Lucie achieve their goal of adopting a child and to assist Gabriella in the adoption process in order to find a suitable and permanent placement for Juanita.

Acting Out of a Sense of Duty: Examining the Situation through the Categorical Rules

As we saw above, Kant asserts that in order to act ethically, a person must act out of a sense of duty to good moral law, as formulated through categorical rules. We shall now examine Mark's dilemma from this perspective.

Course of Action 1: The Placement is Deemed Unviable

We will begin with the first possible course of action described above, in which Mark informs Justina and Lucie that the placement is not viable and that he will be contacting them again soon when another suitable child becomes available. In this way, Gabriella does not revoke her parental consent for Juanita to be adopted, and other potential adoptive parents can be found.

This course of action would emphasise the importance of promoting and respecting the views and wishes of Gabriella. One could claim that this course of action takes into consideration the wishes of all parties, since Justina and Lucie could have another child proposed to them rather quickly, and Gabriella could have her views taken into consideration fully. We must now examine this situation through the categorical rules. To facilitate the process of practical reasoning and to understand the difference between categorical and hypothetical rules, we will begin by providing an example of both types of rules, hypothetical and categorical. We will then examine this course of action more carefully through the principles of universality and respect for the person.

Many rules could be formulated with regard to this dilemma, as long as the rule remains general in nature. We could, for example, begin with the hypothetical rule that "If you want to ensure the best outcome for a person in an intervention, you must do anything in your power to achieve it". However, as we discussed above, Kant believes that a categorical rule will always result in a person being treated as a means to an end (respect for the person) and therefore, a hypothetical rule here is not satisfactory. Indeed, acting on this hypothetical rule would suppose that for the sake of the child, you are ready to use other people as a means to an end, that is, Justina and Lucie. Justina and Lucie's desire to have a child has been voiced for several years now, and acting in this manner would be disrespectful to them. We may wonder, however, if this hypothetical rule fails by the mere fact that it is hypothetical. Would it still fail if we articulated a categorical rule? We shall now turn to this question.

As a categorical rule, we could propose this: "Always put the best interests of the person you are working with first". Let's examine this categorical rule further and test it against the principles of universality and respect for the person set out by Kant. With regard to the former, we must enquire as to whether we could render this rule universal. In other words, are there situations in which we would not want such a moral law to be universal, or could it pass the test of applicability to any situation or context? Would it be possible to find situations in which it is not justifiable to act in such a way as to put a child's interests first? Would it be acceptable, for example, to lie in order to put the interests of a person we are working with first? If it is acceptable in one situation, can we justify that lying is something that we can render universal in order to protect the interests of all service users with whom we will work in the future? Kant would certainly tell us that if everyone lied, for whatever reason, then society could not function, and the notion of trustworthiness would disappear completely. Therefore, in light of this rule, we could assert that lying would not meet the principle of universality because there are situations in which it would be morally wrong to do whatever is needed to uphold the best interests of a person with whom we are working. The end would justify the means, and this is not morally acceptable in Kantian ethics because it does not respect the person intrinsically. Therefore, we need to find a categorical rule that would satisfy both principles. To formulate such a rule, we shall now turn to the other course of action and examine it through another set of commands.

Course of Action 2: To Continue With the Adoption Process

The second course of action is for Mark to continue with the process of working with Justina and Mary regardless of Gabriella's course of action. From Justina and Lucie's point of view, this course of action would emphasise the importance of non-discriminatory and non-oppressive practice, without taking into consideration possible outcomes, even negative ones (i.e. Gabriella removing her parental consent). We mentioned earlier, with regard to Mark's motivation, the importance of clearly identifying the main client. In reality, the categorical rule you use to help resolve a situation should apply to all situations and should not account for the possible consequences of the action. This is because Kantian ethics reminds us not only that "what is good for one is good for all" but also that a means should not justify an end. In this sense, a categorical command that may apply to this possible course of action would be "You should never discriminate against another person".

The next question to ask is whether this command would satisfy the universality principle. Would it be possible to have an example in which discrimination was acceptable and necessary? Would 'positive' discrimination be acceptable, for example? The answer to this is probably yes. For example, would it be acceptable for an agency providing services to ethnic minority women who have experienced domestic violence to positively discriminate in their recruitment strategy in order to appoint a new member who could relate to the main client group? Would this still not count as discrimination? Would our categorical command still satisfy the universality criterion? Or do we only need to formulate it better? Would our command be more universal if we refined it and specified the type of discrimination? The categorical command "You should never discriminate negatively against a person" would probably satisfy the universality criterion since, if discrimination were accepted broadly in society, this same society would go against the principles of human rights. Therefore, the categorical rule would meet this first principle.

Would it also meet the principle of respect for the person? This principle tells us that people should never be treated as a means to an end, but always as an end in themselves. Discriminating negatively against people because of their sexual orientation would not to be treating them as an end in itself, but instead, as a means to an end. Furthermore, this categorical command would also meet the principle of 'respect for the person'. Thus, in this situation, "never discriminate negatively against a person" would be a good moral command to follow. It would follow that one of the duty of Social Workers is also to respect basic human rights (CASW, 2024) as set out in the United Nations Universal Declaration of Human Rights, which specifically asserts in Article 2:

> Everyone is entitled to all the rights and freedoms set forth in this Declaration, without distinction of any kind, such as race, colour, sex, language, religion, political or other opinion, national or social origin, property, birth or other status. Furthermore, no distinction shall be made on the basis of the political, jurisdictional, or international status of the country or territory to which a person belongs, whether it be independent, trust, non-self-governing or under any other limitation of sovereignty.
>
> (United Nations, 1948)

Applied to the case above, this would probably result in Mark deciding to continue his work with Justina and Lucie in order not to discriminate against them, even though Gabriella could decide to retract her voluntary agreement for the adoption result in the process to may take longer in the end.

Reflexion Break

Looking through the code of ethics or code of practice published by the professional association who regulate practice in your jurisdiction, identify which elements would help Mark resolve the ethical dilemma presented in the case study. Which of these elements becomes apparent in terms of Kantian principles? How do they help in a course of action that stresses the importance of self-determination, duty, and autonomy?

This is one possible way of managing the ethical dilemma applying a Kantian approach. You may find the solution acceptable, or perhaps you could think of another categorical rule to test in this particular dilemma. What is important in Kantian ethics is to use your practical reason in examining your motivation for acting, and to always intervene out of a sense of duty, that is, by formulating rules that meet the two principles of universality and respect for the person, and which is coherent with your professional duties, that is those articulated in various codes of ethics in Social Work. If the categorical rule satisfies the two principles of universality and respect for the person, and your motivations are good in the intervention, then it is very likely that your decision is Kantian in essence.

You may realise that many articles found in your Code of Ethics are Kantian in nature. This Kantian legacy had a long history in Social Work, with literature on Social Work from the 1960s already articulating Social Work principles around Kantian principles.

Reflexion Break

Biestek, a Christian priest doing Social Work, had already articulated the following principles for Social Work:

- Individualisation
- Purpose expression of feelings
- Controlled emotional involvement
- Acceptance
- Non-judgemental attitude
- Client self-determination
- Confidentiality.

(Biestek, 1961)

What link can you make between these principles and the Kantian approach to ethics discussed above? Do you feel they are adequate to Social Work contemporary practice? What are the weaknesses of such principles?

The principles articulated by Biestek are mostly Kantian in nature since they are all underpinned by the respect for the person and human dignity and worth. Having said that, to be truly in a Kantian perspective, these principles would need to be articulated in commands that meet the criteria of respect for the person and universability, as we saw above, be subjected to the notion of practical reasoning, and the action be undertaken out of good will.

We have demonstrated above that practical reasoning as a way of weighing different courses of action based on Kantian principles is useful in managing ethical dilemmas. Of course, in practice, Social Workers must adhere to the various laws, policies, guidelines, and procedures of their agencies and governments, not to mention all the practical and mundane pressures that Social Workers must face on a daily basis. Such factors can affect the application of the Kantian approach in practice, a point which Banks (1995) notes when she states that the interpretation of Kant's moral philosophy may pose a problem for practical ethics because principles of self-determination and confidentiality often clash with existing rules and regulations. Warburton (2012) additionally argues that Kant's moral principles do not always yield satisfactory solutions to moral questions. For example, in Quebec, the Youth Protection Act (1984) states, "The interest of the child is the primary consideration in the application of this Act. Decisions made under this Act must be in the interest of the child and respect his rights" (3, P-34.1). Also to be considered in situations such as Justina and Lucie's is the any provincial or nation-wide human rights act – such as the Quebec Human Rights and Freedom Charter (1977) that would apply in Mark's situation above states that

> every person has a right to full and equal recognition and exercise of his human rights and freedoms, without distinction, exclusion or preference based on race, colour, sex, gender identity or expression, pregnancy, sexual orientation, civil status, age except as provided by law, religion, political convictions, language, ethnic or national origin, social condition, a handicap or the use of any means to palliate a handicap and that a distinction on any of those basis would constitute discrimination (Government of Québec, 1977)

Therefore, when applying the different Kantian principles, it is important to take these laws and regulation into consideration and not only reason in terms of Kantian principles, as demonstrated above. However, from a Kantian perspective, you should not take for granted all the rules and regulations that are imposed on you, but instead, reason practically and examine such rules and regulations before applying them to your ethical dilemma. A Kantian perspective is therefore helpful in managing the dilemma, but it cannot be applied without careful thought. You should be ready to challenge, if appropriate, any law or regulation that would be detrimental to a service user, if such a challenge follows Kantian ethics. Thus, it is not simply about applying Kantian principles for the sake of applying them, but about using these principles to help us better understands how to approach the dilemmas that occur in day-to-day practice. As Warburton illustrates, Kantian principles may appear impractical in some situations:

> If, for example, I have a duty always to tell the truth, and also a duty to protect my friend, Kant's theory would not show me what I ought to do when these two duties conflict. If a madman carrying an axe asked me where my friend was, my first inclination would be to tell him a lie. To tell the truth would be to shirk the duty I have to protect my friend. But on the other hand, according to Kant, to tell a lie, even in such an extreme situation, would be an immoral act: I have an absolute duty never to lie.
>
> (Warburton, 2012, p. 45)

In terms of ethical social care practice, Rhodes (1986) tells us that a Kantian legacy would imply that Social Workers should seek the respect of the person. However, because a Kantian approach is based on the ability to reason practically, it is important not to merely apply this principle for the sake of applying it. Using Mark's story as an example, we demonstrated that the Kantian way of resolving the ethical dilemma was not simply to apply the principle of user self-determination in an outright manner, but instead, to carefully think the case through, and examine the various principles underpinning Kantian theory. In practice, we must also balance the various interests of all the parties involved. We demonstrated in the case study that disallowing Justina and Lucie to proceed with the adoption may have shown concern for Gabriella's self-determination but would not have passed the test of universality, nor would it have treated the service users as ends in themselves. Kantian ethics is also useful in that it heightens our awareness of our own self-interest in the particular situations in which we find ourselves (Vardy and Grosch, 1999) and emphasises questions of fairness. As Hugman points out, "Kant's categorical command can be seen as a statement that implies fairness as a moral good, because it asserts that what applies for one person should apply for everyone in similar circumstances" (2005, p. 16). However, even though a Kantian perspective may be applied to a dilemma in practice, it is also important to remember that the situation remains a dilemma and ultimately involves the difficult task of making a decision one way or another. The Kantian perspective will provide you, however, with a framework for analysing your dilemma that is compatible with the values of Social Work as formulated in our codes of practice, in other words, a commitment to the values of an individual's right to dignity, respect, privacy, and confidentiality. These values are directly inspired by Kant's moral philosophy and remain important in everyday Social Work practice.

Conclusion

Kant was one of the most important moral philosophers of the Enlightenment, and his philosophy continues to have a major influence on contemporary moral theory and attitudes, not the least of which is contemporary Social Work practice. Kant based his moral philosophy on the fact that all human beings have the ability to reason, and that as long as actions are taken out of good will and a sense of duty, then they are morally right. For Kant, a good moral law must meet the criteria of two categorical commands, namely, universality and respect for the person. The influence of the Kantian tradition on Social Work today is illustrated by the various codes of ethics and practice that exist in the profession and which are based on the principles of respect for the person and the notion that "what is good for one is also good for all".

9 The Ethics of Mill, Bentham and Rawls

Social justice is an important principle of Social Work. The Code of Ethics in Social Work often identifies social justice as a core value, which, along with the principle of human dignity, serves as a central motivation and justification for Social Work action. The term 'justice' itself is very broad and can be understood differently depending on the many theoretical frameworks applied to it. In fact, like the concept of power discussed in Chapter 3, Scott and Marshall (2009) note that the concept of social justice is subject to wide disagreement among sociologists, social psychologists, and philosophers. In the context of this book, the concept of social justice broadly relates to justice applied to social life. However, what does the term justice mean? What does it imply? What does it mean to intervene within a social justice perspective? How can we make the right decisions when faced with a dilemma that brings to light issues of social justice?

To answer these questions, we will examine two broad sets of theories that articulate different ways of understanding social justice. First, we will look at *utilitarian ethics*, examining the work of John Stuart Mill and, to a lesser extent, the work of Jeremy Bentham. We chose to examine utilitarian ethics because the principles it outlines concern mostly social issues and remain widely used today. Next, we will look at the *theory of justice* developed by John Rawls. Rawls remains one of the most influential philosophers of our time, and his theory continues to form the basis of many laws and policies, especially those of liberal orientations. By examining these two broad theoretical perspectives, we will gain an understanding of what can be considered a 'just' outcome, providing us with a framework for analysing specific situations in Social Work practice as well as more generally to social life.

As in the previous chapters, we will present an analysis of a case study drawing on the two ethical perspectives. We will also establish links with the principle of social justice as formulated in IFSW and BASW codes. The purpose here is to help develop your understanding of the continued influence of these theories on the formulation and management of ethical issues in Social Work and to assist you in the process of 'practical reasoning'. We will conclude this chapter by drawing some conclusions about the meaning of social justice as applied to contemporary Social Work.

Utilitarian Ethics

Utilitarian ethics is often described as a form of *ethical consequentialism*. This means that in order to assess an action as being right or wrong, we examine carefully the different possible consequences that may result from different courses of action (Figure 9.1).

DOI: 10.4324/9781003458715-13

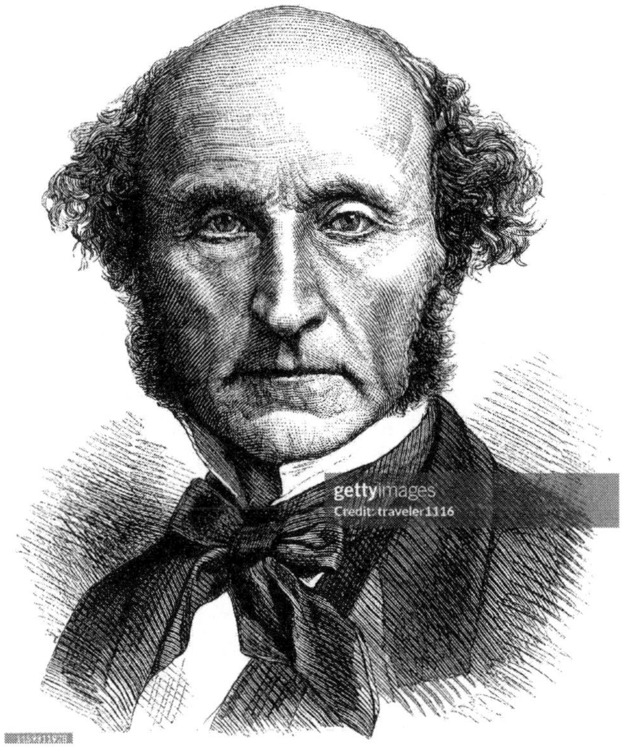

Figure 9.1 John Stuart Mill

So, how does this play out in everyday life? Let's say that you are walking on the street and you cross paths with a homeless person asking for some money. While most people will not spend much time thinking about their decision or the justification for it, there are different reasons you may decide to give or not to give some spare coins to the person in front of you. First, you could say that giving money is the right thing to do because you have many privileges and material resources to survive while the other person is in need, so to share what you have with others is what you have to do. You can probably see from this example that the decision to give money is made on the basis of what you considered to be good, regardless of the consequences of your action. This may remind you of Kantian ethics, whereby the motivation behind the action is central.

Another way of deciding could be to think about the impact of your actions. If you were to adopt a consequentialist perspective, you would think about all the possible consequences of giving money or not giving money to the person in order to make your decision. For example, you could think that giving money may allow them to eat a warm meal at night or to prevent them from going hungry. With this line of argument, you are clearly thinking about the consequences of your action, that is, by preventing negative outcomes for the person or facilitating a better one. This type of justification would fit within the consequentialist perspective. This type of justification aligns with the consequentialist perspective. Whether you agree with this reasoning or not, it highlights the potential positive or negative consequences of an action rather than motivations based on a sense of duty.

Utilitarian Ethics as a form of Consequentialisms

Have you ever heard someone say that a good outcome is an outcome that will facilitate *the greatest happiness for the greatest number?* This catch phrase is, in its simplest form, what utilitarian ethics believe in. As we will see later, utilitarian ethics is more complex, but simply put, an action that is right will maximise the welfare, or the likelihood of achieving the greatest good for the greatest number of people possible.

The Concept of 'Greatest Good'

John Stuart Mill, one of the fathers of utilitarian ethics, suggested that what is considered to be 'greatest good' in fact correlates with the *outcome that will produce the most pleasure* and *the least pain.*

In fact, Mill believes people will always try to maximise their pleasure and minimise their pain. While this may be debatable, Mill thought that the more people have pleasure, the happier they are likely to be. In this sense, the pursuit of pleasure corresponds, in his perspective, to the pursuit of happiness.

But how do we know if a type of happiness is better than another? What leads to more happiness? To finish a marathon? To read a book from your favourite author? To attend a wedding of a dear old friend?

Earlier versions of utilitarian ethics, such as the one proposed by Jeremy Bentham, proposed that pain and pleasures could simply be measured quantitatively according to seven criteria:

- intensity
- duration
- certainty
- extent
- remoteness
- richness
- purity.

According to this earlier version of the theory, the action that would ensure the best outcome and produce the greatest amount of pleasure would meet the most criteria. As such, pleasure was measured in terms of quantity. As such, reading your favourite book might not bring as much happiness as completing a marathon, as the latter requires extensive and rigorous training. However, this could be debatable, as the idea of running a marathon might also bring to mind a lot of pain in preparing for and doing it!

What do you think of this way of calculating pleasure? Do you see any difficulties in applying those criteria to assess the idea of pleasure and pain?

Continuing on this work, Mill warns us to consider that one should not only consider the quantity of pain and pleasure but also its *quality*. For example, a person may have many acquaintances or thousands of 'friends' on social media (quantity) but have no real friends (quality). Is a person with many friends on social media happier than someone who has one or two real friends with whom they can have profound discussions about life? For Mill, it is therefore important to examine both the quality and quantity of pain and pleasure that may result from an action:

> According to the greatest happiness principle, the ultimate end, with reference to and for the sake of which all other things are desirable (whether we are considering our own good or that of other people), is an existence exempt as far as possible from pain, and as rich as possible in enjoyment both in the point of quantity and quality; the test of quality, and the rule for measuring it against quantity, being the preference felt by those, who in their opportunity of experience to which must be added their habit of self-consciousness and self-observation, are best furnished with the means of comparison.
>
> (2004, p. 17)

Thus, the 'greatest good' can be assessed by examining whether the consequences of an action will lead to happiness by providing pleasure, which can be measured both qualitatively and quantitatively. That said, other questions remain: Is happiness not a subjective expression of feeling? How do we make sure – pain and pleasure apart – that an action will lead to more happiness than another? Is happiness always related to experiencing a maximum pleasure and a minimum of pain? Is someone who likes some form of pain (a masochist) necessarily unhappy? An athlete training for their next marathon must go through considerable pain to achieve the goal of a medal. Does this not somehow contradict "pleasure equals happiness"?

These questions can be settled, according to Mill, because the happiness that an action confers also needs to be assessed in terms of its *utility – not just in terms of pain and pleasure*. The greatest good for Mill is, in fact, the course of action that maximises the quantity and quality of happiness by virtue of its usefulness in a given situation. In other words, for a course of action to be right, it must not only promote happiness but also be useful.

But this, again, can pose some problems if you think about that. For example, if you work with a service user who currently lives in the community and requires a high level of care, and her daughter, the only natural carer, is exhausted and demands that her mother be placed in residential care against the wishes of her mother, what course of action will you support based on happiness and utility? This example demonstrates competing demands that often cannot be maximised simultaneously. Of course, you would undertake a thorough assessment of the situation and have in hand all the relevant policies and legislation, but the fundamental question remains: whose happiness should you favour? According to utilitarian ethics, to decide if an action is right or wrong, we must not only look at the results, but also figure out which results will bring the most happiness to the most people thanks to their usefulness. We will now look at the second part of the slogan, the 'greatest number', to further explore the concept of utility.

The Concept of 'Greatest Number'

Put simply, what is considered to be promoting the greatest good, the greatest happiness, or, as we have just seen, the greatest utility, is also what will produce an outcome benefiting the greatest number of people involved in a situation. This is supported by the belief that it is the sum of individual interests that makes up the collective interest. As Almond (1995, p. 7) explains, "For a utilitarian, a multiplicity of individual interests – what is good for each member of society – make up the common interest – what is good for all, or at least the most". For the utilitarian, then, the ethically right action is that which maximises the welfare of the greatest number of people based on utility Of course, this necessitates considering utility when conducting assessments, as the example above illustrates, as we may find ourselves in a situation where one person's needs may be prioritised over those of the caregiver. Vardy and Grosh (2016) provide an interesting example to illustrate this point in their discussion about utilitarian ethics. They explain that abortion is neither good nor bad, as it involves one person against another, but it only becomes a question of rightness or wrongness when we consider its intended purpose, that is, how it satisfies the greatest good for the greatest number in terms of its utility. Therefore, the authors suggest that abortion is morally acceptable when used to control the birth of a tenth child in a low-income family, but immoral when performed on a young married woman because it interferes with her career (Vardy and Grosch, 2016). The concepts of utility and the greatest number are clearly illustrated in this example.

Another important point in the utilitarian theory of justice is that one's decision-making should remain impartial. As Mill explains, "All persons are deemed to have the right to equality of treatment except when some recognised social expediency requires the reverse" (Mill, 2004, p. 93). This means that equal rights should be upheld as much as possible, unless some conditions that promote the greatest good for the greatest number require us to act otherwise. Therefore, according to the utilitarian perspective, in order to act ethically, you may have to compromise your own interests with those of others. In this sense, this theory views justice as balancing private interest with public interest.

The Greatest Good for the Greatest Number as a Method of Ethics

We have seen that the morally right action is defined in terms of its consequences with regard to the utility it brings in a given situation. As such, act-utilitarianism will support an action as morally good as long as the action itself is conducive to general happiness. It is the value of the consequences of one act or another that is then used to examine general happiness. For example, a Social Worker in a food bank has just conducted an assessment and realises that the needs of the service user in question are valid but that the service user's particular situation does not meet the eligibility criteria. Applying the principle of the "the greatest good for the greatest number", as we have seen, would require examining the consequences of action or non-action in this situation in terms of its utility for the various parties.

The two basic actions that could be taken in this situation are as follows: the Social Worker bends the rules and offers food to the person, or the Social Worker does not bend the rules and does not offer food to the person. Applying the utilitarian perspective would mean weighing the different consequences. Simply put, we could argue that bending the rules would result in the family having access to food, and since this only involves one family, the other service users may not feel the effect. On the other hand, not giving food to the family may result in further problems for them. Therefore, through the simple application of the "greatest good for the greatest number", it would be justifiable to bend the rules because it would promote the happiness of most people in this situation, that is, the family. This way of applying "the greatest good for the greatest number" is called the act-utilitarian perspective. Act-utilitarianism, in its simplest form, is founded on the belief that "every action should be taken so as to maximise happiness" (Graham, 2004, p. 144). This means that you must consider the whole situation and weigh each consequence in terms of its utility for all those involved.

As you may have surmised from the above example, the act-utilitarian perspective may present some problems in that it can be too permissive or be used to justify many actions, even unethical ones, if the value of a particular course of action in terms of its consequences can be considered above all others.

For example, as Mill explains in his book *Utilitarianism*:

> It appears from what has been said that justice is a name for certain moral requirements, which regarded collectively, stand higher in the scale of social utility and are therefore of more paramount obligation than any others; though particular cases may occur in which some other social duties are so important as to overrule any one of the general maxims of justice. Thus, to save a life, it may not only be allowable, but a duty, to steal or take by force the necessary food or medicine or kidnap and compel to officiate the only qualified medical practitioner.
>
> (2004, pp. 93–94)

In other words, act-utilitarianism should be used with caution, and it is in this context that we will now look at a variation of this perspective: 'rule-utilitarianism'.

What is the Difference Between 'Act' and 'Rule'-Utilitarianism?

Act-utilitarianism is based on the prediction of the consequence of one particular action. As long as the outcome will produce the greatest happiness for the greatest number, the action can be justified.

Rule-utilitarianism is similar to the 'act' version but claims that the action will only be good if the consequences are good and that the action is universalisable into law.

Rule-Utilitarianism

Rule-utilitarianism suggests that, instead of being determined by the utility of the difference/consequence of one particular action, our actions should be determined by *rules* that, if generally followed, would lead to the greatest happiness (Graham, 2004). Such rules take priority over individual actions and do not allow for exceptions. Therefore, "the greatest good for the greatest number" still applies, but for a *rule* as opposed to a single situation. Indeed, under rule-utilitarianism, rules are developed under utilitarian principles, that is, they promote the greatest happiness for the greatest number: if followed, they will lead to morally right action; if not, they will lead to morally wrong action. Let us now return to the example of the Social Worker who must decide whether or not to bend the rules at a food bank for a particular service user. We saw that under act-utilitarianism, bending the rules may be deemed 'morally right' in such a situation. Let us now consider the same situation under the rule-utilitarian perspective. We now must define a rule that will apply to everyone. We may ask if it is morally right to bend a rule if a service user needs a service that he or she cannot access otherwise. We must now determine whether this rule would lead to the greatest good for the greatest number for all similar cases. Obviously, if rules are bent to meet every exception, the system would soon fall apart. In this sense, the rule applied in this case would become useless and not produce the greatest good for the greatest number, and resources, which are always limited, would not be sufficient to help those who truly need them, i.e., the majority of users. Therefore, under the rule-utilitarian approach, bending the rule would not be morally right since it would not promote the greatest happiness for the greatest number. To achieve the greatest happiness, everyone must obey the rule; for the principle to be utilitarian, it must maximise utility for the greatest number.

Rule-utilitarianism is useful in so far as that instead of simply weighing the consequences of one action, it looks at the rule that, if applied to a given action, would maximise the welfare of the majority. Rule utilitarianism may therefore help to counteract some of the difficulties associated with act utilitarianism.

Reflexion Break

- Try to summarise the two versions of utilitarian ethics.
- What are the main differences between act-utilitarianism and rule-utilitarianism?
- How do you feel they can be applied to ethical deliberation in Social Work?
- Can you see any limitations in applying them to Social Work practice?
- How can these perspectives help you in dealing with ethical dilemmas related to social justice?

The ultimate end of both versions of utilitarian ethics is to serve the majority of people involved in a situation. Therefore, using both approaches in the resolution of an ethical dilemma may help in weighing right and wrong actions by examining the consequences they have on society in general. For the utilitarian,

> Justice is a name for certain moral requirements, which regarded collectively, stand higher in the scale of social utility, and are therefore of more paramount obligation than any others; though particular cases may occur in which some other social duties is so important, as to overrule any one of the general maxims of justice.
>
> (Mill, 2004, p. 54)

As we stated at the beginning of the chapter, the utilitarian tradition largely influences society's rules, crafting many laws to cater to the majority and thereby maximising utility for the greatest number. Anti-Social Behaviour Orders are clearly an example of utilitarian policies that are established so that the majority can live happily without a 'troubling minority'. In addition, various codes of conduct are influenced by utilitarian values (Banks, 2020; Rhodes, 1986).

Although utilitarianism is considered one of the main approaches to ethics in Social Work (and one of the three moral perspectives we have chosen to cover in Part 3 of this book), a chapter on social justice would not be complete without discussing, even briefly, another theory of justice, that of John Rawls. Not only will this theory help us further our understanding of social justice, but it will also address some of the limitations identified above with regard to utilitarian ethics.

Rawls's Theory of Justice

John Rawls (1921–2002), an American born in Baltimore, USA, was one of the most important political philosophers of the twentieth century. His theory of justice was

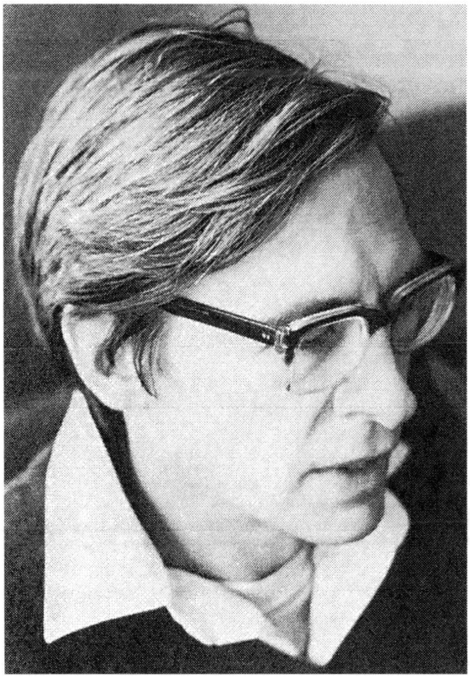

Figure 9.2 John S. Rawls

inspired by many Kantian principles (see Chapter 8) and was developed as an attempt to oppose some of the premises articulated in the utilitarian perspective. The aim of his work was to establish fundamental principles that, if followed, would provide a model for organising social life based on cooperation and consensus (Figure 9.2).

He spent the greater part of his life working at Harvard University, where he published his *Theory of* Justice (1971). Rawls attempted to formulate principles of justice that, instead of favouring the majority (as in utilitarianism), would consider each person equally important and worthy. As such, Rawls proposed a conception of justice equated with fairness. Indeed, by defining a basis for equality and fundamental rights, his theory is an attempt to establish principles in which the rights of individuals are central but in which inequalities are impossible to avoid. Such a conception provides minimal protection for the oppressed and marginalised of society (Rawls, 1971). Rawls's theory of justice also proposes a shift away from utilitarian principles of ethics, in which justice is no longer understood as a matter of utility and majority of interests but instead as a matter of fairness and fundamental liberties.

Rawls (1971) on 'Equality', 'Fairness' and 'Justice'

Rawls understands 'equality' in terms of positions between people, whereas he discusses 'fairness' in terms of procedures in deliberation. 'Justice' is the result contained in the principles that have emerged as a process of equality and fairness in defining principles.

The Conditions for a Theory of Justice: Social Contract, Original Position, and the Veil of Ignorance

The basis of Rawls theory is what he calls a 'social contract'. For Rawls, a social contract involves a set of rules that, through reason, are determined and agreed upon by everyone in any given society. The social contract, once agreed, is to be maintained by the state and its political system, which will then provide the necessary conditions to ensure that people can achieve their goals and live a good life. A social contract in the Rawlsian sense involves basic liberties and equalities. Fundamental to this principle is the respect for individuals and their ability to reason, two concepts borrowed from Kant (see Chapter 8 for further discussion). The notion of social contact is fundamental to Rawls's theory of justice. From this, a first question may be asked: How can we achieve Rawls's notion of social contract, that is,

> **Rawls's Social Contract**
>
> A social contract is a form of agreement that people consent to live by in society.

a contract that is determined and agreed by everyone? Indeed, how can self-interest be controlled in the definition of such a contract? Given that there are many power relationships in society, if a group is made up of individuals with different needs and interests, how can we guarantee that this group will be able to define and agree on rules that suit everyone? Can the interests of an unemployed single mother be represented on the same basis as those of a powerful banker? Indeed, this represents quite a challenge since a social contract is one that is agreed upon by all individuals. Rawls believes that this is possible as long as two conditions are met: the 'original position' and the 'veil of ignorance'. Put simply, these two concepts provide the two necessary conditions for developing the principles of justice that will benefit people both individually and collectively.

The *original position* means that people are placed in a situation of equality, and the *veil of ignorance* implies that people develop the principles of justice without knowing what their condition would be in a hypothetical society; people therefore have no way of knowing how they would be personally affected by such principles.

Let us now take a look at these two conditions.

The 'original position' is a hypothetical situation in which everyone is placed in an equal social position. In the original position, there are no power relationships between the 'rich' and the 'poor', or in terms of race, gender, sexuality, gender role, disability, culture, religion or any other difference that could generate social inequalities. Consequently, the original position requires people to forget about who they are and just 'be' as everyone else. However, given that such a situation is unlikely to occur (we live in a society with many social inequalities, and it is difficult to act against our own interests), Rawls adds a second condition – that people wear a 'veil of ignorance'. Rawls explains that under the veil of ignorance, people "do not know how the various alternatives will affect their own particular case, and they are obliged to evaluate the principles solely on the basis of general considerations" (Rawls, 1971, p. 136) (Figure 9.3).

The 'veil of ignorance' is a concept in which individuals must 'blindly' decide on the rules that make up their 'social contract'. In other words, under the veil of ignorance – i.e., without knowing their future roles, status, position, cultural heritage, general health, religion

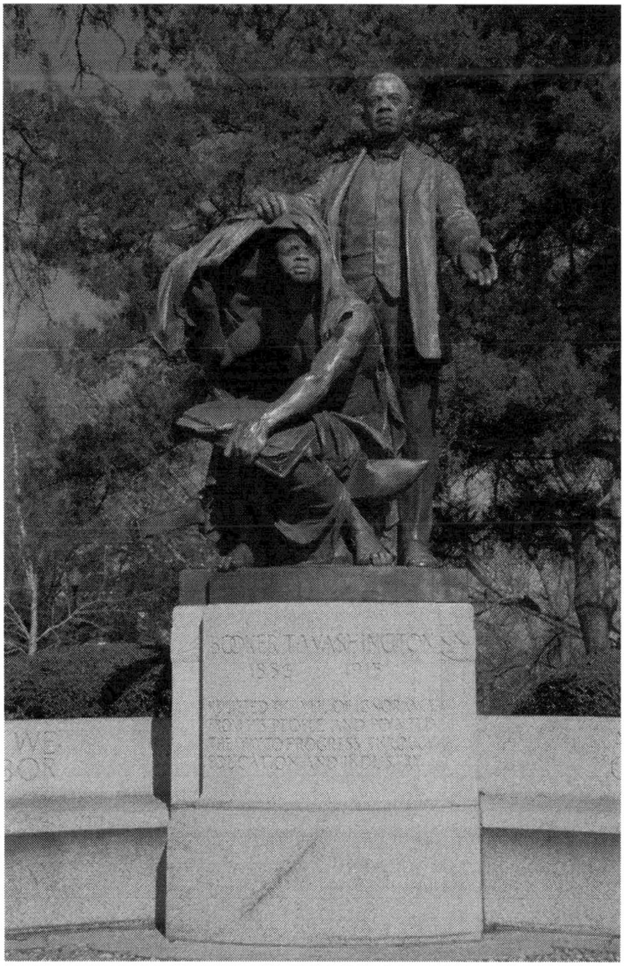

Figure 9.3 Lifting the veil of ignorance

etc. – people must define and agree on rules that are then used to organise social life. Thus, "If the individuals concerned do not know what position they will occupy in society, then it is rational for them to agree that each should receive a 'fair distribution of primary social goods'" (Fives, 2008, p. 46). In other words, this process ensures that people from all walks of life have an equal representation in the definition of the principles of justice. Without an advantage in 'the original position' and wearing 'the veil of ignorance', everyone should end up with the same principles as formulated by Rawls.

Reflexion Break

Imagine you are on a desert island with five other people. You are a recognised leader and have many strategic ideas. The other people are a pregnant woman, a child, a wounded doctor, a healthy man, and a craftsman.

There is only enough food (one goat, two litres of milk, five litres of water, one kilogram of nuts) for three people to survive for one week until you find more resources.

1 Try to imagine how you would share the food. Define the principles you would use to share the food among yourselves. Take some notes about the reasons for your choices.
2 Now imagine you are in the original position and wearing the veil of ignorance. This implies that you are no longer the person who allocates the food and that you could be any of the people described above. Again, try to define some principles for sharing the food and note the reasons for defining such principles
3 Are the principles you came up with the same as those when you were not in the original position and wearing the veil of ignorance?

Let us now explore the principles of justice as formulated by Rawls.

Rawls's Principles of Justice

You may have gathered in the reflection break that it is not any easy task to distribute limited resources or any other 'goods' in the Rawlsian sense. To achieve this task fairly, Rawls proposes two fundamental principles for allocating goods, including liberties, opportunities, and material goods:

1 the principle of equal liberty
2 the principle of equality of opportunity and the difference principle.

As you can see, these principles are numbered. According to Rawls, the order of these principles is important because only when the first principle (liberty) is met can the second principle be applied. There are also certain conditions under which this can happen. We shall now look at these principles in more detail.

Rawls Often Refers to the Concept of 'Goods'. What Does This Concept Mean in Terms of the Principles of Justice?

For Rawls, the notion of 'goods' to be distributed in Box 1 Para includes material goods, public services, wealth, power, etc. However, Rawls makes an important distinction between primary goods such as liberty of expression and political liberty and material goods such as wealth, financial resources and property.

Equal Liberty:

The first principle, related to basic liberties, reads as follows:

> Each person has an equal claim to a fully adequate scheme of equal basic rights and liberties, which scheme is compatible with the same scheme for all; and in this

> scheme the equal political liberties, and only those liberties, are to be guaranteed their fair value.
>
> (Rawls, 1993 in Lamont and Favor, 2007, pp. 5–6)

In other words, this principle dictates the equal distribution of all fundamental liberties: what is permissible for one should also be permissible for all.

How, you may ask, can this be achieved? It is important to note that Rawls did not consider all types of 'goods' to be of equal importance. Included in his first principle are only those 'goods' related to fundamental rights, such as political liberty, liberty of expression and assembly, the freedom of personal property, that is, the liberty to think and to choose what one believes in. Other liberties, such as having the right to own a big house or having a particular social status within a group or community, are not covered by Rawls's first principle of *basic fundamental liberties*. In defining what can be considered an acceptable social contract, Rawls comes to the conclusion that in the original position and under the veil of ignorance, individuals would likely accept this first principle as being fair. Indeed, if you had to define and agree on the principles of liberty but did not know what social position you would occupy in a future society or what religion you would practice (veil of ignorance), you would certainly agree on ensuring maximum rights and liberties.

In the context of Social Work, we can interpret this principle as follows: every individual has the right to fundamental liberties, irrespective of their age, gender, culture, class, ability or any other factor that could distinguish them from others. According to Rawls, this means that no matter whom you provide services to, each person, by law, should be treated in the same way as others. Many of the fundamental liberties that Rawls cites can be found in such documents as the Universal Declaration of Human Rights; for example, Article 1: "All human beings are born free and equal in dignity and rights". You can see in this article that no attention is paid to a person's origin, age, or any other distinctive feature. Clearly, in this principle, everyone is equal in terms of basic rights and liberties.

Now that the question of basic liberties is covered, you must wonder why there are so many inequalities in society. The first answer is that Rawls's principles are not necessarily integrated or even interpreted everywhere the same way. Of course, while Rawlsian principles are recognised as extremely influential, how they are applied in each country may vary. For example, in the UK, some laws are still deemed incompatible with the Universal Declaration of Human Rights. The court has the right to make 'declarations of incompatibility' between home legislations and the Universal declaration of Human Rights. While Article 9 of the Universal Declaration of Human Rights asserts that no one shall be subject to arbitrary arrest, detention, or exile, the Anti-Terrorism, Crime, and Security Act 2001 permits the police to stop and search people arriving at the border without grounds. Those two principles are clearly incompatible. In Canada, while the Federal Government supports the principles of the Universal Declaration of Human Rights through the Canadian Charter of Rights and Freedoms and has ratified the principal conventions and covenants, it is still possible for a provincial government to pass laws that would be deemed incompatible with human rights by using what they call the 'notwithstanding clause'. Using this clause prevents any human rights challenges for a period of up to five years. For example, in the Province of Quebec, the Coalition Avenir Quebec (CAQ) government used the notwithstanding close in 2021 when they adopted Bill 21, *Act Respecting the Laicity of the* State, to ban public service workers and teachers from wearing religious signs such as hijabs, kippahs, and crosses. This bill, now in effect, clearly limits those groups' ability to obtain work if they wear religious symbols, unless they were already employed before the law was passed.

As you can see, not every country applies all of the human rights defined in the Convention, and some countries may enact laws that clearly violate some of the Convention's principles. Therefore, while Rawls's first principle is fundamental to many current acts and legislations in many parts of the world, some of the liberties are not always seen as compatible with regional legislation, and therefore, not everyone's access to these basic rights is always guaranteed.

We shall now turn to the second principle of Rawls's theory of justice and examine how, where inequalities are unavoidable, society can still be based on social justice principles.

Equality of Fair Opportunity and the Difference Principle

How can we equally distribute goods that are not considered fundamental and that are scarce? What principle could we use to help us decide on the distribution of resources in the Reflexion Break exercise above?

Rawls proposes a second principle for achieving justice but also reminds us that to apply this second principle we must ensure that the first principle has been satisfied. Rawls formulates his second principle as follows:

> Social and economic inequalities are to satisfy two conditions: (a) they are to be attached to positions and offices open to all under conditions of fair equality of opportunity; and (b), they are to be to the greatest benefit of the least advantaged members of society.
>
> (Rawls, 1993 in Lamont and Favor, 2007, pp. 5–6)

What Rawls is saying here is that if inequalities must exist in society, they shall not be about basic fundamental liberties, and they shall only be acceptable if they benefit the least advantaged of society. Let us explore what this means in practice.

Imagine a hypothetical situation in which a company wishes to recruit a new employee to perform a series of tasks that no one in the company is able or qualified to perform. The company decides to advertise the job at a higher salary than most employees receive because the job requires a higher qualification and involves many difficult tasks. According to Rawls, it may be acceptable to pay someone a higher salary, even though this could be considered 'unequal'. However, for it to be fair, you would need to satisfy two conditions: first, you would need to make sure that there are procedures that guarantee equal access to the job and that the opportunities for applying are fair. There are many levels at which this principle could be applied. First, there is the obvious equal opportunity strategy to be used in advertising the job, as well as a fair assessment of all candidate profiles. However, we could also apply the principle at a higher level and examine whether everyone of equal ability has the opportunity to develop their skills equally. Given the current social inequalities that exist in most Western countries, it is unlikely that such a situation would pass the first principle of justice as formulated by Rawls. Indeed, there are many inequalities with regard to access to education, for example. One could argue that not every one of the same abilities has equal access to higher education, and therefore, this would not meet the first part of the second principle. Economic inequalities may prevent eligible people from accessing education. A just society, in Rawls's terms, would be one that promotes equal opportunity for equal ability, skills etc. Therefore, if we return to our example above, even if the company put various mechanisms in place to ensure equal opportunity in the hiring process, there would still remain other factors to consider regarding the second principle, that is, ensuring equal opportunity for everyone to meet the requirements of the job (e.g. ensuring higher education or overall life opportunities), but this would need to be analysed at a much higher level.

The second part of the principle explains that if inequalities are to be present in society, they must be for the benefit of the most disadvantaged of society. To illustrate, let's return to our example of having a higher salary for a more skilled job. Rawls would probably argue that a higher salary can only be justified if it benefits everyone, including those who earn less in the company and society as a whole. However, how can this principle be achieved? Again, we would probably need to analyse the situation at a higher level and determine, for example, whether the higher salary means more tax revenues and whether these revenues are reinvested in social programmes to serve the most disadvantaged of society. While this example may be simplistic, it effectively demonstrates how the second principle can allow inequalities while still promoting a society based on fair principles.

Reflexion Break

Placing yourself in the conditions of the original position and the veil of ignorance, would you agree with the principles of justice as formulated by Rawls?

How would you apply these principles to the 'desert island' 'exercise above'? How would you distribute the food?

What would be the difficulties of applying Rawls's theory of justice to the 'desert island' example?

Returning to our desert island exercise, you may begin to realise that Rawls's theory of justice is not quite suited to the management of routine ethical dilemmas but is more useful for defining and developing policies that are just. In fact, one of the critiques of Rawls's theory is that it is more a political philosophy than an ethical perspective. As such, while it helps to understand the concept of social justice in a certain way, it is more useful for examining the notion of justice and defining the principles of justice within institutions and organisations than it is for analysing ethical issues as in the Kantian and utilitarian perspectives.

Having said this, applying Rawls's principle of justice to the desert island situation would require you to define principles for the distribution of the resources. Based on Rawls's principles, you could justify the decision of giving more food to those who are able to cross the island because it would give an advantage in the long term to those who are not able to. Indeed, those who are 'fitter' to cross the island may need more resources to do so, but the inequality of the distribution of resources would be offset by the advantage it would bring to everyone. Therefore, what is considered a priori as 'unfair', that is, giving more food to a few, would be justified, according to Rawls, as fair because such inequalities will eventually benefit the most vulnerable.

One critique of Rawls's theory is whether or not it is possible for individuals to fully detach themselves from their social and historical contexts when defining principles of justice. Indeed, the essence of the veil of ignorance is that individuals will make decisions not knowing where they are located in the socio-political spectrum of society. Another problem with Rawls's theory is that for some moral theorists, it is neither possible nor desirable to separate yourself from your social, cultural, and historical background when trying to understand moral issues. This is something we talked about in the introduction of this book, as well as in Chapter 7 when we presented about decolonial ethics and will talk about again in Chapter 10 when we talk about virtue ethics. Finally, some scholars argue that the concept of justice should not be analysed in terms of resources (or primary goods) but instead in terms of social practises (Mullaly and West, 2018)

In sum, Rawls provides a useful framework for understanding the notion of social justice and proposes, through his theory, a way of achieving a society in which everyone agrees on the principles of justice. Rawlsian principles don't really tell us how to do things in real life, like how to handle an ethical dilemma in Social Work, but they do tell us how to apply justice principles to policies or organisations.

In the first part of this chapter, we examined two different broad ethical theories to understand the concept of social justice. We saw that utilitarian ethics is commonly used in the welfare state and continues to influence some of the articles found in the codes of ethics of the UK and elsewhere. We also saw that Rawls's theory of justice helps to address some of the shortcomings of utilitarian ethics, especially with regard to integrating some of Kant's principles (see Chapter 8). Nevertheless, both theories provide us with two valid frameworks for understanding and applying decisions in terms of justice. We now propose to look at a case study and to see how both the utilitarian and the Rawlsian theories of justice can help us make decisions related to Social Work ethics.

Case Study: Mourad's Story

Mourad is a qualified Social Worker who works for the asylum seekers team in a social services department of the West Midlands. He has been asked to assess Sithembiso, a young woman who arrived unaccompanied from Sudan. The police picked her up two weeks ago at a service station in their local authority area. Since that time, she has been seeking asylum with the authorities. She has no identification papers with her.

Following a thorough psychosocial assessment in cooperation with other agencies, Mourad is of the opinion that Sithembiso is around 15 years old. However, the Council had also asked for the medical report, which states that she is more likely to be 17–18 years old. When Mourad meets with his manager, Helen, to discuss the discrepancy between the team's report and the medical report, including the report of the dental x-ray, Helen takes the view that the medical report is most likely the correct one. When Mourad and Helen discuss the details of the psychosocial assessment, Helen asserts that Sithembiso may be decreasing her real age to qualify for care and support from the local authority under Child Welfare legislation. She also mentions that this claim is likely aimed at gaining more support and enabling her to attend school immediately. Based on the medical report, Helen asserts that the department's official stance must be that Sithembiso is not eligible for any additional support as an unaccompanied minor.

Mourad is concerned not only by this case but also by a number of recent cases in which his team was convinced that the asylum seekers were younger than 18 – always around 15–16 years old, even though the medical methods of age assessment, focusing mainly on dental x-rays, classified them as older. Mourad is perplexed as he has read that an emerging body of evidence points to the questionable reliability of these tests for young people aged between 15 and 20 years, and on that basis, he questions the inappropriateness of using such tests as the sole measure of age assessment at his local authority department. Mourad also feels that her manager's attitude reflects an increasing culture of cynicism and disbelief among the staff team. He asked his manager if he could present his findings as evidence at the next team meeting to initiate a discussion on the age assessment of unaccompanied asylum seekers, but they denied his request. Mourad's manager, Helen, has now asked him to modify his report and close the case.

Reflection Break

Looking back through the case study:

1 Identify the ethical dilemma facing Mourad;
2 Identify the various courses of action Mourad can take;
3 Write down what you feel are the most important elements to consider in each course of action you identified above. Why do you feel these are important?
4 How would you express the issues facing Mark in terms of social justice?

Analysis

The dilemma faced by Mourad raises many controversial issues. The main elements of the case are as follows: (1) Mourad is engaged in a professional relationship with Sithembiso; (2) Mourad estimates Sithembiso's is minor and aged about 15 years old; (3) the medical examination estimates her to be 17–18 years old; (4) the manager is of the opinion that the medical report is correct; (5) Mourad recognise the potential limitation of dental x-rays in estimating the youth between 15 and 20 years old; (6) Mourad is in disagreement with the management position; and (7) Helen asks Mourad to alter his report.

To move forward with the analysis, we will formulate the situation as an ethical dilemma:

- Mourad is faced with the choice between fighting his position and continue to support Sithembiso's claim that she is 15, or,
- Mourad let go of this case and modified his report as demanded by his manager.

Before analysing any ethical dilemma, you should always review the code of ethics published by your professional association or the Social Work regulator in your area. Codes of ethics are always a useful starting point to manage an ethical dilemma, as they can help you to reflect on your professional values during the analysis. Since this book caters to a global readership, we provide below a few excerpts from ethics codes that could aid in analysing Mourad's story. However, we encourage you to carry out this task independently, referencing pertinent codes of ethics to pinpoint articles that could have local relevance to this case (Table 9.1).

It is also important to keep in mind, from consequentialist perspective, that a breach of code of ethics could lead a Social Worker to be subjected to professional discipline in many parts of the world.[1] This could lead to serious consequences, such as being suspended temporarily or striking off the professional register and losing the right to practice your profession. Consequences of a disciplinary action could also ripple to services

Table 9.1 Examples of article from BASW 2021 and IFSW 2018

British Association of Social Workers' Code of Ethics (2021)	*International Federation of Social Workers' Global Social Work Statement of Ethical Principle (2018)*
Responsibility for relieving and preventing hardship and for promoting wellbeing is not always fully discharged by direct service to individuals, families, and groups. Social workers have a duty to: Challenging unjust policies and practices: Social workers are expected to bring to the attention of their employers, policy makers, politicians, and the general public situations where resources are inadequate, and/or where distribution of resources, policies and practice are oppressive, discriminatory or otherwise unfair, harmful or illegal; Challenge oppression on any basis, respect diversity of the community which they practice; Social workers should demonstrate a clear commitment to anti-oppressive practice. Distributing resources: Social workers should advocate for access to, and equitable distribution of, resources. Empowering people: Social workers should make decisions about sharing information legally and ethically. Human rights and social justice serve as the motivation and justification for Social Work action. In solidarity with those who are disadvantaged, the profession strives to alleviate poverty and to work with vulnerable and oppressed people in order to promote social inclusion. Social work values are embodied in the profession's national and international codes of ethics.	Social workers embrace and promote the fundamental and inalienable rights of all human beings. Social work is based on respect for the inherent worth, dignity of all people and the individual and social/civil rights that follow from this. Social workers often work with people to find an appropriate balance between competing human rights. Social workers have a responsibility to engage people in achieving social justice, in relation to society generally, and in relation to the people with whom they work. This means: Challenging discrimination and institutional oppression; Respect for diversity; Access to equitable resources; Challenging unjust policies and practices: Social workers work to bring to the attention of their employers, policymakers, politicians, and the public situations in which policies and resources are inadequate or in which policies and practices are oppressive, unfair, or harmful. In doing so, Social Workers must not be penalized. Promoting the right to self-determination: Social workers respect and promote people's rights to make their own choices and decisions, provided this does not threaten the rights and legitimate interests of others. Promoting the right to participation: Social workers work toward building the self-esteem and capabilities of people, promoting their full involvement and participation in all aspects of decisions and actions that affect their lives.

users, and more broadly, be felt on society, for example, when the trust in the Social Work profession become compromised.

A justice perspective according to utilitarian ethics

Let's now examine the different possible consequences for each possible course of action (Table 9.2):

a Mourad maintains his position that Sithembiso is 15 years of age;
b Mourad accepts the manager's position and modifies his report accordingly.

Table 9.2 The different possible consequences for each possible course of action[2]

	Possible consequences if A		*Possible consequences if B*	
	Positive	*Negative*	*Positive*	*Negative*
Mourad	Maintain trusting relationship with Sithembiso Act in the best interest of the service user Act in accordance with both the code of ethics and the code of conduct: avoid possible professional disciplinary actions	Bring trouble upon himself; challenging the manager could have negative repercussions on his work relationship with the manager and the agency	Protect himself from difficulties with the manager and the agency	Damaging the relationship with Sithembiso May be in breach of code of ethics (BASW /IFSW) May increase Sithembiso's level of distress
Sithembiso	Have access to a package of services more adapted to her identified need Maintain trust towards Mourad and the Social Work profession Decrease anxiety More likely to be continuously engaged in education; to become more socially integrated (Wade et al., 2005)	none	none	Will only have access to a less appropriate level of care May increasingly feel anxious Damaged relationship with Mourad Damage trusting relationship towards other Social Work professionals Will lead to many complications with getting services
Manager	Indirectly, may lead her to review the management style of the department and team	May be perceived as a challenge to her authority and could have an effect on the staff team Could be perceived indirectly as a challenge to Social Work services	Maintain status quo	Maintain status quo
Social services department where Mourad works	Indirectly, may lead to a review of policy and the broader organisational culture	May be perceived as a challenge to management structure May affect the budget of the agency and, indirectly, the distribution of other services	Maintain status quo	Maintain status quo Maintain structure that promotes social injustice
Other service users / the broader environment	May promote fairer access to services for a small number of service users, i.e. unaccompanied child asylum seekers	May affect other services users with regard to resource allocation	Maintain status quo Maintain current level of resources for other services	Maintain status quo Continue to support a culture that does not promote fair access to services or equality of opportunity

The Act-Utilitarian Perspective

You will remember that act-utilitarianism defines an action as morally good as long as the action itself is conducive to general happiness. We also asserted that it is the value of the consequences of one act or another that we then use to examine general happiness. Looking back at Mourad's case and both the positive and negative consequences emerging from the two possible courses of action, we can now begin to apply the principles of the act-utilitarian perspective. As such, we will analyse the dilemma through its consequences in terms of general utility for the greatest number.

In examining the consequences above, it seems that one particular course of action may maximise happiness or utility for the greatest number and therefore be considered a more ethical course of action according to the act-utilitarian perspective. For example, if Mourad decides not to continue supporting Sithembiso despite having access to strong evidence that she is 15, the most important consequence seems to be for Sithembiso, who would still have access to some resources, but more limited than if she were assessed as 15 years old. Another important consequence is that Sithembiso may lose her trust in Mourad and in the Social Work profession. We know, indeed, that trust is an essential component of work with unaccompanied child asylum seekers (Kohli and Mitchell, 2007). A consequence for Mourad is that he could be disciplined by one of the Social Work regulators or professional associations. However, for this to happen, a complaint would need to be filed, and looking at the case study, it is unlikely that this would be carried out by the agency, a colleague, or even Sithembiso, who is in a vulnerable situation. Under utilitarian principles, we must situate and weigh private interests to serve the public interest. Therefore, a regulator's disciplinary action against Mourad is unlikely to justify a different course of action. On the other hand, discontinuing support for Sithembiso by modifying his report could be seen at this time as promoting the greatest utility for the greatest number, considering the consequences for the staff team, the agency, and, more indirectly, the population using all services.

Therefore, in this case, from an act-utilitarian perspective, the right course of action, i.e., the one seen as promoting the greatest utility for the greatest number, could appear to be for Mourad to modify his report.

Reflexion Break

Think back on the criticism of the act-utilitarian perspective. Do you feel that this perspective promotes the principles of social justice in this case? Why or why not? Considering that many decisions are based on act-utilitarian principles, how do you feel the understanding of this perspective influences your view of ethics?

As we discussed earlier, act-utilitarian ethics can sometimes be seen as justifying unacceptable behaviours. Deliberation may be solely based upon a series of predicted consequences, and it is difficult to assess the extent to which our prediction will be correct. Therefore, a simple application of the act-utilitarian perspective, as seen above, may raise important issues. This is primarily due to the fact that the act-utilitarian perspective solely analyses the current situation, which can result in incorrect actions, even if they are theoretically justified. Therefore, while we do not believe that the analysis above constitutes the ethical way forward to manage the dilemma of this particular case study, we felt it was necessary to demonstrate this theory in action: understanding act-utilitarianism and being able to apply its principles may help us see *ethically* more clearly. As in Francis Bacon's famous adage, 'knowledge is power'. Therefore, one can develop a platform for resisting dominant societal principles in practice by understanding how they influence decision-making. Let us now explore how the rule-utilitarian perspective can inform decision-making in this case.

The Rule-Utilitarian Perspective

As we previously noted, rule-utilitarianism counters some of the criticisms of act-utilitarianism by proposing that the rules that would bring the greatest happiness or utility should determine our actions rather than the consequences of the actions themselves. Applying the rule-utilitarian perspective in Mourad's case means finding a rule that, if respected in all cases, would lead to the greatest utility. The question is: What sort of rule would help us achieve the right course of action according to this perspective?

We saw that, according to the act-utilitarian perspective, Mourad may be inclined to modify his report to bring the greatest utility to the greatest number of people. Could we make a universal rule out of this possible course of action? In other words, could we define a rule that, if generally followed, would justify Mourad's action?

We saw above that values expressed in various codes of ethics would be in opposition to modifying the report. Could we then arrive at an ethical rule by saying that "breaching a professional code of ethics is acceptable if it benefits the greatest number of people involved in a given situation"? Upon analysis, it would be difficult to universalise this rule because if codes of ethics can be broken, what is the point of having rules at all? We could argue that it would not be promoting the greatest good for the greatest number because such rules would be useless. Therefore, the rule-utilitarian perspective in this case would not be in favour of Mourad breaching his professional code of ethics because the consequences would be detrimental to the general population. Indeed, professional codes of ethics in Social Work or other disciplines are usually developed, among other things, to protect the population from misconduct. Therefore, according to a rule-utilitarian perspective, it would be wrong to breach the professional code; therefore, this perspective would justify Mourad's continued support of Sithembiso's claim.

We will now examine a final theory to see what, in terms of justice, could be the right action in Mourad's case.

Rawls's Theory of Justice

The situation in which Mourad is placed may stem from broader issues related to social justice and inequalities, two dimensions that are apparent in the views of the staff team and the agency. Looking at Rawls's theory of justice may be useful to further analyse the situation.

First, applying the original position and the veil of ignorance in this case may be helpful in underlining the beliefs that may be at the root of the situation. For example, it would be useful to consider whether the staff team, manager and agency would still maintain a culture of disbelief and cynicism regarding unaccompanied child asylum seekers if they themselves had to define the principles of justice that apply in the case.

Let's now look at the application of Rawl's principles. The first principle, that of *basic liberty for all*, would certainly not be apparent in this case. Indeed, broadly speaking, this principle resonates with Article 2 of the United Nations Declaration of Human Rights, which states:

> Everyone is entitled to all the rights and freedoms set forth in this Declaration, without distinction of any kind, such as race, colour, sex, language, religion, political or other opinion, national or social origin, property, birth or other status. Furthermore, no distinction shall be made on the basis of the political, jurisdictional, or international status of the country or territory to which a person belongs, whether it be independent, trust, non-self-governing or under any other limitation of sovereignty.

Accordingly, and strictly speaking, any asylum seeker should be treated the same way as a UK citizen or permanent resident. From Rawls' perspective, applying this principles would mean that all councils should treat every child equally, using the same rules, regardless of the child's origin or citizenship status. However, because the services are not organised in such a way as to achieve justice in a Rawlsian sense, Mourad would have to at least maintain and defend his position so that Sithembiso could have access to the services she needs. Indeed, as long as Sithembiso a minor, under Rawls's first principle, she should have access to adequate placement and prompt access to school so she can have the best chances in life. Mourad maintaining his position would at least guarantee this. Otherwise, Sithembiso would likely be placed in unsupported housing and experience amplified difficulties, like for many unaccompanied minors who are not ready to live independently (Wade et al., 2005). Recently, there were many reports of asylum-seeking children in the UK who were incorrectly assessed and placed in unsupervised adults' accommodation and detentions, leading them to experience significant risk and harms (Helen Bamber Foundation, Human Rights Network and the Refugee Council, 2024). Rather, Sithembiso should be given access to a placement that provides security and opportunities for building new attachments (Wade et al., 2005). Rawls's first principle of justice would also require Mourad to take the necessary actions to challenge the culture that exists in his organisation so that all unaccompanied minor asylum seekers are treated the same way as UK children in need of care.[3]

Because Rawls's first principle is not met – and, as we have stressed, only when the first principle is met can the second principle be applied – we cannot proceed with the application of the second principle. Indeed, only when basic liberties are applied equally can inequalities be tolerated and utilised in order to benefit the less advantaged. Clearly, in this case study, this first principle is not satisfied. Unaccompanied child asylum seekers are among the most vulnerable in society and are disadvantaged by many policies – from age assessment to detention (Simmonds and Merredew, 2010). Yet, this population is already vulnerable to social and structural detrimental conditions. As Stevens et al., (2024) explain,

> children displaced by war and persecution have increased health needs compared to host populations because of their experiences pre, during and post-migration. Health risks associated with psychological trauma, violence, environmental hazards, and disease exposure are widely recognised. These children also face potential health harm from racism, xenophobia, and discrimination during the journey and after arrival. Racism, xenophobia and discrimination, at interpersonal, institutional

> and structural levels, are profound determinants of health, and are associated with an increase in infectious and non-communicable diseases throughout the life course and intergenerationally (p.1).

The situation presented in this case study and relative to unaccompanied child asylum seekers in the UK generally may be qualified as unjust and therefore unethical according to both Rawlsian and rule-utilitarian principles. From a social justice perspective, Social Workers should challenge oppression, insuring that the rights of unaccompanied asylum seeker are upheld, and providing interventions that aim at building their self-esteem and capabilities.

Conclusion

We have seen that both utilitarian ethics and Rawls's theory of justice propose principles that can be applied to practical situations and help us analyse ethical issues and dilemmas related to social justice and equality. We have seen that utilitarian ethics, as formulated by Mill, provides an understanding of justice that is oriented towards the concept of utility, and that a solution will be considered as long as it benefits the greatest number of people. We have emphasised that utility, which can be explored through an action's consequence, must be assessed both qualitatively and quantitatively. Rawls, on the other hand, proposes an understanding of justice involving an equally shared set of liberties and allowing for inequalities, as long as these inequalities benefit the less advantaged. Compared with other theories presented in this book, both theories provide us with further tools for understanding and managing the many complexities of Social Work practice in a variety of settings and involving populations facing numerous difficulties.

Notes

1 In the UK, it is the four social work regulators (Social Work England, Scottish Social Services Council, Northern Ireland Social Care Council and Gofal Cymdeithasol Cymru – Social Care Wales) that are responsible for the protection of the public. For example, Social Work England can receive complaints from the public about social workers which, if serious enough, can be taken into a procedure to examine their 'fitness to practice', that is, that they behave in line with the professional standards. While BASW (and IFSW) do not have a disciplinary power over social workers in the UK, we made the decision to draw on those code of ethics in order to make the analysis easier to follow from an international perspective.

2 This table is adapted from a deliberation tool proposed by French Canadian scholar Georges A. Legault (1999).

3 This may involve contacting his professional association for support in this process.

10 Virtue Ethics and Ethics of Care

Virtue ethics and the ethics of care are ethical perspectives often referred to as 'relationship-based' approaches. These frameworks are particularly relevant in Social Work, as they emphasize the personal qualities—such as integrity and competence—that underpin professional conduct. Social Workers are expected to embody these values in their interactions with various stakeholders, including service user groups, organizations, communities, and the state. It is therefore through this theme that we will examine this fourth broad perspective in moral philosophy, one that enables the contextualisation of the concept of personal qualities and stresses the importance of relationships.

Character- and Relationship-Based Ethics

Principles-based ethics include ethical perspectives such as Kantian and utilitarian ethics that use principles, or rules to follow that help define the right and wrong action, whereas *character-based and relationship-based ethics* do not rely on rules to follow but instead focus on the sort of person you are or the relationship you have with others. We saw in Chapters 8 and 9 how both utilitarian and Kantian ethics are based on the application of a *set of principles* (e.g. 'universality' for Kant, and "every action should be taken so as to maximise happiness" for some utilitarians). On the other hand, character- and relationship-based ethical theories generally refer to a variety of notions such as virtue ethics and the ethics of care, which do not rely on principles to guide the action, but instead, on the type of person a Social Worker should be, and on the type of relationship a Social Worker should develop with service users. In this case, the ethically good action will not be based on such or such principles to apply, but instead, on the type of person the Social Worker should aim to become. Thus, opposed to principle-based ethics discussed in previous chapters, virtue ethics and the ethics of care do not try to prescribe the principles to follow and consequently the types of behaviour that could be considered right or wrong but instead establish what is considered to be essential qualities of the person facing the dilemma and the context in which action or Social Work intervention takes place.

To illustrate this, lets return to an example already discussed in Chapter 8. Imagine you are about to leave the office at 5 p.m. when one of the service users you already work with arrives at the office appearing very distressed. Your manager asks you if you would stay a little longer to deal with the situation. You know that this situation will probably keep you at the office much longer than what you had accepted. However, you decide to stay and see the service user. Now, try to imagine the reason behind your decision. First, you could say that you are staying late because there is a person in distress and according

DOI: 10.4324/9781003458715-14

to your profession and your work setting; you have the duty to help this person and provide them with a service. Alternatively, you could say that you are staying to see that person simply because you are someone who is caring, professional and committed to your profession and therefore you have to see this person because you do not feel there is any other way of doing it. The former way of making the decision emphasises a principle you are following, that is 'duty of care' and "helping people in distress is part of your role within the agency", whereas the second reason for staying is justified by the sort of person you are.

We shall now consider more in details two ethical traditions related to character-based ethics and explore some of their similarities and differences before examining a case study. We will therefore draw a broad picture of what is virtue ethics and the ethics of care and explore how these traditions can potentially help Social Workers to be more ethical in their work.

Virtue Ethics

Did You Know?

Virtue ethics was the main way of discriminating between good and bad until the eighteenth century, but decreased in popularity with the emergence of modern moral theories such as Kantian and utilitarian theories. However, virtue ethics has started to regain popularity in philosophy, and now in Social Work since early 1980s

Virtue ethics originally derived from the works of Plato and Aristotle, two philosophers of ancient Greece times who lived four centuries before Christ. Virtue ethics is a form of moral perspective, much like Kantian and utilitarian ethics, but emphasising the *type of person* needed for an ethical community to develop. For a life to be ethical, an individual's actions follow from the virtuous character traits that he or she has developed through the course of his or her life. Therefore, a person who strives to live an ethical life will aim at acquiring a set of positive character traits, or personal qualities which help the person to behave morally well at any given time. We shall return to the notions of the good life and positive character traits later in this chapter.

Virtue ethics was very popular as a way of ethics until the development of other ethical perspectives such as Kantian and utilitarian ethics during the Enlightenment period. However, it did regained popularity from the second half of the twentieth century. This return to virtue ethics was driven by philosophers who had a reaction against modern moral philosophy, such as Kantian and utilitarian ethics, which, for them, were no longer adequate for understanding right from wrong. On this, MacIntyre (2007), an influential philosopher in virtue ethics, asserts that the main problem with ethical perspectives that use principles to decide right from wrong is that often, the principles get themselves into conflicts. For example, what would you do in an ethical dilemma where the principle of "respect for the person" (Kantian ethics) gets into conflict with the principle of 'utility' (utilitarian ethics)? Indeed, for MacIntyre (2007), the central problem lies in the question, "How do we know which rules (or principle) to follow?" Let us examine a simple situation involving a young offender who is repeatedly arrested by the police for doing graffiti on walls in the park and causing damage to other people's property. We have chosen this example precisely because graffiti is something that some people see as a form of social expression, while some other sees it as anti-social and causing criminal damage. From a utilitarian perspective (see Chapter 9), the ethically right principle would be to promote the greatest good for the greatest number and, therefore, to take the necessary steps to prevent the young person from visiting the areas where they are carrying out the graffiti through an Anti-Social Behaviour Order. However, the young person, as an individual, deserves respect and should get the support he needs from his family but will not be able to if an Anti-Social Behaviour Order is issued against him. This would go against the principles of the Kantian approach (see Chapter 8). Therefore, in such a situation, which principles should receive priority? While you may have your own opinion as to which course of action should be taken, we must acknowledge that both of these principles could be applied. Unfortunately, many situations like this involve conflicts of principles from different 'families' of perspectives, such as those opposing autonomy with the greater good. This is where virtue ethics can help Social Workers reposition themselves in terms of ethical practice because it does not rely on principles to apply to certain situation, but instead, is based on the sort of person who would act ethically.

The 'Good Life' from the Perspective of Virtue Ethics

True goodness, according to what we have discussed above, relies not so much on which principles to apply in one situation or another, but instead, on what sort of person one ought to be. Virtue ethics, therefore, focuses on the character of a person because, according to this perspective, such personality traits will have, generally speaking, an impact on that person and on others in terms of who they are and what they do. For example, an empathic Social Worker will not display empathy because there is expectation of that quality in her work, but instead, because it is a quality that she has, which transcend all of her behaviours.

But how do we know who is the right type of person that produces 'good' in society? This is where Socrates draws from the concept of *eudemonia*, or supreme good, which is achievable through the finding of happiness. Virtue ethicists talk about the means to an end and the end in itself. Eudemonia is the ultimate end, and all humans strive to achieve it.

Eudemonia

Aristotle believed that *eudemonia* was the ultimate purpose in life. Eudemonia is the ultimate good, which can be achieved through the pursuit of happiness (well-being). Eudemonia also promotes 'human flourishing' (Graham, 2004).

To define the ethical life, the virtue ethicist will therefore focus on examining what kind of person someone should be in order to achieve *eudemonia*. In this sense, a good person would exhibit good qualities, and this would have an effect on the good life in general and on the pursuit of happiness for both one's self and for others. The definition of what constitutes the good life can be found in the concept of 'virtue'.

Virtues

For the virtue ethicist, eudemonia, or the absolute good, can be achieved through the nurturing and cultivating of 'virtues'. A virtue is not "an unthinking habit, but rather involves an intelligent judgement about the appropriate response to the situation you are in" (Warburton, 2013, p. 53). A virtue is therefore a personal quality that you develop over time which will help yourself and others to grow and be happy. In this sense, a virtue is a fine balance between too much and not enough of something. A virtue is a trait or character that has developed to a point of perfection. In this sense, Aristotle, in his book *Nicomachean Ethics*, explains that because a virtue is perfection, people who display this virtue will always produce the perfect result by performing the right action in any given situation. A virtuous practice in Social Work, therefore, consists in the Social Worker cultivating and developing the character traits or personal qualities that will lead to the ultimate purpose – *eudemonia* – or in Social Work terms, a sort of *best ethical practice.*

What Is a Virtue?

From the Greek word 'aretè' (excellence of character), a virtue is a human quality that is displayed appropriately through the use of practical reason in various situations, with the aim of promoting the wellbeing of people in general. A virtue is a quality that is situated between having too much and not having enough of something.

Let us now look at some examples of virtues and the relationship between their excess and lack thereof.

Some virtues and the relationship between their lack and excess

Lack of	Virtue	Excess
Indifference	Compassion	Excessive concern
Intemperance	Self-control	Self-denial
Vanity	Humility	Timidity
Cowardice	Courage	Recklessness
Dishonesty	Trustworthiness	Blind trust
Intolerance	Patience	Resignation

McBeath and Webb (2002) point out, in relation to virtue ethics, that Socrates differentiates between two types of virtues: intellectual virtues and moral virtues. Moral virtues include character traits such as liberality and temperance and provide people with opportunities to examine their experience, whereas intellectual virtues are acquired by instruction and include character traits such as wisdom and understanding. Criticality is another example of intellectual virtue.

Aristotle tells us that a virtuous person will display many virtues at the same time. It is therefore only through a combination of a number of virtues that a person can be considered virtuous, since exhibiting only one virtue would not be sufficient. Therefore, virtues come in sets; one cannot possess a single virtue without possessing others. To illustrate this point, let us examine some virtues that cannot exist without others: A *courageous* person will also be *temperate* because without *temperance*, a person would risk becoming reckless; a Social Worker who is *compassionate* will also be patient because being *compassionate* involves a desire to fully understand the suffering of others, which requires time and patience.

A person who develops a set of virtues (excellence of character) will therefore aim at reaching *perfection* in many aspects of their lives. Thus, a virtuous Social Worker will aim at developing and nurturing these qualities, even though such qualities may never be fully developed. The end result is *eudemonia*, whereas attempting to develop them is a means to an end. For example, the *wise* Social Worker is a person who uses her judgement, sensibility, and comprehension in any given situation. According to the virtue ethicist, this type of person would promote, in general, eudemonia because her actions will be based not so much on plain application of principles but because she precisely displays these character traits needed to excel in her practice. An example of promoting eudemonia in Social Work practice in Britain would be the development of a type of practice that reflects the principles established by the International Federation of Social Workers, that is, a practice that respects the dignity of all humans and is based on the principles of social justice.

We understand, therefore, that a virtue is a personal quality that is developed and displayed in various situations. We now turn to the virtues that are required in Social Work and to the conditions for their development.

Practical Reason

For the virtue theorist, virtuous character can be developed through reasoning. It is through habituation in reasoning that a person can develop virtues or positive character traits such as courage, justice, and temperance. MacIntyre (1999) points to the development of reasoning abilities in people to unlock and cultivate virtues that are appropriate to practice, in this case, Social Work. The process of reasoning can help people make decisions and decide to perform good actions, and it is through reasoning at all times that people can become virtuous. Morse (1999) asserts that only then will a virtuous person perform virtuous acts in any given moral situation.

Practical Reason

Practical reason, in terms of virtue ethics, involves both reflection and self-knowledge. It is an "enquiry that provides us with grounds for the criticism, revision, or even rejection of many of our judgements, our standards of judgement, our relationships, and our institutions" (MacIntyre 1999, p. 157).

To illustrate this point, let us now consider a Social Worker who is asked to comply with a policy that is promoted within the organisation for which she works, but that has the potential of compromising the Social Work value base. For example, the manager may ask her to reduce the size of a service user's care package, purely for financial reason. The Social Worker may decide to implement the policy or not.

Through reasoning, the Social Worker will have to think through the situation in context and consider carefully the different aspects emerging from the situation. The reasoning process, according to the virtue ethicist, will make the Social Worker adept at figuring out what is most appropriate in the situation. Let us imagine that the Social Worker decides that she cannot reduce the care package because it compromises the Social Work value base. Let us also say that the manager and his boss are both in disagreement with the Social Worker and insist that the Social Worker reduces it. If the Social Worker still thinks the action goes against the Social Work value base, and she carefully reasoned about every aspect, she may decide not to implement the policy. On the one hand, just doing what you are asked to do would not be virtuous because it means you lack courage. On the other hand, simply refusing to do something without the support of your colleagues may not necessarily be an act of courage, but one of recklessness or intemperance. The virtuous behaviour in this case would be to reason about the situation, to be wise and consider all possible avenues, and to be courageous enough to carry out the decision without lacking judgement. It may also involve a certain amount of patience from the Social Worker. A virtuous Social Worker may therefore decide to gain some time, to pursue the challenge to the policy by exploring different avenues, such as seeking support from a professional association. What is important to remember is that in virtue ethics, the appropriate behaviour depends on who you are, what the context of the situation is, and your ability to reason while making a decision. Only then can you draw from your intellectual virtues in order to decide what is good or bad, and reason as to the best course of action in a particular situation.

If we examine what, essentially, constitutes a virtue, it becomes clear that practical reasoning can help Social Workers better define their Social Work values. As MacIntyre (2007) points out, a virtue can be developed through strength of character. He explains that virtue is 'an acquired human quality' (MacIntyre, 2007, p. 191) rather than a feeling about rightness or wrongness. These personal qualities or 'virtues' have to be practised in order to become part of one's life, as opposed to a one-off 'act of heroism' (Lynch and Lynch, 2006).

To give a practical example of how virtues can be developed, let's explore an ancient virtue praised in the early Greek community. Although 'physical strength' has nothing to do with Social Work practice today, we nevertheless believe that thinking about this virtue will help you grasp how other virtues, whether moral or intellectual, can be developed and nurtured. Why was physical strength a virtue in ancient Greece? Before the polis was developed, many small communities were living far apart from one another. Therefore, they could not rely on fast protection like people do with the modern police force, or the army. Thus, people, in order to protect their community and village had to develop a certain physical strength to defend themselves. So in context, physical strength was considered as an important virtue to protect the community and do 'good'. Now, imagine that you have to develop this virtue. What do you need to develop physical strength? You will probably need to train regularly, and work very hard and this will not happen overnight. It will also take more than one session at the gym. It may take months or even years before you become strong. As you may realise, developing physical strength will happen over time, with lots of practice and dedication because to achieve excellence, you will have to pursuit that training, even when things are difficult. If you stop training, you will also lose your physical strengths. The same principle applies to develop other kinds of virtues. Whether we are talking about 'patience', 'trustworthiness' or 'humility' or 'criticality', these virtues or personal qualities will not develop overnight. Therefore, to develop patience for example, you will have to be exposed to many situations whereby your patience will be tested. It is through being exposed to these situations, and by reasoning on the way your feelings make you behave that you may develop your patience even further.

Social Work Virtues

While virtue ethics as applied to contemporary Social Work practice has gained in popularity during the last few decades (Banks, 2020; Banks and Gallagher, 2009; Clark, 2005; McBeath and Webb, 2002), there is no formal, exhaustive list of which virtues are most suited to Social Work practice. However, it is through the ability to reason that Social Workers are in a position to identify which set of virtues are appropriate for the context of practice and to develop and nurture these virtues through their experience of working with service users.

Some virtues related to Social Work, such as temperance, magnanimity, gentleness, truthfulness, wittiness, friendliness, modesty, and justice have been identified by Lynch and Lynch (2006), as well as Clark (2006). Banks and Gallagher (2009) also point to another set of virtues appropriate to the fields of health and social care and are thus useful in a Social Work framework: professional wisdom, respectfulness, care, trustworthiness, justice, courage, and integrity. As we can see, therefore, there is no 'official list' of virtues consensually accepted by the Social Work community as 'Social Work virtues'. This can actually be seen as a critique of virtue ethics, as articulated by Houston (2003, p. 819), who asserts that "insufficient attention is given to the problem of how virtue is defined and established in the first instance". While the topic of virtue ethics is still in the development stages, it is essential to remember that the notion of 'reason' is indispensable in virtue ethics since it enables the Social Worker to explore and identify which set of virtues is important to achieve *eudemonia* in a given Social Work context. The Social Worker will then have to develop and nurture these virtues. We can now begin to understand the rationale behind the use of reasoning in determining what constitutes a virtue or set of virtues. The centrality of using reason needs to govern the practice and should not be considered merely a theoretical option. On this, Aristotle reminds us that a set of virtues is a "voluntary acquired disposition which is defined under the guidance of a thoughtful person" (Aristotle, 1999).

From Virtue Ethics to the Ethics of Care

We have seen that the focus of virtue ethics lies in the development of an individual's excellence of character and in the pursuit of happiness through the use of practical reason. Another critique of virtue ethics, however, is that most virtue theories have been developed and furthered by men, and that 'feminine' traits of personality have been all but ignored (Banks, 2020). As we saw above, virtue ethics is related to practical reason and does not emphasise the role of emotions, which are more the realm of women than they are of men. As Jaggar (2013, p. 433) confirms, "throughout the history of Western ethics, the moral status of women has been a persistent though rarely central to the topic of debate". It thus becomes clear that virtue ethics could be enhanced by taking into consideration a more feminine mode of ethical deliberation, which is the main thrust of this section on the ethics of care. Indeed, given that one of the views of virtue ethics is that it can complement other types of ethics (Banks and Gallagher, 2009), we now propose to examine another character-based ethical theory that we believe can be successfully combined with virtue ethics to render the latter more compatible with 'feminine' character traits.

What Is Ethics of Care?

Ethics of care, as developed by feminists such as Gilligan and Noddings, argues that "traditional ethical perspectives such as Kantian, utilitarian, and virtue ethics lack the values and qualities that are usually associated with women, for example, caring and responsibility".

Essential Features of Ethics of Care

Ethics of care was born out of a critique of Kohlberg's stages of moral development, which according to Gilligan, are not entirely adaptable to women. Indeed, based on a critique of Kohlberg's methodology, and her own research with women, Gilligan came to the conclusion that there were fundamental differences in the way men and women morally deliberate and as such, Kohlberg's stages of moral development are not universally applicable. Such criticism is still relevant today, and the point here is not to say that men reason in one way and that women reason in another. However, we want to stress that there are many times that a person may not feel comfortable applying a particular moral theory to his or her life precisely because such a theory does not account for relationships with others, which are central to the context in which a decision is made. For example, in terms of virtue ethics, justice may be an important virtue (always give to others their due), but this may not be so simple to apply in practice. A person may be confronted with a situation in which she must decide between what is right for her family and what is right for someone else's family and may very well decide in favour of her own family. But can we affirm that such a person is acting unethically or without virtue? Is it not because of her relationship with her family? This is where the ethics of care can contribute significantly to Social Work.

What Are Kolhberg's Stages of Moral Development?

Kolhberg defined six universal stages of moral development, which, according to his research, are applicable to everyone. These involve three different levels, from 'obedience and punishment' to 'application of ethical principles', the latter being the highest level of moral development. According to Kolhberg, not everyone progresses to the highest level.

In this book, we shall use the foundation of the ethics of care as an approach in ethics that emphasises the importance of relationships, responsibility, and caring in its definition of ethical behaviour. Indeed, we understand Social Work as involving "people in relationships of commitment to each other's well-being, often sanctioned by the state" (Dominelli, 2009, p. 7). We therefore believe that the concept of relationships between people is an essential feature of Social Work practice and requires a type of ethics that can account for it.

Thus, an ethics of care based on this understanding is one that emphasises the importance not only of character (as in virtue ethics) but also of the relationships in which the ethical issues take place and the centrality of such concepts as responsibility and caring in the definition of the morally right action. As such, the ethics of care emphasises the roles of *mutual Interdependence and emotional response,* as noted by Beauchamp and Childless (2001, p. 373):

> (...) many human relationships involve persons who are vulnerable, dependent, ill, and frail (...) [and] the desirable moral response is attached attentiveness to needs, not detached respect for rights (...) The person who acts from rule-governed obligations without appropriately aligned feelings such as worry when a friend suffers seems to have a moral deficiency. In addition (...) insight into the needs of others and considerate alertness to their circumstances often come from the emotions more than reason.

Consequently, while virtue ethics does not emphasise the importance of emotion in defining virtues and deciding on the morally good action, the ethics of care emphasises that emotions can have a cognitive role and allow us to deal with situations that are not immediately resolvable using practical reasoning alone.

During the last decade, there has been increasing debate about the resemblances between virtue ethics and the ethics of care. For example, Halwani (2003) asserts that the ethics of care should be subsumed under virtue ethics by constructing care as an important virtue, while Hugman (2005, p. 71) states that the ethics of care is more a framework for understanding ethics within concrete experiences of relationships than it is a 'grand moral theory'.

Reflection Break

Thinking back on what you have just read about virtue ethics and the ethics of care:

1 Summarise what you consider the main point of virtue ethics theory
2 Summarise what you consider the main point of the ethics of care
3 How might these principles be used in Social Work practice?

Virtue ethics and the ethics of care both stress the importance of the character of the Social Worker and the nature of the relationship in which the intervention or ethical dilemma takes place. Virtue ethics emphasises that it is through practical reasoning and the nurturing of appropriate virtues or character traits that a person will promote eudemonia or perfect happiness. The ethics of care complements virtue ethics because it asserts that it is the nature of the relationship that determines what type of person one ought to be.

The rest of this chapter will thus be devoted to combining our understanding of virtue ethics with that of the ethics of care, with particular attention not only to the context of practice but also to the relationship between the Social Worker and the service user, an approach which we feel is promising. Let us now examine a case study to which we will apply both the perspectives of virtue ethics and the ethics of care. As such, we will explore the case study by considering 'care' as one of many virtues relevant to Social Work practice, paying particular attention to the relationship between the Social Worker and the service user. Although virtue ethics and the ethics of care may not be considered as part of the larger family of principle-based approaches, we will nevertheless examine their application in light of the various codes of ethics and practice of Social Work. In this regard, we will not consider these codes as principles to follow in the Kantian or utilitarian sense, but instead as a reminder of a set of values that can help us develop the virtues that are relevant to our profession.

Case Study: Ruth's Story

Ruth is a 45-year-old white British Social Worker who works with a disability team in Scotland. She has two daughters, one who lives abroad, and another, with cerebral palsy, who lives nearby in a housing resource provided by another disability team. Ruth's experience as a mother of a child with a long-term illness and physical disability is what motivated her in her late thirties to study Social Work and obtain her qualification in order to help other families in similar situations.

Samantha is a 19-year-old white British woman living in a council estate near Glasgow. She accesses a number of services through her local learning disability team. Ruth is her Social Worker and case manager and has been working with Samantha since she moved to adult care 18 months ago. Samantha was born with Down syndrome and is currently waiting for the result of an assessment for autism. She has mild to moderate learning disabilities. Samantha attends a special school three days a week and a mainstream community college the rest of the week. The teachers at her mainstream school say that she is integrating well overall. She lives semi-independently in a small block of self-contained flats that include a bedroom, bathroom, and kitchen. The block also includes an on-site support worker who provides ad-hoc support to all residents, as well as a warden. Even though Samantha is very different from Ruth's daughter, Ruth sometimes feels that Samantha reminds her of her daughter, and this somehow affects her relationship with her. Last month, Samantha, who is a keen chat room user, tells Ruth that she has met a man through Facebook. During the last three meetings of the disability team, Samantha has told Ruth that her new boyfriend plans to come and visit her at the week-end. By the way she describes him, it would appear that the man is considerably much older than her. Samantha says that she is in love, and that deep down in her heart, she feels he is the one. Ruth, who wants to support Samantha appropriately, uses the opportunity to discuss notions of sexuality and respect of self and others. At the following meeting, Ruth notices that Samantha is not as dynamic as usual. When asked about the week-end, Samantha changes topic. A few weeks later, Ruth notices that Samantha has a bruise on her arm. When asked about it, Samantha appears shy and does not know what to say. However, the bruise appears to have been caused by someone grabbing her arm because of the appearance of finger marks. When Ruth asks Samantha about her relationship with her boyfriend, Samantha says that he sometimes gets 'stressed' while with her, but she prefers not to say anything because he said he would leave her, and deep down she is in love with him. Ruth is beginning to feel concerned about the situation. When the warden of the block calls Ruth's supervisor to report that a man has been visiting Samantha regularly for three weeks, Ruth is asked to take appropriate measures to end Samantha's relationship with her boyfriend.

Analysis

The dilemma facing Ruth underlines many aspects of Social Work practice that relate to professionalism. Central to the case are elements that relate to setting appropriate boundaries and positioning oneself correctly between protecting and supporting the service user. Issues of confidentiality and respect for the person are also present in the case.

We now propose to examine how different virtues help shed light on the definition of an ethically good action. We will also observe how the role of emotions and the nature of the professional relationship can shape ethical practice. We will do this by examining some of the relevant virtues proposed by Banks and Gallagher (2009) and McBeath and Webb (2002) and how they impact on our comprehension of Ruth's story and the notion of professionalism overall. In particular, we will explore how the virtues of 'respectfulness', 'care', 'trustworthiness', 'justice', 'courage', 'integrity' and 'criticality' can help Social Workers become better professionals in their practice and maintain the Social Work value base.

Reflection Break

Looking back thought the case study:

1 Identify the ethical dilemma facing Ruth.
2 Identify the conflicting values and the various courses of action Ruth might take.
3 Write down what you feel are the most important elements to take into consideration in each course of action you identified above. Why do you feel they are important?
4 How would you express the issues facing Ruth in terms of virtue ethics and the ethics of care?

Respectfulness

Respectfulness, in its simplest form, is showing respect for another person. For a Social Worker, this would mean respecting the values and views of the service user, even if these differ from one's own beliefs or personal experiences of similar situations. This means that Ruth would respect Samantha's desire to share (or not) her story with her and to continue seeing (or not) her boyfriend. In the case presented above, Samantha is deemed autonomous, since she is living independently in a resource facility in which she can access the services she needs. She also attends mainstream school three days a week and therefore has sufficient ability to make her own decisions with regard to the relationships she engages in and to other areas of her life. In this sense, she is apt to make her own decisions, despite needing support to do so elsewhere. Even if she is deemed having more difficulties to make her own decision in certain areas, and final decisions must be made for her, she would still have to be respected. She expresses to Ruth that she loves her boyfriend, and Ruth therefore needs to respect Samantha's feelings.

Care

The word 'care', whether in terms of 'care plans', 'care management' or simply 'social care', has different meanings in different contexts. This observation is echoed by Banks and Gallagher (2009), who assert that 'care' as a virtue is difficult to define because there are so many meanings attached to the term. As such, we will propose a definition of care that stresses the characteristic of Social Workers involved in relationships with service users and that includes aspects of responsibility and concern. The notion of caring also involves emotions that affect the relationships between carers and persons cared for.

In the above case study, Ruth and Samantha have been working together for 18 months. As such, it is likely that their experience of 'care' has changed during this period. At the beginning of the relationship, the notion of responsibility may have been devoid of emotions, more formal, and probably more policy-orientated. Furthermore, Ruth now acknowledges that Samantha tends to remind her of her own daughter. This has the potential of creating a range of emotions in the caring relationship. As the helping relationship developed, it may also have changed in nature and fostered a deeper relation of trust.

So what does 'caring' mean in this situation? Care, as a virtue, would bring Ruth to recognise her emotions while working with Samantha. Despite her emotions, caring here would require Ruth to intervene with Samantha professionally, and with the best interest of the service users in mind. A caring relationship between Ruth and Samantha would imply that Ruth takes the appropriate means to ensure that Samantha is aware of the risk to which she may be exposing herself. Indeed, barriers in understanding and communication may mean that people with learning disabilities are more at risk of manipulation and exploitation crime and abuse (Wiseman and Watson, 2022). Moreover, Ruth should ensure that Samantha understands her right to be treated with dignity and respect as a human being.

Trustworthiness

Trustworthiness is a central quality of Social Work and is clearly recognised in each of the Council's codes of practice. In the case of Ruth's story, Samantha has trusted her Social Worker by confiding in her that her boyfriend was doing something when 'stressed' in her company. While it is not clear, in this case study, what is happening when Samantha and her boyfriend are together, Ruth has some concerns about Samantha being at risk of physical violence. When Social Workers engage in a relationship with a service user, they have the duty to explain the policy regarding confidentiality, as well as its limits, before anything is disclosed to the Social Worker. Therefore, Samantha should be aware that Ruth, as a Social Worker, should not disclose this information or any other information shared during the intervention to anyone else, except where there is clear evidence of serious risk to the service user or to others in the community. In these exceptional circumstances, Social Workers, on the basis of professional consideration and consultation, must limit any such breach of confidence to the needs of the situation at the time (BASW, 2021).

With regard to the case study, Ruth therefore must ask herself whether she considers this a serious threat to the service user and whether it warrants compromising her relationship with the service user. In this particular situation, it is clear that the service user may be exposed to some risk, but the Social Worker needs to ask herself about the seriousness of the risk involved. For example, Samantha, because she has discussed her private life with her Social Worker, must feel, to a certain extent, that she has developed a relationship of trust with her. Otherwise, she may not feel the need to disclose personal information to her Social Worker. Simply put, this kind of disclosure about boyfriends is not what is usually expected as part of the Social Work services of an adult disability team. Therefore, a trustworthy Social Worker will make sure that she explains the limits of confidentiality to the service user at the beginning of the relationship and that she will remain open as to how she will perceive the situation. The Social Worker will want to reason based on the evidence she has regarding the situation and will carefully analyse its seriousness. In this case study, we can identify a presence of risk, but we must reason and deliberate as to whether the risk is imminent and serious enough to compromise the relationship with the service user by taking further action that directly involves her private life. In this particular case, and based on the perspectives of virtue ethics and the ethics of care, Ruth should continue to develop the relationship of trust with Samantha so that she can continue to share her concerns with her and support her in her decisions regarding the situation.

Justice

Much like for 'care', there are many ways of understanding the notion of 'justice'. For example, justice could be understood from a Rawlsian or utilitarian perspective (see Chapter 9), or as a Kantian principle of universality (see Chapter 8). While we are aware that there are many definitions and perspectives regarding justice, we shall understand justice in this chapter as being a virtue or character trait that allows a person to treat others equally and to promote a situation in which everyone can flourish and exercise their rights.

In this context, for Ruth to be a 'virtuous' Social Worker who embodies justice, she must, on the one hand, inform Samantha of her rights as a service user, and on the other hand, treat Samantha within a the perspective of human rights.

As to informing Samantha of her rights, the policy regarding learning disabilities in the United Kingdom is clear:

> (...) a commitment to enabling people with learning disabilities to live as equal citizens in the community alongside their non-disabled peers, with choice and control over their lives, and the support they need to enable this (...) and that *Valuing People* explicitly name that good services will help people with learning disabilities develop opportunities to form relationships, including ones of a physical and sexual nature.
>
> (Joint Committee on Human Right, 2008)

Therefore, in acting with a sense of justice, Ruth will make sure that Samantha is aware of her rights and that these rights will be upheld during the intervention. In practical terms, this means that Ruth must support Samantha in understanding that, as a woman, she is free to choose with whom she engages in a relationship; at the same time, however, Samantha should be treated with respect in that relationship, despite her learning disability.

On the other hand, Ruth will also need to make sure that she treats Samantha with dignity and respect during the intervention. This echoes one of the principles of the Ethical Document of the International Federation of Social Workers: "Respecting the right to self-determination – Social workers respect and promote people's right to make their own choices and decisions, provided this does not threaten the rights and legitimate interests of others" (2018). This means that Ruth must not treat Samantha differently because of her learning disability. If Samantha's relationship with her boyfriend becomes violent, Ruth should discuss with Samantha the different options and services available. Rather than taking unilateral action, Ruth should support Samantha in her own decision and help her look at the different possibilities of "ending her relationship with her boyfriend".

Integrity

The BASW (2021) asserts that integrity comprises honesty, reliability, openness, and impartiality, and is an essential value in the practice of Social Work. What does acting with integrity mean from a virtue ethics and ethics of care perspective in relation to Ruth's story?

Honesty means that Ruth should be open with Samantha and tell her that she is concerned about her safety. This was discussed more extensively above with regard to 'trustworthiness'. Ruth should also make sure that she explores her own value base and ensure that her judgement is not clouded by certain personal values that she may hold which would affect her reading of the situation. This would help Ruth avoid placing her own beliefs before Samantha's needs and interests (BASW, 2021). While it is unlikely that Ruth has any prejudices against people with disabilities, since her own daughter has a long-term illness, behaving with integrity would also mean believing that everyone has the ability, when supported appropriately, to make decisions for themselves. Acting with integrity here would be to consider Samantha's needs and wishes about the situation, and although Samantha may express herself in a way that Ruth disagrees with, Ruth should not try to coerce Samantha into making a decision. The IFSW (2004) states that acting with integrity also includes not abusing the relationship of trust with service users, recognising the boundaries between personal and professional life, and not abusing one's position for personal benefit or gain. In Samantha's situation, Ruth must act in such a manner as to recognise the limits between her personal and professional life, and because of the nature of the relationship, she must avoid treating Samantha like her own daughter, but as an adult needing services with regard to her disability. Ruth should also seek to discuss the situation with her supervisor and seek support if needed.

Criticality

Criticality is an important element of Social Work and is discussed in the National Occupational Standards for Social Work (2002) as a significant aspect of Social Work practice. Criticality, according to Adams et al. (2002, p. xxi) is the faculty that

> enables us to question the knowledge we have and our own involvement with clients, including our taken-for-granted understanding. It enables us to assess situations so as to make structural connections that penetrate the surface of what we encounter and locate what is apparent within wider contexts. Criticality therefore involves a process of reflection, an ability to reassess our own judgement and stresses a particular emphasises on the structural analysis of the situation we are observing or involved in.

To be critical in Samantha's situation, therefore, requires that Ruth examine her knowledge and explore it in relation to the work she is undertaking with the service user. For example, she may want to check that the relevant policy and theory she is using are indeed relevant to the situation; she should not simply apply guidelines that seem to fit in the first instance. She should explore, for example, best evidence regarding women who are victims of violence and the risks to which certain vulnerable groups may be more exposed. Being critical also means examining Samantha's situation using a more structural analysis and repositioning issues of gender, disabilities, and socio-economic conditions central to this analysis and reasoning of the case. Is Samantha really at risk, or are Ruth's own prejudices affecting her professional judgement? Would it be possible that the marks on Samantha's arm have been caused by someone else? What policy is the agency trying to enforce? What is the supervisor's reading of the situation? What are the reasons behind the warden's telephone call? Are there any signs of disabilism? What is the view of the support health worker? Does he or she also have concerns about the situation? What is, indeed, Samantha's perception of the situation? A critical Social Worker will take the time to think about how structural elements and issues of power that are identified can shape the analysis of the situation.

Courage

The last virtue we wish to explore in relation to the above case study is 'courage'. Courage as a virtue has been considered important since ancient times and is still relevant to contemporary Social Work practice. Courage, according to Aristotle, can be developed firstly by being able to recognise situations that need to change, and secondly, by being able to stand our ground. We can therefore understand courage as a quality that, on the one hand, allows us to recognise practice that needs to be challenged, and on the other, give us the strength of character to carry the decision forward, regardless how difficult things may get.

In Ruth's story, the Social Worker must be able to recognise that Samantha reminds her of her own daughter and that this may affect her analysis of the situation and potentially cloud her judgement as to the best way to intervene. Furthermore, the Social Worker must be able to acknowledge the possible obstacles facing her should she decide to leave the situation as is, i.e. supporting Samantha as an adult who is able to make her own decisions. The Social Worker will also have to take into consideration the course of action the organisation is endorsing and how this might affect her own course of action. For example, issues of risk management may have become dominant from the agency's point of view, and this may potentially affect Ruth's judgement in making her decision in ways that are not compatible with the virtues discussed above. As O'Brian explains,

> professional judgment becomes circumscribed [...], the social worker's role is somewhat different than ones that are based on the two values of personal caring and social justice. A third value base appears to have emerged that we might call 'resource and risk management'.
>
> (2003, p. 391)

As seen in the case study, Ruth is working for an organisation who wants her to intervene more directly in the case. A courageous Social Worker will take appropriate means to resist such pressure if her chosen course of action is to not follow the advice of her supervisor. Courage can therefore be an important virtue here in that it may help the Social Worker carry her decision forward even as things become more difficult. Ethical issues of this type, that is, involving a conflict of loyalty between the user's interest and agency policy, has been identified by the IFSW (2004) as an important area for the emergence of ethical dilemmas and problems in practice. A courageous Social Worker will therefore have the strength to recognise possible conflicts and to carry through with the decision she has made despite the odds.

Professionalism in Social Work: The Virtuous, Caring Social Worker

The above virtues, as we have seen, are not always mutually exclusive and contain certain shared elements. For example, the theme of honesty was included in discussions about 'trustworthiness' and 'integrity'. This is a good example of how virtues are not exhibited alone and illustrates the need for developing them in sets. This is why, in a Virtue Ethics perspective, it is so important to develop a combination of different character traits. In the case study explored above, it is clear that Ruth could not have reached the best course of action based on a single virtue such as 'care'. Instead, it is the combination of all the different virtues explored above that made Ruth position herself as a more ethical Social Worker. This demonstrates that ethics based on virtue must include a combination of character traits to be effective, and that no single virtue will lead to happiness.

As to which course of action would arise from virtue ethics and the ethics of care in this particular case, it is clear that Ruth may want to continue working with Samantha while respecting the latter's relationship with her boyfriend, as well as the decision she has made. Professionalism, in this sense, will require Ruth to continue monitoring the situation from a care perspective and critically analyse and re-evaluate it in light of new elements. She will also be aware of her own values and emotions and the impact they may have on her perception and analysis of the situation. She will respect Samantha in her choices and show compassion throughout. Even if the situation becomes difficult to manage and Ruth feels pressure from her agency to act in a particular way, she will have the courage and strength to persevere if she believes that it is the best way forward for Samantha and is compatible with the Social Work value base. More importantly, Ruth will continue to reason practically with regard to the situation as it unfolds and will remain flexible as her analysis of it evolves.

The virtuous Social Worker will then become habituated to reason and will exhibit the appropriate virtues necessary to maintain the best ethical Social Work practice at all times. This brings us to the conclusion of the chapter, in which we will briefly explore the application of virtue ethics and the ethics of care to modern Social Work practice.

Professionalism in Context: The Role of Virtue Ethics and the Ethics of Care in Different Organisations

We have seen throughout this book, and as illustrated in the above case study, that the organisational work context can greatly impact the way ethical practice is constructed, interpreted and maintained within Social Work. Indeed, the organisational work context often contributes to the development of relationships of power between the organisation and the Social Worker, and between the Social Worker, service users, groups, and communities. In some situations, these relationships of power may result, for example, in the enactment of a particular legislation to protect a young person, or in limiting the application of a policy related to resource allocation, which may seriously affect preventative Social Work intervention for a particular service user.

How then can character-based ethics such as virtue ethics and the ethics of care help Social Workers in different organisational contexts? Some authors believe that a combination of virtue ethics and the ethics of care can help Social Workers operate ethically regardless of the work context. Indeed, MacIntyre (1999) asserts that cultivating virtues through practical reasoning is an effective mechanism for counteracting organisational contexts that may be detrimental to service users. If we truly understand what essentially constitutes a virtue, it becomes clear that practical reasoning can help Social Workers better identify their Social Work values and the nature of Social Work practice in general, without having to restrict themselves to the dominant forms of ethics seen in previous chapters, in which ethical principles are simply applied. Applying these principles without possessing the appropriate character traits or without having an awareness of the relationships in which we are involved can lead Social Workers to become technocrats instead of professionals capable of ethical judgement and reasoning.

As MacIntyre points out, a virtue is "an acquired human quality" (2007, p. 191) rather than a feeling about rightness or wrongness. These personal qualities or 'virtues', when practised, will become part of the person instead of a one-off "act of heroism" (Lynch and Lynch, 2006). Understanding the primary concept of virtues, and developing them through 'practical reasoning', will help practitioners to feel more confident about their decisions and, consequently, to challenge, when necessary, the power relationships that exist in their organisational work context, between themselves and their employers, and between themselves and service users. A note of caution, as MacIntyre (2007) explains: 'virtue ethics' is not always compatible with effectiveness and therefore does not always go hand in hand with the aims of organisations. To accomplish virtuous acts, Social Workers must exhibit many virtues at once; they must possess practical reasoning abilities in order to exhibit the right virtue at the right time and avoid succumbing to organisational pressure and bureaucracy. We acknowledge, however, that the impact of the organisational work context is significant for Social Workers and that challenging this context is not always an easy task.

Conclusion

We have explored in this chapter the major tenets of virtue ethics and the ethics of care, and how these perspectives can be relevant to modern Social Work practice. We have also seen that it is through practical reasoning that virtues can be developed and cultivated to the point that they become habits and integrated into all aspects of one's life. The ethics of care complements virtue ethics by emphasising the importance of the intervention relationship and the role of emotions in ethical reasoning. By examining Ruth's story, we observed how combining practical reason with the right character traits can help Social Workers act ethically and find the appropriate responses to ethical dilemmas in practice. Furthermore, by considering the application of various codes of ethics and conduct, we have seen how character-based ethics can use the various principles of Social Work practice and values to complement ethical reasoning as one of many ways to arrive at ethical decision-making. We have also seen how certain virtues, such as courage and criticality, can help Social Workers challenge inappropriate use and abuse of power within organisations, and how these virtues can help Social Workers act ethically regardless of the context in which they practice.

11 The Ethics of Recognition

The ethics of recognition was proposed by Axel Honneth, a contemporary German philosopher born in 1945. To this day, Axel Honneth continues to work as a professor of philosophy at Columbia University in the United States.

Similar to virtue ethics (see Chapter 10), the ethics of recognition gives attention to the relationships between a person or a group of people and their environment (Pullen Sansfaçon and Bellot, 2016). However, the ethics of recognition focuses not only on the relationship between people but also pays attention to how the broader environment, including the social and the political contexts, affects the experience of a person or a group. The idea of a just society is also very important for Honneth, but as we will see in this chapter, it takes a different form for Honneth than what is considered 'just' by Bentam, Mills or Rawls, covered in Chapter 9. You may remember that for Bentham and Mills, justice results from applying principles that help to determine the right course of action. For Honneth, experiences of justice and injustice instead take form within the relationship one has with their loved ones, and with society and the institutions that compose it. Honneth's notion looks at how those relationships contribute to the experience of being recognised as person or not. Hence, for Honneth, justice is the result of a process of recognition. Conversely, social injustice emerges when a person or a group of people are denied recognition by others, or by society or its institutions (Honneth, 2007).

At the centre of his proposal, Honneth asserts that human identity cannot be separated from the experience of recognition, which, as we will see later in this chapter, can be manifest in everyday lives (Houston, 2015). As such, the ethics of recognition require that we understand ethical action as being rooted in the recognition of all human beings in different dimensions of one's life. An analysis of the experience of recognition, or of disrespect, can then be used as a framework to understand how a situation can be ethical or not and help to identify directions to move forward to work towards a more socially just society, that is, one that produces recognition for everyone.

Reflection Break: Understanding Recognition and Non-recognition at an Individual Level

Think about a situation when you felt recognised. This could be when you achieved something, received an award or any other situation that you can relate to when thinking about being recognised.

DOI: 10.4324/9781003458715-15

Now think about another situation, one where you felt disrespected. It could be a situation that you experienced with your family, for example, or even a situation where you felt that your needs or even your rights were not taken into consideration or upheld.

How did you feel? What emotions did you experience? What did you do? Write down your thoughts about those two experiences of recognition and non-recognition.

Recognition and Disrespect

Based on his theory, Honneth posits that the value or worth that each of us can recognise in ourselves depends on how people and institutions around us value us, and our perception of that. For example, let's say you are learning to play the violin. You may have practised for many years, and believe you are getting good at it. But if you think about this, how do you self-assess your skill level? It may be by having a goal and meeting this goal; it may also be by the feedback you are receiving from your violin teacher or mentor. You may feel good about your progress because people around you are telling you that you are doing great. Or you may self-assess by comparing the sound you make to the sounds made by other violinists you know. But can you develop this feeling of worth or value about your violin-playing if no one is there to give you feedback, or if there is no one around to compare your skills to? Would your feelings be the same if people around you told you that you are not very good at playing the violin?

If that happened, you might not feel so good about it, and you might even decide to abandon your violin practice. But what if, for everything you try, you get that same negative feedback? You might feel good about something, but if the feedback you receive is constantly minimising your success or skill, it may well affect the way you think about yourself in the long run.

A reflection like this one can be a good start to understanding the idea of recognition and disrespect. For Honneth, the idea of recognition is understood as an intersubjective experience – that is, a subjective experience you have in relation to others. Recognition, in this sense, is only possible in the context of relationships between people.

If you look for a synonym of *recognition* in a reference book like a thesaurus, you will find words like *acceptance, appreciation, realisation, respect* and *understanding*. We can see that winning a prize makes you feel recognised, because prizes are usually awarded to people who have distinguished themselves for a specific achievement or a skill. But having the right to vote is also a form of recognition because this specific right means that you are recognised as someone who can self-determine, who is autonomous and can make decisions regarding what sort of society you want. Being told by someone you love that you are important in their life is also a form of recognition because it contributes to this feeling of worthiness that is important in each relationship.

So far, you can see that recognition can take various forms and is shaped, to a certain extent, by the relationships you have with others and the feedback you receive from them. In the examples we have just examined, you can see that, to a different degree in each case, you would feel appreciated, recognised and respected for who you are or for a particular skill you have. This, in its simplest form, is how we can experience recognition.

But for Honneth, recognition is not only individual and does not happen only in relation to other people. The experience of recognition, while subjective, is also integrated into social norms and practices, which set the conditions that underlie this mutual intersubjectivity (Pada, 2017). Otherwise, how do you know that your particular skill is to be praised and not put down? To feel recognised is an individual experience that requires first the capacity to be autonomous in your judgement about yourself. When it is examined in relation to social norms, the feeling or recognition can lead you to develop a feeling of legitimacy (Pada, 2017).

Norms are informal rules that people follow. Rules, and to a certain extent, the laws, are often manifestations of norms that have been formalised. Norms, rules and laws all contribute to reinforcing the social order, which benefits people who are in positions of power (Mullaly, 2010). It is important to remember at this point that social norms can influence both individual and social behaviours. Accordingly, to take into consideration the personal and the social experience of recognition, Honneth proposes three interlinked forms, namely: love or caring appreciation; recognition in the form of rights and equal treatment under the law; and social recognition, that is, acknowledgement in the community or society (Honneth, 2004; Houston, 2009).

We will now look at these three forms of recognition in detail to understand how they manifest, as well as the experiences of disrespect that people can also have in each area. We will see that those experiences of recognition can lead to the development of self-confidence, self-respect, self-worth and self-esteem (Brown and Murphy, 2011). We will also examine how a lack of recognition in even just one area can result in experiences of disrespect and contempt. In these experiences, relationships with others and the importance of self-other recognition are both key:

> Self-confidence develops when one is recognized by significant others in terms of love and care, as an individual with needs and desires, possessing a unique value to others. Self-respect develops out of recognition by others that one is just as responsible for one's actions as all others in society—one is recognized by others as a morally accountable member of that society. Self-esteem emerges from the gaze and recognition of others who acknowledge one's capabilities and qualities as making a significant contribution to a community. Honneth links this to a sense of community solidarity—a sense of wellbeing founded on respect and recognition of the contribution being made to common goals.
>
> (Brown and Murphy, 2011, p. 47)

Love

Love, which supports the development of self-confidence, is the first level whereby someone can experience recognition. From Honneth's perspective, and in many Western societies, love takes form in the context of affective relationships, often experienced within primary relationships. By primary relationships, we mean the relationships we have with our parents, our siblings and other people we are in close relationships with (lover, partner, close friend and so on). These relationships usually require that primary needs, meaning physical and emotional needs, be fulfilled. Feeling recognised, through love and affective relationships, means that one feels cared for, important and worth it. Experiences of recognition at that level are linked to the development of self-confidence, which is the basis for social autonomy. As Honneth explains,

> The positive attitude to oneself that arises from such affective recognition is that of trust in oneself. It refers to the fundamental layer of emotional and bodily self-assurance in the expression of one's needs and feelings, which forms the psychological preconditions for the development of all the other aspects of self-respect (...) [This type of recognition can only be achieved] through primary social relationships, apparent in affective ties such as family, friendship or love.
>
> (Honneth, 2001, p. 49)

Did You Know?

While the notion of self-confidence is often used interchangeably with the concept of self-esteem in the literature, they are considered different. Self-confidence relates to a person's capacity to believe in their ability to achieve something, whereas self-esteem relates more to the idea of self-appreciation.

An intersubjective experience of love therefore allows a person to develop their emotional safety, which, in turn, enables the person to trust their own emotions and articulate them to other people (Le Goff, 2008). To illustrate this, imagine a five-year-old child who dropped a glass of milk on the floor. If the child feels that their parents' love is strong, it will be natural for the child to tell the parent about this spill. The child who is loved should not be too worried about telling their parent, and their worth should not be negatively affected by such a small incident. The experience and the feedback the child receive from the interaction with the parent should be overall positive and should contribute to building the child's confidence because they continue to feel that their parents love and respect them for who they are even though they spilled a glass of milk on the floor.

Imagine, now, an alternative scenario where the child spills a glass of milk, but instead of taking care of the child, the parent severely reprimands them. Imagine that every time that the child encounters a small accident like this one, or does something the parent does not appreciate, the parent strongly criticises them or even calls them names, like 'clumsy' or 'worthless'. This type of situation will quickly have a negative impact on the child's self-confidence. They will internalise the negative labels and they will start doubting their capacity to be autonomous.

In the first example, the experience of self-other recognition will enable the child to develop self-confidence as well as autonomy, knowing that even when they make a mistake, it does not challenge who they are. In the second example, the child will grow more wary, will doubt their feelings and, if the situation continues, may grow up as an adult who lacks self-confidence. According to an ethics of recognition perspective, child neglect and abuse are considered severe forms of disrespect which "[violate] autonomy and self-realization within the developing infant" (Houston, 2009, p. 1282).

Rights

A second level of recognition happens within the realms of a person's right to be treated equally and to self-determine. For Honneth, a person can develop a feeling of self-respect when they enjoy the same rights and responsibilities as other members of society. Having access to equal rights affects a person's self-respect because it allows a person to see themselves as morally competent, with all the rights and obligations that this entails. It is also through rights that people can participate in society. Not enjoy the same rights as others is a form of disrespect (Honneth, 1995):

> We are here dealing with the denial of rights and with social exclusion, where human beings suffer in their dignity through not being granted the moral rights and responsibilities of a full legal person within their community. Accordingly, this type of disrespect has to have, as its corresponding relation, the reciprocal recognition through which individuals come to regard themselves as equal bearers of rights from the perspective of their fellows.
>
> (Honneth, 2001, p. 49)

In Honneth's perspective, having rights is essential for a person to feel validated, and must be interpreted as inclusive of legal, political, cultural and material privilege (Houston, 2009). The right to have shelter, the right to be treated equally and with respect, the right to vote and express your thoughts freely, and the right to practice your religion or your culture freely are all illustrative of essential rights.

To be denied those rights directly affects a person's moral autonomy because it constrains their capacity to decide for themselves. Research also shows that human rights violations have an important effect on the mental health of people affected by them. For example, human rights violations such as torture or being displaced as a refugee can have significant consequences, such as developing a higher rate of post-traumatic stress disorder and depression (Steel et al., 2009). This is also true of other forms of rights restrictions and violations.

Reflection Break

During pandemics, many populations have seen their rights restricted, sometimes for long periods of time. For example, in the Province of Quebec, Canada, populations were subjected to strict lockdowns for five months, with the imposition of a curfew where people were not allowed to leave their homes between the hours of 8 p.m. and 5 a.m. While some of the restrictions implemented in different places may have been necessary at the time, they may still have had some impacts on the people who were subjected to them.

Think about some of the restrictions that were imposed in your area during the early phases of COVID-19, and answer the following questions, taking care to write down your answers:

What restrictions were imposed?
How did they affect you? Why?
What helped you navigate this period of restriction?

During the early phases of the COVID-19 pandemic, many countries implemented restrictions on populations to prevent the spread of the virus (Rahman et al., 2021). National lockdowns and all the consequences that came with them (e.g., loss of income, being prevented from attending school, being isolated, and so on) have been shown to have effects on mental health, including suicidality, and this was particularly true among populations that were already vulnerable before the pandemic, such as children, girls, elderly people and racial and ethnic minority groups (Rahman et al., 2021).

We have just seen that a person who has their rights denied can experience many negative consequences. You can probably also see how having your rights upheld is a basic condition that allows you to feel capable of making decisions for yourself, and to feel self-determined.

We will now turn to the last dimension of recognition, that of solidarity.

Solidarity

It is not enough for a person or a group to be recognised through rights under the law. It is also essential that these rights be accepted and recognised more widely in the community and in society at large. This is the basis for solidarity. This last form of recognition pertains to the social world and helps create a person's feeling of worth and a sense that they can contribute to society. It is through feeling recognised socially that a person can develop their self-esteem. Through solidarity, a person can feel acknowledged in their community for who they are and what they do (Houston, 2009). For example, in a study about the social inclusion of young refugees in Australia, researchers showed that when the refugees felt a sense of belonging to their family and their community, this was linked to a greater feeling of well-being and specifically to greater self-esteem (Correa-Velez et al., 2010). More generally speaking, research has shown that feeling connected to a community is correlated to having higher self-esteem, but this link also creates a feedback loop, in the sense that your self-esteem may also affect your experience of engaging in social relationships (Harris and Orth, 2019). Honneth (2001, pp. 49–50) suggests that the "solidaristic acceptance and social regard of an individual's abilities and way of life" is fundamentally how people experience social recognition.

What Is the Ethics of Recognition?

The ethics of recognition state that social order cannot exist if individuals or groups are not recognised fully (Pullen Sansfaçon and Bellot, 2016). In this sense, ethics of recognition is a framework that helps identify where recognition is lacking, and how society can produce more recognition for all human beings. According to Honneth (1995), a just society will ensure that everyone is recognised because feeling positively recognised by others through love, rights and solidarity can promote a society that allows all human beings to flourish through self-confidence, self-respect and self-esteem.

A society that fails to provide recognition to all human beings is what Honneth would describe as a socially unjust society, which in his view provides "the justificatory impetus for struggle, contest and social change" (Houston, 2009). In other words, lack of recognition, while generally leading to negative consequences for those who experience it (as we have already seen), also constitutes grounds for confronting oppression. Indeed, Honneth believes that those experiences of disrespect may inspire resistance and lead people or groups to demand greater recognition individually, socially and legally.

Reflection Break

While trying to apply the ethics of recognition to any given social situation, you may want to ask yourself the following questions:

1 Are certain individuals or groups differently valued in society on the basis of who they are?
2 Are individuals usually treated with respect in their primary relationships (e.g. by their parents, close friends and lovers)?
3 How are the differences in the way people are treated expressed in social interactions, and more broadly, in society (e.g. are they experiencing disrespect)?
4 How are these interactions reflected in larger social policies, laws, institutions and belief systems?

(Adapted from Dotolo et al., 2018, pp. 150–151.)

So, in terms of ethics, recognition theory provides a framework to understand whether or not social injustices are occurring, how they are occurring and how they can be challenged (Doloto et al., 2018). In Social Work, this framework can be particularly relevant, especially in guiding interventions that aim to promote the empowerment of people and groups who are experiencing oppression, as we covered in Chapter 6 about empowerment.

We will now examine a case study, that of Riley, a 13-year-old trans youth. We examine how trans youth like Riley experience of various forms of recognition, and we will discuss what a more ethical society could look like according to the ethics of recognition.

Case Study: Riley

Riley is a 13-year-old transgender girl (assigned male at birth) who resides in a small town in Nova Scotia, Canada. She attends her local high school and is currently completing her second year. In response to growing challenges at home and school, her parents asked to speak to a Social Worker.

At the first meeting, Riley's parents reported that her grades had dropped dramatically and that she was increasingly isolated herself. The past three weeks have been particularly difficult for Riley, who has refused to go to school because she was being bullied. Previously, Riley had a supportive network of friends, mostly girls. However, since she started to express her gender identity in a more feminine manner (she is now wearing nail polish and is growing her hair longer, and she has asked her teacher to use she/her pronouns), she has reported that her friends have started distancing themselves from her. Riley also says that boys, with whom she never felt a natural affinity, have begun to threaten her. Riley's parents also say they have noticed small cuts on her forearms, which the Social Workers identify as possible self-harming.

The parents also explain that since early childhood, Riley has shown a keen interest in activities such as dance, gymnastics and visual arts. Riley's parents recall that at a younger age, their child always played with a cousin's old Barbie. They explain that about a month ago, they caught Riley dressing up in a nightgown, which felt like too much for them to handle. The parents say that they didn't mind their child playing with Barbies, but dressing like a girl 'was unacceptable'. Riley's parents expressed being very uncomfortable with Riley's recent gender expression and mentioned feeling increasingly embarrassed by their child in public. They want the behaviour to stop, and they clearly express their frustration with it.

After a few sessions with a psychologist, Riley receives a diagnosis of 'gender dysphoria', which means an experience of distress stemming from a feeling of incongruence between her sex assigned at birth and her gender identity. They recommend that Riley be referred to the local gender clinic and receive continued follow-up with a Social Worker to identify her needs and discuss possible transition care.

Analysis

Trans youth like Riley are at great risk of experiencing many forms of rejection and violence by one or more family members or friends due to the stigmatisation of their gender identity (Weinhardt et al., 2019). These experiences can be a good illustration of various individual and social forms of disrespect. Even though coming out about one's gender identity or sexual orientation can lead to a positive feeling (e.g., relief), many young people are afraid to come out and fear being rejected, threatened or abused by their family and their peers. Families can be supportive and foster resilience, but can also be a source of difficulties for trans youth (Fuller and Riggs, 2018) as these youth often experience rejection. The road to family acceptance can be arduous and time-consuming, leading to conflict within the family sphere (Pullen Sansfaçon et al., 2015). For example, a study of trans youth in 10 Canadian clinics has shown that on average, they realised that their gender was different from their sex assigned at birth at the age of 9.9, but only began living in their affirmed gender around age 12.3. This study highlights the significant gap between the moment a young person realises what their gender identity is and the moment they start to live in their gender, i.e., a gap of 2.4 years (Lawson et al., 2024). The negative attitudes the family can have after their youth comes out can have various consequences on the youth, such as feeling rejected and disrespected in their identity, in addition to being subjected to open violence and hostile behaviours (Pullen Sansfaçon et al., 2020).The discrimination and violence trans youth suffer can take extreme forms, such as physical assault or blocking access to gender-affirming medical care (Katz-Wise et al., 2018). In a recent study of trans youth in Quebec, Canada, Ladry et al., (2024) found that nearly half of the trans youth in their study had experienced sexual violence (44.1%) and nearly 20% of the sample had been physically injured by a family member, a phenomenon more frequently encountered among 14- to 18-year-olds.

In Riley's situation, it is clear that her parents are struggling with accepting their child's behaviours. These challenges are clear in the way they express themselves to the Social Worker as well as to Riley. Indeed, they tell Riley not to express her gender identity. According to Honneth, in wanting her to stop expressing her gender identity, they are engaging in a form of disrespect, which will contribute to Riley feeling low self-confidence and perhaps even shame about herself.

But the situation could change if Riley's parents were more accepting of her. In a study led by Olson and colleagues which examined the mental health outcomes of 73 prepubertal trans children who had socially transitioned, their results show that children who socially transitioned had the same levels of mental health outcomes compared with their siblings and cisgender peers, except for anxiety, which was slightly higher than for the other groups (Durwood et al., 2017; Olson et al., 2016). Being socially transitioned involves people from all spheres of one's life using the correct name and pronoun. Another study of 148 trans youth found similar results (Gibson et al., 2021). The results of these studies differ significantly from previous work that reported higher rates of anxiety and depression. This underlines the importance of respecting and recognising young people's gender identity and shows the positive impact this can have on their lives.

This case study illustrates how experiences of recognition can lead to positive outcomes. In Riley's situation, Social Workers who adopt an ethics of recognition framework would try to work with the parents to help them accept their child, to increase the recognition Riley experiences in her family.

That said, the Social Worker will also need to be aware that it may be difficult for parents to come to accept their youth and that they may experience disrespect in the process of accepting their child, such as being subjected to indirect stigmatisation and rejection from their friends and family, which may lead to challenging emotions (Pullen Sansfacon et al., 2015). The Social Workers will need to be equipped to work with the parents and understand that they may lack knowledge about their child's experience. For example, parents need to understand that not supporting a child who experiences gender dysphoria will not make the behaviour change. Instead, not supporting a trans child's gender identity is linked to higher odd of suicidal ideation (Jin et al., 2020). This makes sense from an ethics of recognition standpoint, in that disrespect leads to a lack of self-respect. Indeed, trans youth who have been experiencing emotional neglect (not feeling loved, important or special) were two and a half times more likely to experience lifetime suicide attempts (Austin et al., 2022). We also know that a feeling of being a burden and low self-esteem are linked to suicide (Teismann et al., 2024).

To increase Riley's experience of recognition, the Social Workers could affirm her identity and address her by the correct name and pronoun so that she feels validated. The Social Workers could also work by helping her parents accept their child by providing information to them, as well as referring them to a resource so they can feel supported. Adopting an ethics of recognition standpoint would therefore require Social Workers to ensure that Riley feels recognised by her family, and that will necessarily require that they intervene with her parents.

The Social Worker will also need to address the question of social and legal recognition. Being recognised and feeling loved by your family is very important, but Riley will also need to experience other forms of recognition. According to Honneth, experiences of recognition – or conversely, of disrespect – are often deeply anchored in a much broader context than within intimate relationships.

In terms of social recognition, we can see that Riley is also experiencing bullying and is being isolated at school. Unfortunately, trans young people are the most likely to experience harassment based on gender and sex at school and these experiences are directly correlated to having poorer mental health (Sares Jäske et al., 2023). Yet research shows that these problems, in school and in the broader social context, are often caused by a lack of social acceptance. As a result, many of the challenges experienced by youth like Riley are not attributable to how they identify, but rather how they are perceived and treated socially. School for a young trans person can become terrorising if no support is provided. Not only can they be subjected to bullying, but they may also experience challenges related to using the bathroom and changing rooms, which can be particularly complicated.

Fortunately, school boards can play an important role in the lives of trans youth by implementing inclusive policies to ensure their well-being and protection. A school can draw on antibullying policies to clearly state that bullying based on gender identity or expression is not tolerated, just like bullying on other grounds. With Riley's consent, the Social Worker could set a meeting with the school to discuss how the learning environment could be improved and make a plan with them to help increase the experience of recognition in this setting. From an ethics of recognition standpoint, this will help Riley to be more recognised and should have a positive impact on her well-being. This can start by having the school use the right name and pronoun when addressing her. Gender affirmation – including the correct use of a name and pronoun and recognition of a person's authentic gender identity – is an important protective factor for the wellbeing of trans youth. Conversely, failure to use the correct pronoun or name has been shown to negatively affect young people's well-being (Pullen Sansfaçon et al., 2018).

However, broader social recognition may also be lacking, and this can have a direct impact on the school context. In Canada, anti-trans rhetoric has also been on the rise lately (Boynton, 2023; Lebel, 2023), even leading the Canadian Security Intelligence Service to issue a report pointing out that the current anti-trans movement poses a risk of extreme violence to gender-diverse people, including trans youth. The negative social and geopolitical context can lead gender-diverse people to experience distress, which again negatively impacts mental health and contributes to the experience of marginalisation (Dubois and Juster, 2022). In other words, a deleterious social climate is also likely to adversely affect the mental health of trans young people. Again, thinking of the ethics of recognition, the Social Worker takes into consideration and develops an understanding of the context and how it can create experiences of non-recognition and disrespect. An ethics of recognition standpoint will also orient some of the interventions that the Social Worker could put in place, such as facilitating community organisation or social action with trans youth like Riley, and with parents of gender-diverse youth, if possible.

In terms of rights and legal recognition, gender identity is protected in federal and provincial human rights charters in Canada. This context can help Riley to feel recognised. However, it may be a challenge for her to access a clinic, even with a diagnosis, if her parents are not supportive of her. Access to medical and social care is also a right, and when trans youth express their needs and have a diagnosis like Riley's, they need to be able to access these types of care. An ethics of recognition standpoint would direct the Social Worker to work with the parents again and support them in their education about the needs of trans young people like Riley. Living in the Atlantic region of Canada, it is often difficult to access mental health care, and Canada-wide, over the past 12 months, 43% of trans youth have not been able to access the physical health care they need (Taylor et al., 2020). This figure shows that access remains a problem. Worldwide we can observe a trend whereby access to gender-affirming medical care to help with gender dysphoria is being banned or restricted (see Chapter 8 – the importance of practical reasoning – for discussion on the reasons for this). From an ethics of recognition standpoint, not being offered care for a situation that is recognised by the World Health Organization could be seen as a form of non-recognition.

The ethics of recognition also suggest that experiences of disrespect at different levels can become fertile ground for resistance. Considering that Social Work "promotes social change and development, social cohesion, and the empowerment and liberation of people" (IFSW, 2014), Social Workers like the one intervening in Riley's situation should be well equipped to develop interventions that could facilitate a process to achieve greater recognition and confront oppressions. The same applies in situations where services users and groups are experiencing non-recognition in any of the three dimensions: love, solidarity and rights.

In doing so, it will be important that the Social Worker involves the people who are concerned by the experience of disrespect. Indeed, planning intervention *for* but *without the involvement of* the people who are concerned by a given issue could manifest itself as a form of disrespect in Honneth's sense because it would treat service users who are cognisant of their own experience as unable to act on their own behalf. Hence, developing interventions, whether at individual, community or social level, based on an ethics of recognition standpoint, should fully involve service users and groups of people concerned with the experience of disrespect, and aim to facilitate anti-oppressive and empowering action so that the intervention not only confronts the oppression but also, by the process itself, produce recognition. Approaches such as the Pedagogy of Liberation, proposed by Brazilian Educator Paulo Freire (Gibson, 1999) or based on self-directed groupwork (Mullender et al., 2013), could be particularly helpful to challenge oppression and facilitate the empowerment of service users.

Conclusion

Through his theory of recognition, Honneth proposed that a just society will be one that produces recognition, not only at the individual level, but also at the social level and in the form of laws. Honneth's theory helps us understand how each of these levels are linked – for example, how a lack of social acceptance may have a negative impact on a young person's experience of acceptance by their parents as well as in terms of legal protections. In this sense, Honneth's theory provides a very helpful framework for analysis that takes into consideration the person in their environment. Such a framework is particularly helpful in a profession like Social Work. It also helps identify how intervention can be oriented to create more recognition for everyone, and helps us understand how experiences of non-recognition, while extremely challenging for those who experience them, can be mobilised to support action aimed at challenging oppression.

Conclusion

The Challenges Facing Social Work

Throughout this book, we have been concerned to open up the ways in which Social Work students and practitioners can engage with ethical issues as they present in contemporary Social Work practice. Inevitably, this has led us into a discussion of many of the difficulties and challenges facing Social Work. For example, we have examined issues of power and bureaucracy, as well as the problems of radicalisation and the rise of the Extreme Right, both in the form of political movements and as parties of government. Through the book, we have presented complex cases and issues in which social workers often have to be involved. We have argued throughout the book that social work is a profession that is inherently complex, both ethically as well as practically. Firstly, the people who social workers work with are disproportionately from those sections of the community with the lowest incomes, the poorest educational outcomes, the poorest health outcomes and the highest levels of unemployment. In the current context, social workers will continue to observe a rise in hardship for these individuals and communities, which will inevitably lead to pressures on family relationships, various forms of social exclusion and criminalisation. It is also the case, as we discussed earlier in the book, that following the Banking Crisis of 2007–2008, we have seen both a huge increase in social inequality and a decrease in the resources available to the Social Work profession. This can influence not only the accessibility of social work but also the type of social work that practitioners will engage in during such a period.

In Part 1 of this book, we examined aspects of Social Work's historic legacy, and one of the most important points we sought to express here was the idea that Social Work never has been and never will be just one thing – there have always been crucial value conflicts within Social Work; we characterised these as the 'two souls' of Social Work. As the chapters in the Part II of the book seek to make clear, one of the most fundamental aspects of neoliberal dominance in economics, politics and policy has been to change "the meanings of welfare and the state as well as the policy and organizational structures to which they refer" (Clarke et al., 2000, p. 3). Many have wondered whether the present politics of austerity process places Social Work itself under threat. However, given the publics' demand for the authorities to 'do something' with regard to the social problems which catch public interest, and given the role Social Work plays in relation to these, it is probably the case that if Social Work was ever abolished it would need to be reinvented under another name. At the same time, one of the most significant impacts on Social Work in the present atmosphere of austerity and financial restrictions is, as we noted, about the kind of Social Work likely to be practised under these conditions. The world we are living

DOI: 10.4324/9781003458715-16

in at the moment is one where political movements of the Right are speaking to the social crisis, insecurity and anxieties people feel through a politics of blame. In situations where people can no longer envisage compassionate and hopeful solutions to problems such as increasing social and economic inequality, global migration and the climate crisis, then they can turn to the politics of despair and blame. We have spent the last 20 years working with practitioners and teaching social work students. We know that the profession of Social Work all over the world is a huge resource of skills and insight. We know that Social Work is a profession that shows that it has the capacity to work creatively with individuals and communities who are experiencing abuse, marginalisation and exclusion. But the progressive legacy of Social Work can never be taken for granted – and it is for this reason that we see the reconstruction and strengthening of ideas of ethical practice in Social Work as so important.

The Social Worker as Intellectual

In Chapter 1, we also discussed two different definitions of Social Work; one from the IFSW and one from Jacqui Smith, former UK Minister of Social Care. We noted that the IFSW definition represented the progressive and democratic impetus within social work, while Jacqui Smith's definition understood Social Workers' skills as 'practical' rather than 'theoretical'. Indeed, it is interesting to note when one looks at the many different conceptualisations of Social Work, how this difference in understanding the Social Work role often focuses on whether Social Work is seen as a synthesis of the theoretical and the practical, as in the IFSW definition, or whether it represents the practical as opposed to the theoretical, as in Jacqui Smith's definition. Our argument is that if Social Workers are to make the link between an immediate presenting situation and its roots in the wider social structure, then, they need to engage their conceptual and intellectual capacities. In an article that makes a definitive argument for Social Workers to see themselves as 'transformative intellectuals', Cowden and Singh argue:

> Central to reconstructing this sense of the social worker as a 'transformative intellectual' lies an understanding of the significance of the way social workers are witnesses to abuses of power and authority in society. The question of how social workers might respond to this is central to social work's 'praxis'; that is, the way it brings together the theoretical conceptual aspect of these situations with the practical tasks involved in attempting to deal with them.
>
> (2009, p. 8)

To talk about "Social Workers as Intellectuals" is not to imply a coldly unemotional response to people's problems and difficulties. However, it is argued that sympathy alone is insufficient in social work. The writer Oscar Wilde put this with characteristic wit when he argued "the emotions of man [sic] are stirred much more easily than intelligence, and… it is much easier to have sympathy with suffering than with thought" (1973, p. 19). When we are confronted by the suffering of service users and their families that we see in practice, it is right that we respond emotionally, but not only so. True empathy and compassion come from the ability to theorise and thereby make sense of the issues that we see service users facing – and it is this intellectual understanding that forms a central tenet of Social Work's practical humanitarianism, as well being that which distinguishes Social Workers from being a good friend or a neighbour to the service user. It is therefore essential that we develop the ability to understand and name the wider structures and hidden assumptions that frame the conditions in which people live.

The Social Worker as Practical Reasoner

One of the concepts which links all the themes explored in the book together in a useful way is the concept of the 'practical reasoner'.

We see a Social Worker committed to practical reasoning as someone who speaks with their own voice and is not simply, in Payne's phrase, "travelling along guidelines and conventions" (Payne, 2005, p. 126). A Social Worker committed to practical reasoning will be someone who looks beneath the surface – of course they must respond to immediate events, but they will also be situating these in a wider context; thinking beyond and through the immediate presenting situation. A Social Worker committed to practical reasoning will be someone who is prepared to think again and think differently, because flexibility of understanding and capacity to deal with complexity are at the essence of dealing with human problems, such as those involving displacement, violence, oppression, loss, trauma or transition. But thinking differently does not mean simply thinking by yourself according to your own likes and dislikes.

Instead, practical reasoning which is achieved through critical awareness and refection must take place within what MacIntyre calls a 'practice' or a community of people sharing similar skills, values and ability. In other words, for ethical action to take place, the process must happen with other people who belong to the same practice community.

Throughout the book, we highlighted the importance of being aware of our value base and our social location, as this can have an important impact on understanding a situation, but also about what we consider the best way to move forward when faced with ethical dilemmas. We have also argued that social workers should engage in a constant process of critical reflection about the norms and laws that underpin practice, and learn to question and sometimes challenge them, in order to contribute to the development of a more ethical society based on practical reason. In the third section of the book, we have examined and discussed how different ethical theories can help in managing ethical dilemmas and issues in practice. Each of these ethical theories, when applied to a case, guides our reflections by highlighting potential assumptions and focusing on specific dimensions presented by each theory. We have talked about how decolonial ethics, for example, asks social workers to think about their social position when they work with Indigenous people and communities. It can also help non-Indigenous social workers who work with Indigenous people to decolonise their institutions in a meaningful way while also getting to know the people who are affected by colonial policies and institutions on a deeper level. While we have specifically applied this ethical theory to working with Indigenous populations, it can nevertheless be helpful for any social workers working in colonial institutions or aiming to facilitate engagement and empowerment of groups and communities. By applying the ideas of decolonial ethics to situations where there is social injustice, we can better understand it and come up with ways to make the process of achieving a greater balance between groups easier. Chapters 8 and 9 have facilitated our understanding of how to apply various principles to a decision-making process, and how each of Kantian, utilitarian, and Rawlsian ethics focuses on specific aspects that lead to a decision. In Kantian ethics, we have highlighted the importance of the person, of their self-determination, and of their intention, which, if good, should always direct the person to take the 'appropriate' decision. In utilitarian ethics, we have discussed the idea of the greatest happiness for the greatest number, how each possible consequence must be taken into account in deliberation, and the importance of maximising social utility. We have seen how Rawlsian ethics allows to analyse a situation or a context and that everyone can seek their own good, as long as the principles proposed are respected and that the reflection happens in the context of a social contract. We have also examined virtue ethics, which, instead of examining which principles should be applied in a given situation, is the character of the person, or their virtues, that need to be emphasised. We have seen that the virtues facilitate human flourishing – the person making the decision as well as all the other people involved – and that virtues are developed through habituation. Finally, we have discussed how the ethics of recognition enables us to analyse various situations of injustice, with particular attention to the various spheres of recognition that manifest in our relationships with our loved ones, in society, and within the laws. This ethical stance requires us to engage in interventions that give voice to the oppressed by transforming an unjust social order. According to this perspective, this transformation itself produces experiences of recognition for those affected by injustice.

So where does this leave us? How do we know which ethical theory should be applied in a practical social work situation?

A practical reasoner bases their decisions on their practice values and considers the relational aspect of social work by reflecting on their own social location and the historical legacy of the profession. We believed it was crucial to incorporate all these ethical theories in the book, as their combination enables us to consider all the crucial aspects of making sound decisions in the Social Work. If we consider these ethical theories and draw from them more holistically, we can then make decisions that not only critically take into account the context and its history of colonisation, but also, to consider the consequences of an act, the unique aspect of the person, and the society's interests –while remaining critical of the power and dynamics that operates through it and that contributes to the oppression of people. By drawing on theories of recognition and decolonial ethics, we can better work toward promoting a just society, meaningfully engaging services users and groups in the process. Furthermore, recognising that some experience of oppressions – or denial of recognition, can themselves be an opportunity to work with people towards their empowerment and foster experiences of recognition at individual, social and political levels. Drawing on these ethical theories also centres the importance of cultivating the character traits needed in social work. As we have seen in the first two parts of the book, Social Work operates within in a broader context that is saturated in oppressions and power relations. This is, in our sense, the ethical foundations of social work. A type of social work that can be critical, empowering and transformative.

By becoming social workers that are practical reasoner, we can integrate those principles and analytical framework to the point where they become an acquired human quality (Macintyre, 2007). This also points to the links between practical reasoning and the importance of Social Workers valuing their intellectual capacities. The challenges that will face social workers in the years to come may be great, but social worker's skills, knowledge, critical understanding of social dynamics, capacity for self-reflection and strong anchorage in social work values can lay strong foundations for ethical social work practice that are necessary to not only intervene in their daily practice but also contribute to other broader and necessary changes in society.

References

Adams, R. (2008) *Empowerment, Participation and Social Work*. BASW/Palgrave Macmillan, London.

Adams, R., Dominelli, L. and Payne, M. (2002) *Critical Practice in Social Work*. Palgrave, Basingstoke.

Afzal, N. (2018) The Manchester bombing was an attack on women and girls' in *New Statesman* 23/5/2018. https://www.newstatesman.com/politics/2018/05/nazir-afzal-s-diary-manchester-bombing-was-attack-women-and-girls. Accessed 10 October 2023.

Alfred, T. (2009) *Peace, Power, Righteousness: An Indigenous Manifesto* (2nd edition). Oxford University Press, New York.

Allen, C. (2008) *Housing Market Renewal and Social Class*. Routledge, London.

Almond, B. (1995) *Introducing Applied Ethics*. Blackwell American Psychiatric Publishing, Oxford.

American Association of Clinical Endocrinology (2022) AACE Position Statement: Transgender and Gender Diverse. Patients and the Endocrine Community. https://pro.aace.com/recent-news-and-updates/aace-position-statement-transgender-and-gender-diverse-patients. Accessed 14 April 2022.

Amnesty International. (2021) 'You don't look Indigenous' and other prejudices. https://amnistie.ca/sites/default/files/2024-04/livretEN.pdf

Amnesty International. (2024) Israel Appartheid Against Palestinians. 1st February 2022. Online. https://www.amnesty.org/en/latest/campaigns/2022/02/israels-system-of-apartheid/. Accessed 19 November 2024.

Amnesty International Press Release (10/1/2024) 'After 22 years of Human Rights Abuses, the US Government Must Closed the Detention Camp at Guantanamo Bay' https://www.amnestyusa.org/press-releases/after-22-years-of-human-rights-abuses-the-u-s-government-must-close-the-military-detention-camp-at-guantanamo-bay/

Anthias, F. (2013) Intersectional what? Social divisions, intersectionality and levels of analysis. *Ethnicities*, 13(1), 3–19.

Aristotle. (1999) *Nicomachean Ethics* (Translated by W.D. Ross). Batoche Books, Kitchener.

Arnstein, S.R. (1969) A ladder of citizen participation. *Journal of the American Institute of Planners*, 35(4), 216–224. https://doi.org/10.1080/01944366908977225

Assembly of First Nations. (2019) AFN Fact Sheet: What Is Bill C-31 and Bill C-3? https://www.afn.ca/wp-content/uploads/2020/01/16-19-02-06-AFN-Fact-Sheet-Bill-C-31-Bill-C-3-final-revised.pdf

Assiter, A. (2021) *A New Theory of Human Rights. New Materialism and Zoroastrianism*. Rowman & Littlefield, London.

Austin, A., Craig, S.L., D'Souza, S. and McInroy, L.B. (2022) Suicidality among transgender youth: Elucidating the role of interpersonal risk factors. *Journal of Interpersonal Violence*, 37(5–6), NP2696–NP2718. https://doi.org/10.1177/0886260520915554

Baistow, K. (1994) Liberation and regulation? Some paradoxes of empowerment. *Critical Social Policy*, 14(42), 34–46. https://doi.org/10.1177/026101839401404203

Bannerji, H. (2011) Building from marx: Reflections on "race," gender, and class. In S. Carpenter and S. Mojab (Eds.), *Educating from Marx: Race, Gender and Learning* (pp. 41–60), Stanford University Press, Stanford.

Banks, S. and Gallagher, A. (2009) *Ethics in the Professional Life*. Palgrave-Macmillan, Basingstoke.

Banks, S. (1995) *Ethics and Values in Social Work*. Macmillan, Basingstoke.

Banks, S. (2020) *Ethics and Values in Social Work* (5th edition). Bloombury, London.

Bar-On, A. (2002) Restoring power to social work practice. *British Journal of Social Work*, 32(8), 997–1014.

Bartholomew, J. (2020) Decoloniality as an ethical challenge. *TRANSMODERNITY: Journal of Peripheral Cultural Production of the Luso-Hispanic World*, 9(5). https://doi.org/10.5070/T495051214

Beauchamp, T.L. and Childress, J.F. (2001) Principles of Biomedical Ethics (5th edition). Oxford University Press, New York.

Beauchamp, T. (2001) Internal and external standards for medical morality. *Journal of Medicine and Philosophy*, 26(6), 601–619.

Bennoune, K. (2010) 'Why I spoke out on Anwar al-Awlaki' Guardian 19 November 2010. https://www.theguardian.com/commentisfree/cifamerica/2010/nov/19/human-rights-usa#comment-8453210. Accessed 4 June 2023.

Bennoune, K. (2013) *Your Fatwa Does Not Apply Here: Untold Stories from the Fight Against Muslim Fundamentalism*. W.W. Norton & Co., New York.

Bennoune, K. (2014) *Your Fatwa Does Not Apply Here* [online] TED Talk. https://www.youtube.com/watch?v=XLi6iYnnsGc. Accessed 4 June 2023.

Bilge, S. (2009) Théorisations féministes de l'intersectionnalité. *Diogène*, 225(1), 70–88. https://doi.org/10.3917/dio.225.0070

Billard, T.J. (2023) "Gender-critical" discourse as disinformation: Unpacking TERF strategies of political communication. *Women's Studies in Communication*, 46(2), 235–243. https://doi.org/10.1080/07491409.2023.2193545

Black, W (2016) *Daesh and other psychopathic cultures*. https://www.opendemocracy.net/en/transformation/daesh-and-other-psychopathic-cultures/. Accessed 1 September 2023.

Borrows, J. (2019) *Law's Indigenous Ethics*. University of Toronto Press, Toronto.

Bowie, A. (2003) *Introduction to German Philosophy: From Kant to Habermas*. Polity Press, Cambridge.

Boynton, S. (2023, janvier 8) As anti-LGBTQ2 hate grows in Canada, advocates say it's 'never been as scary'. *Global News*. https://globalnews.ca/news/9393280/canada-lgbtq-hate-trans-west-block/

British Association of Social Workers. (2021) *The BASW Code of Ethics for Social Work*. BASW, Birmingham.

British Association of Social Workers. (2024) Climate change is changing social work. *21 mai 2024*. Online. https://basw.co.uk/about-social-work/psw-magazine/articles/climate-change-changing-social-work. Accessed 19 novembre 2024.

Brown, W. (2019) *In the Ruins of Neoliberalism: The Rise of Antidemocratic Politics in the West*. Columbia University Press, New York.

Brown, L.A. and Strega, S. (2015) *Research as Resistance: Revisiting Critical, Indigenous, and Anti-Oppressive Approaches* (2nd edition). Canadian Scholars' Press, Toronto.

Brown, T. and Murphy, M. (2011) Self-Respect, self-confidence and self-esteem: Psychoanalytic and philosophical implications for higher education. *Cliopsy*, 6, 43–51. https://doi.org/10.3917/cliop.006.0043

Butler, J. (1990) *Gender Trouble: Feminism and the Subversion of Identity*. Routledge, New York.

Canadian Association of Social Workers. (2024) Code of Ethics, Values and Guiding Principles. https://www.casw-acts.ca/files/attachements/CASW_-_Code_of_Ethics_Values_Guiding_Principles_-_2024.pdf

Canel-Çınarbaş, D., & Yohani, S. (2019) Indigenous Canadian university students' experiences of microaggressions. *International Journal for the Advancement of Counselling*, 41(1), 41–60. https://doi.org/10.1007/s10447-018-9345-z

Carey, M. (2008a) Everything must go? The privatisation of state social work. *British Journal of Social Work*, 38, 918–935.

Carey, M. (2008b) The quasi-market revolution in the head: Ideology, discourse, care management. *Journal of Social Work*, 8(4), 341–362.

Case-Con Manifesto. https://socialworkfuture.org/case-con/. Accessed 14 August 2009.

Cass, H. (2024). The Cass Review - Independent review of gender identity services for children and young people: Final report. https://cass.independent-review.uk/home/publications/final-report/

Clark, C. (2000) *Social Work Ethics: Politics, Principles and Practice*. Macmillan, Basingstoke.

Clark, C. (2005) The deprofessionalisation thesis, accountability and professional character. *Social Work and Society*, 3(2), 182–190.

Clark, C. (2006) Moral character in social work. *British Journal of Social Work*, 36, 75–89.

Clark, T.C., Lucassen, M.F.G., Bullen, P., Denny, S.J., Fleming, T.M., Robinson, E.M., Rossen, F.V. (2014) The health and well-being of transgender high school students: Results from the New Zealand adolescent health survey (Youth'12). *Journal of Adolescent Health*, 55(1), 93–99.

Clarke, J., Gewirtz, S. and McLaughlin, E. (2000) *New Managerialism, New Welfare?* SAGE Publications Ltd, London.

Clarke, J. (2005) New labour's citizens: Activated, empowered, responsibilized, abandoned?. *Critical Social Policy*, 25(4), 447–463. https://doi.org/10.1177/0261018305057024

Coleman, E., Radix, A.E., Bouman, W.P., Brown, G.R., de Vries, A.L.C., Deutsch, M.B., Ettner, R., Fraser, L., Goodman, M., Green, J., Hancock, A.B., Johnson, T.W., Karasic, D.H., Knudson, G.A., Leibowitz, S.F., Meyer-Bahlburg, H.F.L., Monstrey, S.J., Motmans, J., Nahata, L. ... Arcelus, J. (2022) Standards of care for the health of transgender and gender diverse people, version 8. *International Journal of Transgender Health*, 23(S1), S1–S259. https://doi.org/10.1080/26895269.2022.2100644

Collins, P.H. (2000) *Black Feminist Thought: Knowledge, Consciousness, and the Politics of Empowerment* (2nd edition). Routledge, Abingdon.

Conference of Socilist Economists (CSE) (1980) *In and Against the State*. Pluto Press, London.

Constitution of India. https://www.constitutionofindia.net/articles/article-38-state-to-secure-a-social-order-for-the-promotion-of-welfare-of-the-people/

Conway, Jill Kathryn (ed.) (1992) *Written by Herself: Autobiographies of American Women*. Vintage Books, London.

Correa-Velez, I., Gifford, S. and Barnett, A.G. (2010) Longing to belong: Social inclusion and wellbeing among youth with refugee backgrounds in the first three years in Melbourne, Australia. *Social Science and Medicine*, 71, 1399–1408.

Cowden S. (2021) *Social Workers Working with the Prevent Duty: Interim Report for Research Dissemination Meeting* - Friday 26 February 2021. https://www.researchgate.net/publication/356442563_Social_Workers_working_with_the_Prevent_Duty_Interim_Report_for_Research_Dissemination_Meeting

Cowden, S. and Singh, G. (2007) The 'User': Friend, foe or fetish?: A critical exploration of user involvement in health and social care. *Critical Social Policy*, 27(1), 5–23. https://doi.org/10.1177/0261018307072205

Cowden, S. and Singh, G. (2009) Social workers as intellectuals: Reclaiming a critical praxis. *European Journal of Social Work*, 12(4), 479–493.

Cowden, S. and Yuval-Davis, N. (2022) Contested narratives of the pandemic crisis: The far right, anti-vaxxers and freedom of speech. *Feminist Dissent* (6), 96–132. https://journals.warwick.ac.uk/index.php/feministdissent/article/view/1264

Craib, I. (1997) *Classical Social Theory*. Oxford University Press, Oxford.

Crenshaw, K. (1991) Mapping the margins: Intersectionality, identity politics and violence against women of colour. *Stanford Law Review*. 43(6), 1241–1299.

Crocker, R.H. (1992). *Social Work and Social Order: The Settlement Movement in Two Industrial Cities*, 1889–1930. University of Illinois Press, Urbana.

Crotty, M. (1998). *The Foundations of Social Research*. Sage Publications, London and New Delhi.

Cruikshank, B. (1999) *The Will to Empower: Democratic Citizens and Other Subjects*. Cornell University Press, New York.

Dale, H. (1998) Child labour under capitalism. [1908] In S. Alexander (Ed.), *Women's Fabian Tracts*. Routledge, London.

Davies, C. (2021, December 10) Police homophobia: the issue Stephen Port jurors couldn't consider. *The Guardian*. https://www.theguardian.com/law/2021/dec/10/police-homophobia-stephen-port-case

Devji, F. (2005) *Landscapes of the Jihad: Militancy, Morality, Modernity*. Hurst Publishers, London.

Dean, M. (2010) *Governmentality: Power and Rule in Modern Society* (2nd edition). Sage Publications, London.

De Beauvoir, S. (1972) *The Second Sex*. Pengiun Books Australia, Melbourne.

Dennis, S. (2018) *From India to Birmingham: A Social Worker Keeping Rights at the Heart of Her Practice across Continents*. Community Care.

De Simone, D. (2021, December 10) Stephen Port: How Met failings contributed to the deaths of three men. https://www.bbc.com/news/uk-59576717

Dhaliwal, S. (2019) Respecting and ensuring rights: Feminist ethics for a state response to fundamentalism. *Feminist Dissent*, 4, 16–54. https://doi.org/10.31273/fd.n4.2019.409

Dixon, T. (2008) *The Invention of Altruism: Making Moral Meanings in Victorian Britain British Academy*. London.

Dominelli, L. (2009) *Introducing Social Work*. Polity Press, Cambridge.

Dotolo, D., Lindhorst, T., Kemp, S.P. and Engelberg, R.A. (2018) Expanding conceptualizations of social justice across all levels of social work practice. *Recognition Theory and Its Contributions*, 92(2), 143.

Dubois, Z.A. and Juster, R.P. (2022) Lived experience and allostatic load among transmasculine people living in the United States. *Psychoneuroendocrinology*, 143, 105849.

Du Gay, P. (2000) *In Praise of Bureaucracy: Weber - Organization - Ethics*. Sage, London.

Dunne, F.J. (2009) Psychiatry in decline. *BJMP*, 2(4), 59–61.

Durwood, L., McLaughlin, K.A. and Olson, K.R. (2017) Mental health and self-worth in socially transitioned transgender youth. *Journal of the American Academy of Child and Adolescent Psychiatry*, 56(2), 116–123.e112. https://doi.org/10.1016/j.jaac.2016.10.016

Epistemic Injustice. (2021, April 27). Dans *BBC - Arts & ideas*. https://www.bbc.co.uk/programmes/p09fwjst

Evans, R (2019) Shitposting, Inspirational Terrorism, and the Christchurch Mosque Massacre. https://www.bellingcat.com/news/rest-of-world/2019/03/15/shitposting-inspirational-terrorism-and-the-christchurch-mosque-massacre/. Accessed 10 October 2023.

Fanon, F. (1952) *Black Skins, White Masks*. Pluto Press, London.

Fanon, F. (2004 [1961]) *The Wretched of the Earth* (Translated by R. Philcox). Grove Press, New York.

Fantz, A. and Shubert, A. (2015) From Scottish Teen to ISIS Bride and Recruiter: The Aqsa Mahmood Story. CNN, 24th February. https://www.cnn.com/2015/02/23/world/scottish-teen-isis-recruiter/index.html. Accessed 10 October 2023.

First Nations of Quebec and Labrador Health and Social Services Commission (FNQLHSSC). (n.d). We are part of a tradition: A guide on Two-Spirited people for First Nations communities. 2-Spirited People of the 1st Nations. https://indigenousto.ca/wp-content/uploads/2018/10/Research_2Spirit_1f.pdf

Fives, A. (2008) *Political and Philosophical Debates in Welfare*. Palgrave Press, Harmondsworth.

Fleming, J. and Ward, D. (2004) Methodology and practical application of the Social Action Research model. In F. Rapport (Ed.), *New Qualitative Methodologies in Health and Social Care Research* (pp. 162–178). Taylor & Francis, Abingdon.

Foucault, M. (2009) *Security, Territory, Population: Lectures at the Collège de France 1977--1978* (vol. 6; edited by M. Senellart, F. Ewald, A. Fontana and A.I. Davidson, translated by G. Burchell). Picador, London.

Foucault, M. (1967) *Madness and Civilisation*. Tavistock Publications, London.

Foucault, M. (1977) *Discipline and Punish*. Penguin Press, Harmondsworth.

Freire, P. (1972) *Pedagogy of the Oppressed*. Penguin, Harmondsworth.

Fricker, M. (2007) *Epistemic Injustice: Power and the Ethics of Knowing*. Oxford University Press, Oxford.

Fukuyama, Francis. "The End of History?" *The National Interest*, no. 16, 1989, pp. 3–18. JSTOR, http://www.jstor.org/stable/24027184. (Accessed 21 Nov. 2024).

Fuller, K.A. and Riggs, D.W. (2018) Family support and discrimination and their relationship to psychological distress and resilience amongst transgender people. *International Journal of Transgenderism*, 19(4), 379–388.

Ghosh, S. (2009) Sexuality, Gender Identity. Emedecine. Last Updated: May 19, 2009. https://emedicine.medscape.com/article/917990-overview. Accessed 16 December 2010.

Gibson, R. (1999) Paulo freire and pedagogy for social justice. *Theory & Research in Social Education*, 27(2), 129–159. https://doi.org/10.1080/00933104.1999.10505876

Gibson, D.J., Glazier, J.J. and Olson, K.R. (2021) Evaluation of anxiety and depression in a community sample of transgender youth. *JAMA Network Open*, 4(4), e214739. https://doi.org/10.1001/jamanetworkopen.2021.4739

Gilligan, C (1982) *A Different Voice*. Harvard University Press, Cambridge MA.

Goffman, E. (1961) *Asylums*. Anchor Press, Harlow.

Government of Québec. (1977) Charter of Human Rights and Freedoms. https://www.legisquebec.gouv.qc.ca/en/document/cs/c-12

Gov.uk. (2021) *Safeguarding and radicalisation: children's social care learning*. https://www.gov.uk/government/publications/safeguarding-and-radicalisation-childrens-social-care-learning

Graham, G. (2004) *Eight Theories of Ethics*. Routledge, London.

Guyer, P. (1998, 2004) Kant, Immanuel. In E. Craig (Ed.), *Routledge Encyclopedia of Philosophy*. Routledge, London.

Hall, S. (2011) Interview with Stuart Hall. In *Cote, Day and de Peuter Utopian Pedagogy: Radical Experiments Against Neoliberal* Globalization University of Toronto Press, Toronto.

Hall, S. (2011) The neoliberal revolution. *Soundings*, (48), 9–28. https://doi.org/10.3898/136266211797146828

Halwani, R. (2003) Care ethics and virtue ethics. *Hypatia*, 18(3) (Autumn, 2003), 161–192.

Harrington, A. (2005) *Modern Social Theory: An Introduction*. Oxford University Press, New York.

Harrington, D. and Dolgoff, R. (2008) Hierarchies of ethical principles for ethical decision making in social work. *Ethics and Social Welfare*, 2(2),183–196.

Harris, J. (1999) State social work and social citizenship in Britain: From clientilism to consumerism. *British Journal of Social Work*, 29, 915–937.

Harris, M.A. and Orth, U. (2019, September 26) The link between self-esteem and social relationships: A meta-analysis of longitudinal studies. *Journal of Personality and Social Psychology*, 119(6):1459–1477. https://doi.org/10.1037/pspp0000265. Epub 2019 Sep 26. PMID: 31556680.

Harvey, D. (2007) *A Brief History of Neo-Liberalism*. Oxford University Press, Oxford and London.

Hauskeller, C., Artinian, T., Fiske, A., Schwarz Marin, E., González Romero, O.S., Luna, L.E. … Sjöstedt-Hughes, P. (2022) Decolonization is a metaphor towards a different ethic. The case from psychedelic studies. *Interdisciplinary Science Reviews*, 48(5), 732–751. https://doi.org/10.1080/03080188.2022.2122788

Hawkins, L., Fook, J. and Ryan, M. (2001) Social workers' use of the language of social justice. *The British Journal of Social Work*, 31(1), February 2001, 1–13. https://doi.org/10.1093/bjsw/31.1.1

Hegel, G. (1991 [1821]) *Elements of the Philosophy of Right*. Cambridge University Press, Cambridge.

Helen Bamber Foundation, Humans for Rights Network et Refugee Council. (2024) *Forced Adulthood: The Home Office's incorrect determination of age and how this leaves child refugees at risk* ([Analysis]). https://www.helenbamber.org/resources/reportsbriefings/forced-adulthood-home-offices-incorrect-determination-age-and-how-leaves

Henrickson, M. (2022) *The Origins of Social Care and Social Work: Creating a Global Future*. Policy Press, Bristol. https://doi.org/10.56687/9781447357377

Hindess, B. (1996) *Discourses of Power: From Hobbes to Foucault*. Blackwell, Oxford.

Hochschild, A. (1989) *The Second Shift*. Penguin Books, Harmondsworth.

Holmes, A.G.D. (2020) Researcher positionality–A consideration of its influence and place in qualitative research–A new researcher guide. *Shanlax International Journal of Education*, 8(4), 1–10.

Honneth, A. (1995) *The Struggle for Recognition. The Moral Grammar of Social Conflicts*. MIT Press, Massachusetts.

Honneth, A. (2001) Recognition or redistribution? Changing perspectives on the moral order of society. *Theory, Culture, Society*, 18, 43–55.

Honneth, A. (2004) Recognition and justice: Outline of a plural theory of justice. *Acta Sociologica*, 47(4), 351–364. https://www.jstor.org/stable/4195049

Honneth, A. (2007) *Disrespect: The Normative Foundations of Critical Theory*. Polity Press, Cambridge.

Horner, N. (2018) *What is Social Work?: Contexts and Perspectives* (5th edition). Learning Matters, London.

Houlgate, S. (2005) *Introduction to Hegel: Freedom*. Truth and History Blackwell, Oxford.

Houshmand, S., Spanierman, L. B., & De Stefano, J. (2019) "I have strong medicine, you see": Strategic responses to racial microaggressions. *Journal of Counseling Psychology*, 66(6), 651–664. https://doi.org/10.1037/cou0000372

Houston, S. (2003) Establishing the virtue in social work: A response to McBeath and Webb. *British Journal of Social Work*, 33, 819–824.

Houston, S. (2009) Communication, recognition and social work: Aligning the ethical theories of Habermas and Honneth. *The British Journal of Social Work*, 39(7), 1274–1290. https://doi.org/10.1093/bjsw/bcn054

Houston, S. (2015) 'When I look I am seen, so I wxist to change': Supplementing Honneth's recognition model for social work. *Social Work & Society*, 13(2). https://ejournals.bib.uni-wuppertal.de/index.php/sws/article/view/437

Howitt, R. (1998) Recognition, respect and reconciliation: Steps towards decolonisation? Australian Aboriginal Studies. https://www.semanticscholar.org/paper/Recognition%2C-respect-and-reconciliation%3A-Steps-Howitt/52a73f3680af125dff5a576c5825f127106b332a

How Police Missed the Grindr Killer. (2017) In *BBC*. https://www.bbc.co.uk/programmes/p04s38l8

Hugman, R. (2005) *New Approaches in Ethics for the Caring Profession*. Palgrave-Macmillan, Basingstoke.

Huntington, S. P. 'The Clash of Civilisations' in *Foreign Affairs*, Summer 1993, volume 72, number 3, pp.22–49 https://www.grip.org/wp-content/uploads/2003/05/THE-CLASH-OF-CIVILIZATIONS_1993_Huntington.pdf (Accessed 21 Nov. 2024).

Hurley, E., & Jackson, M. (2020). Msit No'kmaq: An Exploration of Positionality and Identity in Indigenous Research. Witness: The Canadian Journal of Critical Nursing Discourse, 2(1), 39–50.

International Federation of Social Workers. (2018) Global Social Work Statement of Ethical Principles. https://www.ifsw.org/global-social-work-statement-of-ethical-principles/. Accessed 3 July 2024.

IASSW and IFSW. (2004) Global Standards for the Education and the Training of the Social Work Profession. Adelaide, Australia, https://www.ifsw.org/global-standards-for-social-work-education-and-training/. Accessed 11 September 2009.

Ioakimidis, V. and Wyllie, A. (2023) *Social Work Histories of Complicity and Resistance: A Tale of Two Professions*. Bristol University Press, Bristol.

Ishchenko, V., & Varga, M. (2021) Focusing on extremism won't counter far-Right violence. OpenDemocracy. https://www.opendemocracy.net/en/north-africa-west-asia/focusing-on-extremism-wont-counter-far-right-violence/

Jaggar, A.M (2013) Feminist ethics. In H. Lafolette and I. Persson (Eds.), *The Blackwell Guide to Ethical Theory* (pp. 433–460). Blackwell Press, Oxford.

James, C.L.R. (1963) *The Black Jacobins*. Penguin, London.

Johnson, B (2021) 'Warning issued to parents after 'extremely concerning' rise in number of children arrested for far-right terrorism offences' *Sky News 1/12/21*. https://news.sky.com/story/warning-issued-to-parents-after-extremely-concerning-rise-in-number-of-children-arrested-for-far-right-terrorism-offences-12483953. Accessed 1 December 2023.

Johnsson, S. (2010) The ideology of universalism. *New Left Review*, (63), 115–126.

Jin, H., Restar, A., Goedel, W C., Ogunbajo, A., Biello, K., Operario, D., Kuhns, L., Reisner, S.L., Garofalo, R. and Mimiaga, M.J. (2020) Maternal support is protective against suicidal ideation among a diverse cohort of young transgender women. *LGBT Health*, 7(7), 349–357.https://doi.org/10.1089/lgbt.2020.0219. Epub 2020 Sep 4. PMID: 32897809; PMCID: PMC7578185.

Jones, C. (2002) Social work and society. In R. Adams, L. Dominelli and M. Payne (Eds.), *Social Work: Themes, Issues and Critical Debates* (2nd edition). Palgrave Macmillan, London.

Jones, G.S. (2014) *Outcast London: A Study in the Relationship Between Classes in Victorian Society*. Verso Books, London.

Jordan, B. (2001) Tough love: Social work, social exclusion and the third way. *British Journal of Social Work*, 31(4), 527–546.

Jordan, B. (2004) Emancipatory social work? Opportunity or oxymoron. *British Journal of Social Work*, 34(1), 5–19. https://doi.org/10.1093/bjsw/bch002

Joseph, B. (2018) *21 things you need to know about the Indian Act*. Indigenous Relation Press, Toronto.

Kalberg, S. (2005) *Max Weber: Readings and Commentary on Modernit*. Wiley-Blackwell Oxford. "Karl Marx: The Eighteenth Brumaire of Louis Bonaparte,"

Kant, I (1785) Groundwork of metaphysics of morals. https://www.justiceharvard.org/resources/immanuel-kant-groundwork-for-the-metaphysics-of-morals-1785/. Accessed 19 August 2011.

Kant, I. (1991) *"The Conflict of Faculties" in Political Writings*. Cambridge University Press, Cambridge.

Katz-Wise, S.L., Ehrensaft, D., Vetters, R., Forcier, M. and Austin, S.B. (2018) Family functioning and mental health of transgender and gender-nonconforming youth in the trans teen and family narratives project. *The Journal of Sex Research*, 55(4–5), 582–590.

Kazi, T. (2019) Jihadi Brides, Prevent and the Importance of Critical Thinking Skills. *Feminist Dissent*, 4, pp. 132–145. https://doi.org/10.31273/fd.n4.2019.218

Keay, L. (11/9/202) '*9/11 anniversary: Who were the September 11th attackers and what are the links with the new Taliban regime?*' https://news.sky.com/story/9-11-anniversary-who-were-the-september-11th-attackers-and-what-are-the-links-with-the-new-taliban-regime-12402917 (Accessed 21 Nov. 2024).

Khan, K. (2019) *Countering Extremisms* [online]. http://sister-hood.com/khadija-khan/countering-extremisms/. Accessed 10 October 2023.

Khosrokhavar, F. (2017) Radicalization. The New Press, New York.

Kirkness, V.J., & Barnhardt, R. (1991) First nations and higher education: The four R's — Respect, Relevance, Reciprocity, Responsibility. *Journal of American Indian Education*, 30(3), 1–15. http://www.jstor.org/stable/24397980

Knapp, P. and Spector, A. (2011) *Crisis and Change Today: Basic Questions of Marxist Sociology*. Rowan and Littlefield, Maryland and Plymouth.

Kohler, A. (2024) 'The Housing Crisis Is Global: What Are Other Countries Doing About It.' *Guardian* 28 September 24. https://www.theguardian.com/books/2024/sep/28/the-housing-crisis-is-global-what-are-other-countries-doing-about-it

Kohli, R.K.S. and Mitchell, F. (Eds.) (2007) *Working with Unaccompanied Asylum Seeking Children: Issues for Policy and Practice*. Palgrave Macmillan, London.

Kundnani, A. (2014) *The Muslims Are Coming!* Verso, London.

Kundnani, A. (2015) Violence comes home: an interview with Arun Kundnani. Open Democracy 22 November 2015. https://www.opendemocracy.net/arun-kundnani-opendemocracy/violence-comes-home-interview-with-arun-kundnani. Accessed 20 April 2023.

Ladry, N.-J., Pullen Sansfaçon, A., Chadi, N., London-Nadeau, K., Taylor, A.B., Chan, A., Chiniara, L. and Saewyc, E.M. (2023) Abuse and violence experienced by trans and nonbinary youth in Quebec. *Criminologie*, 56(2), 295–322. https://doi.org/10.7202/1107607ar

Lamont, C. and Favor, C. (2007) Distributive Justice. Stanford Encyclopedia of Philosophy. https://plato.stanford.edu/entries/justice-distributive/. First published Sun September 22, 1996; substantive revision Mon March 5, 2007. Accessed 12 August 2011.

Langan, M. (1998) *"Radical Social Work" in Dominelli et al. Social Work: Themes, Issues and Critical Debates*. Palgrave, Basingstoke.

Lawson, Margaret L., Gotovac, S., Couch, B., Gale, L., Vandermorris, A., Ghosh, S. and Bauer, Greta R. (2024) Pathways to care for adolescents attending a first hormone appointment at Canadian gender affirming medical clinics: A cross-sectional analysis from the trans youth CAN! Study. *Journal of Adolescent Health*, 74(1), 140–147. https://doi.org/10.1016/j.jadohealth.2023.07.021

Leckey, R., Schmieder-Gropen, R., Nnebe, C. and Clouthier, M. (2022) Indigenous parents and child welfare: Mistrust, epistemic injustice, and training. *Social & Legal Studies*, 31(4), 559–579. https://doi.org/10.1177/09646639211041476

LeBel, J. (2023, septembre 23) Anti-trans rallies met with counter-protests across Ontario. *Global News*. https://globalnews.ca/news/9973504/anti-trans-rallies-met-with-counter-protests-across-ontario/

Le Goff, A. (2008) Care, empathie et justice : Un essai de problématisation. *Revue du MAUSS*, 32(2), 203–241. https://doi.org/10.3917/rdm.032.0203

Legault, G.A. (1999) *Professionalisme et Deliberation Ethique*. Presse de l'Université du Québec, Montréal.

Lewis, G. (1998) Coming apart at the seams: The crisis of the welfare state. In G. Hughes & G. Lewis (Eds.), *Unsettling Welfare: The Reconstruction of Social Policy*. Routledge, Open University, London.

Liebenberg, L., Ungar, M. and Ikeda, J. (2015) Neo-Liberalism and responsibilisation in the discourse of social service workers. *The British Journal of Social Work*, 45(3), 1006–1021.

Lipsky, M. (1980) *Street Level Bureaucracy: Dilemmas of the Individual in Public Service Russel*. Sage Foundation, New York.

Lukes, S. (2005) *Power: A Radical View* (2nd edition).Palgrave Macmillan, Basingstoke.

Lukes, S. (2021) Power and domination. *Journal of Political Power*, 14(1), 97–108. https://doi.org/10.1080/2158379X.2021.1878408

Lynch, D.T. and Lynch, C.E. (2006) Aristotle, macIntyre and virtue ethics. *Public Administration and Public Policy*, 116, 55–74.

Macey, D. (2012) *Frantz Fanon: A Biography* (2nd edition). Verso, London.

MacIntyre, A. (2007) *After Virtue: A Study in Moral Theory* (3rd edition). University of Notre Dame Press, Notre Dame.

MacIntyre, A. (1999) *Dependant Rational Animals*. Duckworth, London.

Manitoba College of Social Workers. (2021) Ethical Decision-Making Framework. https://mcsw.ca/wp-content/uploads/2024/12/Ethical-Decision-Making-Guide-FINAL.pdf

Marx, K. (1975) Critique of Hegel's philosophy of right. In K. Marx (Ed.), *Early Writings*. Penguin, Harmondsworth.

Marx, K. (2004) *"Theses on Feuerbach" in Marx and Engels: Collected Works*. Lawrence and Wishart, London.

Marx, K. and Engels, F. (2012) *The Communist Manifesto: A Modern Edition*. Verso Books, London.

Mashford-Pringle, A. and Shawanda, A. (2023) Using the medicine wheel as theory, conceptual framework, analysis, and evaluation tool in health research, SSM – *Qualitative Research in Health*, 3, 2023, 100251, ISSN 2667-3215, https://doi.org/10.1016/j.ssmqr.2023.100251.

Matheson, K., Seymour, A., Landry, J., Ventura, K., Arsenault, E. and Anisman, H. (2022) Canada's colonial genocide of indigenous peoples: A review of the psychosocial and neurobiological processes linking trauma and intergenerational outcomes. *International Journal of Environmental Research and Public Health*, 19(11), 6455. https://doi.org/10.3390/ijerph19116455

Mayhew, H. (1968) *London Labour and the London Poor, with a New Introduction by John D. Rosenberg*. Dover Publications, New York.

McBeath, G. and Webb, S. (2002) Virtue ethics and social work: Being lucky, realistic, and not doing ones duty. *In British Journal of Social Work*, 25, 423–39.

McDonald, K. (2018) *Radicalization*. Cambridge, Polity Press.

McKendrick, D and Finch, J (2017) 'Under heavy manners?': Social work, radicalisation, troubled families and non-linear war. *British Journal of Social Work*, 47 (2), 308–324. https://doi.org/10.1093/bjsw/bcv141

McLaren, P. and Tadeu da Silva, T. (1993) Decentering pedagogy: Critical literacy, resistance, and the politics of memory. In P. McLaren and P. Leonard (Eds.), *Paulo Freire: A Critical Encounter* (pp. 47–89). Routledge, London.

McLaughlin, H. (2012) *Understanding Social Work Research* (2nd edition). SAGE, London.

Meyer-Cook, F. and Labelle, D. (2004) Namaji: Two-spirit organizing in montreal, Canada. *Journal of Gay & Lesbian Social Services*, 16(1), 29–51.

Mill, J.S. (1989) *On Liberty and Other Essays*. Cambridge University Press, Cambridge.

Mill, J.S. (2004) *Utiitarianism* (1863 edition). Parker Son and Bourn, West Strand, London.

Millaire, K. and Pullen Sansfacon, A (2023) Guide to inviting Indigenous Elders and Knowledge Keepers and Making Land Acknowledgement. Centre de echerché interdisciplinaire sur la justice intersectionnelle, la décolonisation et l'équité (CRI-JaDE). Montreal. Online: https://crijade.com/mL4eP8sA/wp-content/uploads/2024/03/Guide-to-inviting-indigenous-elders-and-knowledge-keepers-and-making-land-ackwoledgements-version-11.03.24.pdf

Moosa-Mitha, M. (2022) Decolonial ethics as a framework for anti-islamophobic social work praxis. *International Journal of Social Work Values and Ethics*, 19(2), 24–46.

Morse, J. (1999) The missing link between virtue theory and business ethics. *Journal of Applied Philosophy*, 16, 47–58. https://doi.org/10.1111/1468-5930.00107

Mullaly, R. (2002) *Challenging Oppression: A Critical Social Work Approach*. Oxford University Press, Ontario.

Mullaly, B. and West, J. (2018) *Challenging Oppression and Confronting Privilege* (3rd edition). Oxford University Press, Ontario

Mullender, A. and Ward, D. (1991) *Self-Directed Groupwork: Users Take Action for Empowerment*. Whiting & Birch, London.

Mullender, A., Ward, D. and Fleming, J. (2013) *Empowerment in Action: Self-Directed Groupwork*. Bloomsbury Publishing, London.

Munro, E. (2011) Munro Review of Child Protection: Interim Report https://www.education.gov.uk/munroreview/downloads/Munrointerimreport.pdf. Accessed 16 May 2011.

Nambiar, D. and Mathew, B. (2022) Roles played by civil society organisations in supporting homeless people with health care-seeking and accessing the social determinants of health in Delhi, India: Perspectives of support providers and receivers. *SSM - Qualitative Research in Health*, 2, 2667–3215. https://doi.org/10.1016/j.ssmqr.2022.100157

Nicholls, T. (2011) Colonialism. In: D.K. Chatterjee (Ed.), *Encyclopedia of Global Justice*. Springer, Dordrecht. https://doi.org/10.1007/978-1-4020-9160-5_229

Novell, R.J. (2014, December 10) I want to fight for social work but I will not fight for bureaucracy. *The Guardian*. https://www.theguardian.com/social-care-network/social-life-blog/2014/dec/10/social-work-bureaucracy-paperwork-stifling

Olson, K.R., Durwood, L., DeMeules, M. and McLaughlin, K.A. (2016) Mental health of transgender children who are supported in their identities. *Pediatrics*, 137(3), 2015–3223. https://doi.org/10.1542/peds

O'Sullivan, T. (2010) *Decision Making in Social Work* (2nd edition). Palgrave Macmillan, London.

Pada, R.T. (2017) *Axel Honneth's Social Philosophy of Recognition: Freedom, Normativity, and Identity*. Cambridge Scholars Publishing, Newcastle upon Tyne.

Pampel, Fred C. (2000) *Sociological Lives and Ideas: An Introduction to the Classical Theorists*. Macmillan, Basingstoke.

Pang, K.C., Hoq, M., and Steensma, T.D. (2022) Negative media coverage as a barrier to accessing care for transgender children and adolescents. *JAMA Network Open*, 5(2), e2138623. https://doi.org/10.1001/jamanetworkopen.2021.38623

Parkin, F. (2002) *Max Weber* (2nd edition). Routledge, London.

Parton, N. and Kirk, S. (2009) The nature and purposes of social work. In I. Shaw, K. Briar-Lawson, J. Orme and R. Ruckdeschel (Eds.), *The Sage Handbook of Social Work Research*. SAGE Publication, London.

Pascoe, K.M., Waterhouse-Bradley, B., and McGinn, T. (2023) Social workers' experiences of bureaucracy: A systematic synthesis of qualitative studies. *The British Journal of Social Work*, 53(1), 513–533. https://doi.org/10.1093/bjsw/bcac106

Patel, P. (2019) Prevent: Safeguarding and the gender dimension. *Feminist Dissent* (4), 55–68. https://doi.org/10.31273/fd.n4.2019.311

Payne, M. (2005) *The Origins of Social Work*. Palgrave Macmillan, Basingstoke.

Picard- Sioui, H.L.K. (2016) *La Femme Venue du Ciel, Myth Wendat de la Création*. Editions Hannenorak, Wendake.

Pitt, V. (2010, December 3rd). Are day centres outdated in the personalisation era? Community Care. https://www.communitycare.co.uk/2010/12/03/are-day-centres-outdated-in-the-personalisation-era/

Polyani, K. (2001) *The Great Transformation*. Beacon Press, Boston.

Porter, R. (1990) *The Enlightenment*. Macmillan, Basingstoke.

Power, A., Coverdale, A., Croydon, A., Hall, E., Kaley, A., Macpherson, H. and Nind, M. (2022) Personalisation policy in the lives of people with learning disabilities: A call to focus on how people build their lives relationally. *Critical Social Policy*, 42(2), 220–240. https://doi.org/10.1177/02610183211004534

Pullen Sansfaçon, A. (2011) Ethics and conduct in self-directed groupwork: Some lessons for the development of a more ethical social work practice. *Ethics and Social Welfare*, 5(4), 361–379. https://doi.org/10.1080/17496535.2011.563749

Pullen Sansfaçon, A. (2013) When the ethical may be illegal: Student movement and resistance in a context of repression. *Critical and Radical Social Work*, 1(1), 117–123. https://doi.org/10.1332/204986013X666018

Pullen Sansfaçon, A., Robichaud, M.J. and Dumais-Michaud, A.A. (2015) The experience of parents who support their children's gender variance. *Journal of LGBT Youth*, 12(1), 39–63. https://doi.org/10.1080/19361653.2014.935555

Pullen Sansfaçon, A. and Bellot, C. (2016) L'éthique de la reconnaissance comme posture d'intervention pour travailler avec les jeunes trans. *Nouvelles pratiques sociales*, 28(2), 38–53. https://doi.org/10.7202/1041178ar

Pullen Sansfaçon, A., Hébert, W., Lee, E.O.J., Faddoul, M., Tourki, D. and Bellot, C. (2018) Digging beneath the surface: Results from stage one of a qualitative analysis of factors influencing the well-being of trans youth in Quebec. *International Journal of Transgenderism*, 19(2), 184–202. https://doi.org/10.1080/15532739.2018.1446066

Pullen Sansfacon, A., Boivin, J., Partridge, P.A., Labelle, D. and Lee, E.O.J. (2024) Mamu: Trans indigenous and two-spirit youth coming together to define their needs and to take action. *Journal of LGBTQ+ Youth Studies*, 22(2), 227–245. https://doi.org/10.1080/19361653.2024.2309520

Pullen Sansfaçon, A., Gelly, M.A., Faddoul, M. and E.O.J. Lee. (2020) Parental support and non-support of trans youth: towards a nuanced understanding of forms of support and trans youth's expectations. Enfances Familles Générations. https://journals.openedition.org/efg/10477

Pullen Sansfacon, A. and Gelly, M.A (2024) Discourses on detransition: how detrans youth perceive and receive it ? Presentation given in the mini symposia: Unity Over Division: Understanding and Caring for People who Detransition. 28th Scientific Symposium of the World Professional Association for Transgender Health, of Lisbon, 25-30th September 2024.

Rachels, J. and Rachels, S. (2023) *The Elements of Moral Philosophy* (10th edition). McGraw Hill, Toronto.

Rahman, M., Ahmed, R., Moitra, M., Damschroder, L., Brownson, R., Chorpita, B., Idele, P., Gohar, F., Huang, K.Y., Saxena, S., Lai, J., Peterson, S.S., Harper, G., McKay, M., Amugune, B., Esho, T., Ronen, K., Othieno, C. and Kumar, M. (2021) Mental distress and human rights violations during COVID-19: A rapid review of the evidence informing rights, mental health needs, and public policy around vulnerable populations. *Front Psychiatry*. Jan 8;11, 603–875. https://doi.org/10.3389/fpsyt.2020.603875. PMID: 33488426; PMCID: PMC7820171.

Ramazanoglu, C. and Holland, J. (2002) *Feminist Methodology*. Challenges and Choices Sage Publications, London.

Rawls, J. (1971) *A Theory of Justice*. Harvard University Press. Cambridge, MA.

Rhodes, M. (1986/1991) Ethical Dilemmas in Social Work Practice Family Service America Press, Milwaukee, WI

Robitaille, E. (2024) Annual study finds support for immigration has dropped for second year in a row. 19 octobre 2024. Online. https://www.cicnews.com/2024/10/annual-study-finds-support-for-immigration-has-dropped-for-second-year-in-a-row-1047442.html#gs.hu4iqa. Accessed 19 Novembre 2024.

Rojek, C., Peacock, G. and Collins, S. (1988) *Social Work and Received Ideas*. Routledge, London.

Rousseau, J. (1998) *The Social Contract*. Wordsworth Classics, Hertfordshire.

Said, E. (1978) *Orientalism*. Penguin Books, Harmondsworth.

Samuel, M. (2022, March 9th) Most social workers happy in role despite unpaid overtime, cuts and Covid mental health toll. Community Care. https://www.communitycare.co.uk/2022/03/09/most-social-workers-happy-in-role-despite-unpaid-overtime-cuts-and-covid-mental-health-toll/

Sares-Jäske, L., Czimbalmos, M., Majlander, S., Siukola, R., Klemetti, R., Luopa, P. and Lehtonen ,J. (2023) Gendered differences in experiences of bullying and mental health among transgender and cisgender youth. *J Youth Adolesc*, Aug, 52(8),1531–1548. https://doi.org/10.1007/s10964-023-01786-7. Epub 2023 May 18. PMID: 37199852; PMCID: PMC10276116.

Schwartz, S.H. (1992) Universals in the content and structure of values: Theoretical Advances and Empirical tests in 20 Countries. In M. Zanna (Ed.), *Advances in Experimental Social Psychology* (pp. 1–65). San Diego: Academic Press.

Scott, J. and Marshall, G. (2009) *Dictionary of Sociology* (3rd edition). Oxford University Press, Oxford.

Simmonds, J. and Merredew, F. (2010) *The Health Needs of Unaccompanied Asylum Seeking Children and Young People EP23 - LAC 9.4 Unaccompanied Asylum Seeking Children*. BAAF, London.

Singh, S. (2020) Social Work in India: My Field-Work Experience with People living on the Streets. https://www.globaalisosiaalityo.org/social-work-in-india-my-field-work-experience-with-people-living-on-the-streets/

Skinner, G.C.M., Bywaters, P.W.B. and Kennedy, F. (2022) A review of the relationship between poverty and child abuse and neglect: Insights from scoping reviews, systematic reviews and meta-analyses. *Child Abuse Review*, 32(2), 1–16. https://doi.org/10.1002/car.2795

Slothouber, V. (2020) (De)trans visibility: moral panic in mainstream media reports on de/retransition. *European Journal of English Studies*, 24(1), 89–99. https://doi.org/10.1080/13825577.2020.1730052

Smart, B. (2003) Michel Foucault. In G. Ritzer (Ed.), *The Blackwell Companion to Major Contemporary Social Theorists*. Blackwell, Oxford.

Smith, R. (2008) *Social Work and Power*. Palgrave Macmillan, Basingstoke.

Social Work England. (2019, July) Professional standards. Social Work England. https://www.socialworkengland.org.uk/standards/professional-standards/

Spolander, G., Engelbrecht, L., Martin, L., Strydom, M., Pervova, I., Marjanen, P., Tani, P., Sicora, A. Adaikalam, F. (2014) The implications of neoliberalism for social work: Reflections from a six-country international research collaboration. *International Social Work*, 57(4), 301–312. https://doi.org/10.1177/0020872814524964

Standing Committee On Aboriginal Affairs, Northern Development And Natural Resources. (2002) Committee Evidence. 37th Parliament, 1st Session. March 12, 2002. Online https://www.ourcommons.ca/DocumentViewer/en/37-1/AANR/meeting-43/evidence. Accessed June 13 2024.

Steel, Z., Chey, T., Silove, D., Marnane, C., Bryant, R.A. and van Ommeren, M. (2009) Association of torture and other potentially traumatic events with mental health outcomes among populations exposed to mass conflict and displacement: A systematic review and meta-analysis. *JAMA*, Aug 5;302(5), 537–549. https://doi.org/10.1001/jama.2009.1132. PMID: 19654388.

Stein, S., Andreotti, V., Hunt, D., and Ahenakew, C. (2021) Complexities and challenges of decolonizing higher education: Lessons from Canada. In S.H. Kumalo (Ed.), *Decolonisation as Democratisation: Global Insights into the South Africa Experience*. UKZN Press.

Stevens, A.J., Boukari, Y., English, S., Kadir, A., Kumar, B.N. and Devakumar, D. (2024) Discriminatory, racist and xenophobic policies and practice against child refugees, asylum seekers and undocumented migrants in European health systems. *The Lancet Regional Health – Europe*, 41, 1–14. https://doi.org/10.1016/j.lanepe.2023.100834

Strega, S. and Brown, L. (2015) Research as resistance: Revisiting critical, indigenous, and anti-oppressive approaches. Canadian Scholars Press, Toronto.

Strom-Gottfried, K. and D'Aprix, A. (2006) 'Ethics for academics'. *Social Work Education*, 25(3), 225–244, April 2006

Suveren, Y. (2022) Unconscious bias: Definition and significance. *Current Approaches in Psychiatry*, 14(3), 414–426. https://doi.org/10.18863/pgy.1026607

Tangney, M. and Mendes, P. (2023) Should social work become a registered profession? An examination of the views of 15 Australian social workers. *Australian Journal of Social Issues*, 58(2), 343–359. https://doi.org/10.1002/ajs4.222

Taylor, A.B., Chan, A., Hall, S.L., Saewyc, E.M., and the Canadian Trans & Non-binary Youth Health Survey Research Group. (2020) Being Safe, Being Me 2019: Results of the Canadian Trans and Non-binary Youth Health Survey. Vancouver, Canada: Stigma and Resilience Among Vulnerable Youth Centre, University of British Columbia.

Teismann, T., Joiner, T.E., Robison, M. and Brailovskaia, J. (2024) Self-burdensomeness, self-esteem and suicidal ideation. *Cognitive Therapy and Research*. https://doi.org/10.1007/s10608-024-10477-x

Thane, P. (1982) *Foundations of the Welfare State*. Longman, London.

The United Nations Declaration on the Rights of Indigenous Peoples (UNDRIP) (2007) https://social.desa.un.org/sites/default/files/migrated/19/2018/11/UNDRIP_E_web.pdf. Accessed 13 June 2024.

The Joint Council for the Welfare of Immigrants. (2024) *Windrush Scandal Explained*. https://jcwi.org.uk/reportsbriefings/windrush-scandal-explained/

Townsend. (1998) The case against the charity organisation society [1911]. In S. Alexander (Ed.), *Women's Fabian Tracts*. Routledge, London.

Truth and Reconciliation Commission of Canada. (2015a) Canada's residential schools: The final report of the Truth and Reconciliation Commission of Canada.

Turner, B.S. (1996) *For Weber: Essays on the Sociology of Fate*. Sage Publications, London; Thousand Oaks, CA. https://archive.org/details/forweberessayson0000turn_o7m8

United Nation. (1989) International Convention of the Rights of the Child. https://www.ohchr.org/en/instruments-mechanisms/instruments/convention-rights-child

United Nations. (1948) The Universal Declaration of Human Rights. https://www.un.org/en/about-us/universal-declaration-of-human-rights. Accessed 19 August 2011

US Department of Homeland Security (2021) '*Domestic Violent Extremism Poses Heightened Threat in 2021*. https://www.dhs.gov/publication/domestic-violent-extremism-poses-heightened-threat-2021. Accessed 10 January 225.

Vandermorris, A. and Metzger, D.L. (2023) An affirming approach to caring for transgender and gender-diverse youth. *Paediatrics & Child Health*, 28(7), 437–448. https://doi.org/10.1093/pch/pxad045

Vardy, P. and Grosch, P. (2016) *The Puzzle of Ethics* (3rd edition). Routledge, London.

Wade, J., Mitchell, F. and Baylis, G. (2005) *Unaccompanid Asylum Seeking Children: The Response of Social Work Services*. BAAF, London.

Walsh, J. (2021) The use of self. In J. Walsh (Ed.), *The Dynamics of the Social Worker-Client Relationship* (pp. 48–66). Oxford University Press. https://doi.org/10.1093/oso/9780197517956.003.0004

Warburton, N., andNigel, W. (2012) *Philosophy: The Basics* (5th edition). Routledge, London. https://doi.org/10.4324/9781315817224

Ward, D. and Mullender, A. (1991) Empowerment and oppression: An indissoluble pairing for contemporary social work. *Critical Social Policy*, 11(32), 21–30. https://doi.org/10.1177/026101839101103202

Weber, M. (2005) On the Difficulty of Destroying the Bureaucracy in Max Weber (ed. Kahlberg, S.) Blackwell, Oxford.

Weinberg, M. (2018) The politics of ethics in human services: Dueling discourses. *Ethics & Behavior*, 28(6), 497–509. https://doi.org/10.1080/10508422.2017.1389280

Weinhardt, L.S., Xie, H., Wesp, L.M., Murray, J.R., Aochemengich, I., Kioko, D., Weinhardt, C.B. and L. Cook-Daniels. (2019) The role of family, friend, and significant other support in well-being among transgender and non-binary youth. *Journal of GLBT Family Studies*, 15(4), 311–325.

West, C. (2000) *The Cornell West Reader.* Basic Civitas Books, New York.

Wilde, O. (1973) The soul of man under socialism. In *De Profundis and Other Writings*. Penguin, Harmondsworth.

Wilson, K. (2018) *Pulling Together: Foundations Guide*. BCcampus, Victoria, BC. https://opentextbc.ca/indigenizationfoundations/

Wiseman, P. and Watson, N. (2022) Because I've got a learning disability, they don't take me seriously: "Violence, wellbeing, and devaluing people with learning disabilities". *Journal of Interpersonal Violence*, 37(13–14). https://doi.org/10.1177/0886260521990828.

Witkin, S.L. (2000) Ethics-R-Us. *Social Work*, 45(3), 197–200 (May 2000). https://doi.org/10.1093/sw/45.3.197. PMID: 10803074.

Woodrofe, K. (1962) *From Charity to Social Work*. Routledge Kegan Paul, London.

Wollstonecraft, M. (1792) A Vindication of the Rights of Woman.

World Association For Sexual Health et European Federation of Sexology. (2024, June 14). WAS/EFS Statement on Healthcare for Transgender and Gender-Diverse Individuals | World Association for Sexual Health (WAS). World Association for Sexual Health. https://www.worldsexualhealth.net/declarations/was-efs-joint-statement-trans-healthcare

World Professional Association of transgender Health et United State Professional Association of transgender Health. (2024, May 17). WPATH and USPATH comment on the Cass Review.

Yu, N. (2019) Interrogating social work: Australian social work and the stolen generations. *Journal of Social Work*, 19(6), 736–750. https://doi.org/10.1177/1468017318794230

Yu, N., Morgenshtern, M. and Schmid, J. (2024) Social Work's Colonial Past with Indigenous Children and Communities in Australia and Canada: A Cross-National comparison. *Child & Family Social Work*, 29(1), 229–238. https://doi.org/10.1111/cfs.13070

Zippay, A. (1995) The politics of empowerment. *Social Work*, 40(2), 263–267.

Zizek, S. (2009) *First as Tragedy*. Then as Farce Verso, London.

Zizek, S. (2009) *Violence*. Profile Books.

Index

Note: **Bold** page numbers refer to tables; *italic* page numbers refer to figures and page numbers followed by "n" denote endnotes.

Kolibri 360 GmbH
Ferdinand-Jühlke-Straße 7
99095 Erfurt, Deutschland
produktsicherheit@kolibri360.de